**MOLECULAR BIOLOGY INTELLIGENCE UNIT**

# E-Cell System

## Basic Concepts and Applications

Satya Nanda Vel Arjunan, PhD
RIKEN Quantitative Biology Center
Suita, Osaka, Japan

Pawan K. Dhar, PhD
Centre for Systems and Synthetic Biology
University of Kerala
Kerala, India

Masaru Tomita, PhD
Institute for Advanced Biosciences
Keio University
Tsuruoka City, Yamagata, Japan

LANDES BIOSCIENCE
AUSTIN, TEXAS
USA

SPRINGER SCIENCE+BUSINESS MEDIA
NEW YORK, NEW YORK
USA

# E-CELL SYSTEM: BASIC CONCEPTS AND APPLICATIONS

**Molecular Biology Intelligence Unit**

Landes Bioscience
Springer Science+Business Media, LLC

ISBN: 978-1-4939-4761-4 Printed on acid-free paper.
DOI: 10.1007/978-1-4614-6157-9



Springer Science+Business Media, LLC, 233 Spring Street, New York, New York 10013, USA
http://www.springer.com

Please address all inquiries to the publishers:
Landes Bioscience, 1806 Rio Grande, Austin, Texas 78701, USA
Phone: 512/ 637 6050; FAX: 512/ 637 6079
http://www.landesbioscience.com

The chapters in this book are available in the Madame Curie Bioscience Database.
http://www.landesbioscience.com/curie

9 8 7 6 5 4 3 2 1

E-cell system : basic concepts and applications / [edited by] Satya Nanda Vel Arjunan, Pawan K. Dhar, Masaru Tomita.
p. ; cm.
Includes bibliographical references and index.
ISBN 978-1-4614-6156-2
I. Arjunan, Satya Nanda Vel. II. Dhar, Pawan K. III. Tomita, M. (Masaru),
[DNLM: 1. Cellular Structures--metabolism. 2. Cell Physiological Phenomena. 3. Computer Simulation. 4. Metabolic Networks and Pathways--physiology. 5. Models, Biological. QU 350]

572--dc23

2012043388

## About the Editors...

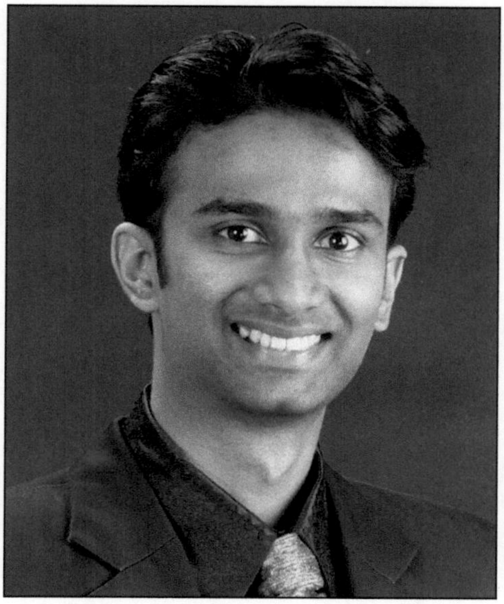

SATYA ARJUNAN is a Postdoctoral Researcher at the RIKEN Quantitative Biology Center, Japan. He received his PhD in Systems Biology from Keio University (2009), BEng in Electronics Engineering (2000) and MSc (2003) in Computer Science from Universiti Teknologi Malaysia. He is also the recipient of the Texas Instruments Malaysia Scholarship (1997) and the Monbukagakusho Scholarship (2003). As part of his PhD work, he developed a multicompartmental spatiotemporal stochastic simulation method, called Spatiocyte, with applications in molecular systems biology.

## About the Editors...

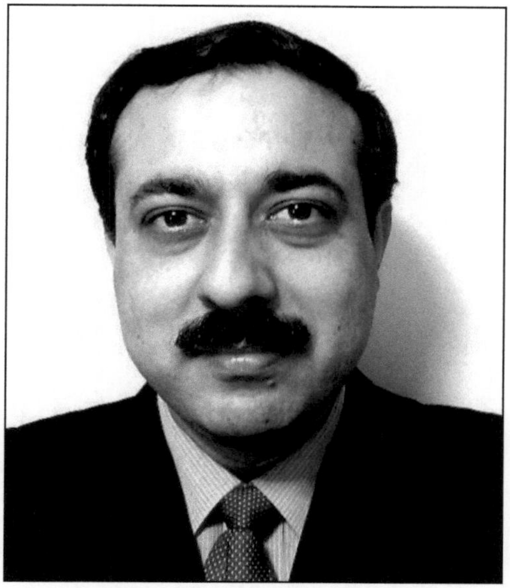

PAWAN K. DHAR is the Director of the Centre of Systems and Synthetic Biology, University of Kerala. Prior to this he held senior scientific positions at RIKEN Genomics Sciences Centre, Japan, Bioinformatics Institute, Singapore and the E-Cell group, Keio University in Japan and Manipal University. One of his key recent contributions has been to make functional proteins from non-coding genome. Dr. Dhar is the Founding Editor-in-Chief of the Springer's *System and Synthetic Biology Journal*. Dr. Dhar heads active research programs on synthetic proteins, virtual cell and BioCAD platform.

## About the Editors...

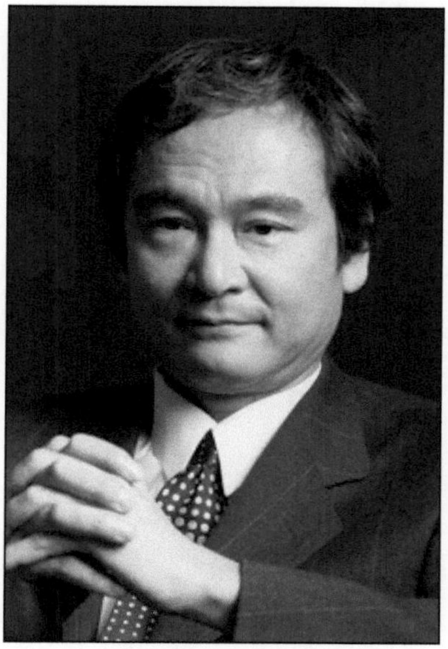

MASARU TOMITA is a Professor and the Director General of the Institute for Advanced Biosciences, Keio University. He received PhD in Computer Science from Carnegie Mellon University (1985), PhD in Electrical Engineering from Kyoto University (1994) and PhD in Molecular Biology from Keio University (1998). He is a recipient of Presidential Young Investigators Award from National Science Foundation of USA (1988) and various other awards. His current research field includes Systems Biology, Metabolomics, and Computational Biology.

# CONTENTS

# EDITORS

**Satya Nanda Vel Arjunan**
**RIKEN Quantitative Biology Center**
**Suita, Osaka, Japan**
*Chapter 4*

**Pawan K. Dhar**
**Centre for Systems and Synthetic Biology**
**University of Kerala**
**Kerala, India**
*Chapter 1*

**Masaru Tomita**
**Institute for Advanced Biosciences**
**Keio University**
**Tsuruoka, Yamagata, Japan**
*Chapter 11*

# CONTRIBUTORS

Nathan Addy
Molecular Sciences Institute
Berkeley, California, USA
*Chapter 2*

Sankar Ghosh
Yale University School of Medicine
New Haven, Connecticut, USA
*Chapter 10, Guest Editor*

Bin Hu
Institute for Advanced Biosciences
Keio University
Tsuruoka, Yamagata, Japan
and
Genome Sciences Group (B-6)
Bioscience Division
Los Alamos National Laboratory
Los Alamos, New Mexico, USA
*Chapter 11*

Hitomi Itoh
Institute for Advanced Biosciences
Keio University
Fujisawa, Kanagawa, Japan
*Chapter 6*

Ayako Kinoshita
Department of Biochemistry
Integrative Medical Biology
School of Medicine
Keio University
Shinjuku-ku, Tokyo, Japan
and
Institute for Advanced Biosciences
Keio University
Fujisawa, Kanagawa, Japan
*Chapter 7*

Yuri Matsuzaki
Institute for Advanced Biosciences
Keio University
Tsuruoka, Yamagata, Japan
*Chapter 5*

Matthias P. Mayer
ZMBH
University of Heidelberg
Heidelberg, Germany
*Chapter 11*

Yasuhiro Naito
Institute for Advanced Biosciences
Keio University
Tsuruoka, Yamagata, Japan
and
Department of Environment
and Information Studies
Graduate School of Media
and Governance
Keio University
Fujisawa, Kanagawa, Japan.
*Chapter 9*

Kumar Selvarajoo
Bioinformatics Institute
Singapore
and
Institute for Advanced Biosciences
Keio University
Tsuruoka, Yamagata, Japan
*Chapter 10*

Masahiro Sugimoto
Institute for Advanced Biosciences
Keio University
Tsuruoka, Yamagata, Japan
and
Department of Bioinformatics
Mitsubishi Space Software Co Ltd
Amagasaki, Hyogo, Japan
*Chapter 3*

Koichi Takahashi
Molecular Sciences Institute
Berkeley, California, USA
*Chapter 2*

Katsuyuki Yugi
Department of Biophysics
and Biochemistry
University of Tokyo
Tokyo, Japan
*Chapter 8*

# PREFACE

The interdisciplinary field of molecular systems biology aims to understand the behavior and mechanisms of biological processes composed of individual molecular components. As we gain more qualitative and quantitative information of complex intracellular processes, biochemical modeling and simulation become indispensable not only to uncover the molecular mechanisms of the processes, but to perform useful predictions. To this end, the E-Cell System, a multi-algorithm, multi-timescale object-oriented simulation platform, can be used to construct predictive virtual biological systems. Gene regulatory and biochemical networks that constitute a sub- or a whole cellular system can be constructed using the E-Cell System to perform qualitative and quantitative analyses.

The first version of the E-Cell System was developed by Koichi Takahashi in 1997, as part of the E-Cell Project in the laboratory of Masaru Tomita at Keio University. Currently at its third version, the E-Cell System consists of the following three major parts: (i) E-Cell Simulation Environment, (ii) E-Cell Modeling Environment, and (iii) E-Cell Analysis Toolkit. The core of the E-Cell System, the E-Cell Simulation Environment allows multiple simulation algorithms with different timescales to coexist. To represent models, the E-Cell System supports the Systems Biology Markup Language (SBML), a standard modeling language adopted by leading publications and scientific grant issuing agencies. The E-Cell System is distributed under the GNU General Public License (GPL) and runs on both Microsoft Windows and Linux operating systems.

The purpose of *E-Cell System: Basic Concepts and Applications* is to provide a comprehensive guide for the E-Cell System version 3 in terms of the software features and its usage. While the publicly available E-Cell Simulation Environment version 3 User's Manual provides the technical details of model building and scripting, it does not describe some of the underlying concepts of the E-Cell System. The first part of the book addresses this issue by providing the basic concepts of modeling and simulation with the E-Cell System. An overview of whole cell modeling and its fundamental concepts are described in the first chapter. In the second chapter, the details of the E-Cell Simulation Environment is provided. This chapter can be used as a reference for both developers and users interested in the algorithm and software architecture of the E-Cell Simulation Environment. Modelers attempting to run multiple instances of their models and utilize distributed computing resources would be interested in the third chapter. The author provides an overview of the E-Cell Session Manager with sample scripts that concurrently distribute multiple E-Cell Sessions to the available processors and cores. The fourth chapter describes the Spatiocyte lattice-based simulation method which is developed as a set of E-Cell System plug in modules. Several reaction-diffusion model examples are also given to familiarize the reader with spatially resolved model building.

The second part of the book provides examples of actual modeling applications that use the E-Cell System. The fifth chapter presents three well-known models of the *Escherichia coli* chemotaxis system that are reimplemented as E-Cell models. In the sixth chapter, changes that take place in the action potential during rodent ventricular cell development are shown using E-Cell electrophysiological model simulations. Different aspects of human red blood cell metabolism under both physiological and pathological conditions are presented using E-Cell model simulation and analysis in the seventh chapter. The eighth chapter gives the simulation results obtained from kinetic models of mitochondrial energy metabolism. Some parameters of the models were estimated using the genetic algorithm module of the E-Cell System. With the aid of a kinetic model of liver ammonia metabolism and E-Cell simulations, the ninth chapter suggests that the enzyme gradients in the lobule model are regulated by gene expressions to reduce energy consumption. In the tenth chapter, the interactions between two toll-like receptor 4 signaling pathways in the innate immune system are investigated using E-Cell System modeling and simulations. The final chapter provides analysis of the kinetic properties and robustness of a heat shock protein chaperone system during folding of an unfolded protein.

The chapters in this book have been critically read and reviewed by experts in the field. We thank the reviewers for their constructive comments and suggestions to improve the quality of the chapters.

*Satya Nanda Vel Arjunan, PhD*
*Pawan K. Dhar, PhD*
*Masaru Tomita, PhD*

# Part 1
# Basic Concepts

# CHAPTER 1

# Introduction to Whole Cell Modeling

**Pawan K. Dhar***

## Introduction

An offshoot of classical bioinformatics, whole cell modeling integrates information from metabolic pathways, gene regulation and expression. This new area of in-silico biology converges disciplines as varied as mathematics, computers, physics and chemistry. Scientific advancements have reached a position where it is possible to create virtual replicas of games that genes play to keep the organism alive. The traditional reductionistic science is slowly but surely giving way to integrative science.

The main purpose of this chapter is to examine the nuts and bolts of whole cell modeling, especially for the non-initiates.

## Modeling Fundamentals

Three elements are necessary to make a good model:

1. Precise knowledge of the phenomenon
2. An accurate mathematical representation
3. A good simulation tool.

Let us discuss each step in detail.

### 1. The Phenomenon

A cell represents a dynamic environment of interaction among nucleic acids, proteins, carbohydrates, ions, pH, temperature, pressure and electrical signals. Many cells with similar functionality form tissue. Each type of tissue uses a subset of this cellular inventory to accomplish a particular function. For example, in neurons electro-chemical phenomena take precedence over cell division, which itself is the domain of skin, lymphocytes and bone marrow cells. Thus, an ideal virtual cell not only represents all the information but also exhibits the potential to differentiate into mission-oriented tissues. The first step in creating a whole cell model is to divide the entire network into pathways and pathways into individual reactions. Any two reactions belong to a pathway if they share a common intermediate. The job of a modeler is not only to decompose events into manageable units but also to assemble these units into a unified framework. As is evident, one needs both reductionist and integrative strategies. Let us discuss the reductionist approach first.

### *1.1 Map*

#### (a) General Introduction

A map uses arrows to represent interactions between substances in a static way. While substances may participate in the primary pathway or activate a side branch, arrows represent the flow of material and are more complex to portray. Arrows must accommodate the flow of matter for forward

*Pawan K. Dhar—Centre for Systems and Synthetic Biology, University of Kerala, Kerala, India. Email: pawan@cssb.res.in

*E-Cell System: Basic Concepts and Applications*, edited by Satya Nanda Vel Arjunan, Pawan K. Dhar and Masaru Tomita. ©2013 Landes Bioscience and Springer Science+Business Media.

and reversible reactions, divergence, convergence, inhibition and activation reactions. Mapping cellular networks is a particularly challenging job, especially in the presence of a large number of crosstalking pathways. To avoid confusion, standard terminologies and graphic representations are followed (Voet 2000). In metabolism there is a tendency to form chains consisting of a minority of forward reactions and majority of reversible reactions. A cell uses a combination of forward/reverse reaction logic to create four basic patterns of linkages (Fig. 1).

I. Linear chains: represent a unidirectional flow of flux.
II. Branched chains: two enzymes metabolize one substance, resulting in different products.
III. Loops: two branches unite, giving rise to inherent dependencies between them.
IV. Cycles: larger loops composed of many intermediates, having one overall entry and one exit point (minimum requirement).

## (b) Tools for Construction and Visualization of Pathways

A number of tools are available for drawing cellular pathways. The basic strategy is to devise a specific algorithm for a specific portion of the pathway instead of creating an all-purpose algorithm, as pathways comprise a mixture of cyclic, linear and hierarchical information. Some of the currently available prominent pathway drawing tools are:

### *(i) PathFinder*

This tool is no longer available online.
Contact: Dr. Alexander Goesmann
Email: agoesman@cebitec.uni-bielefeld.de

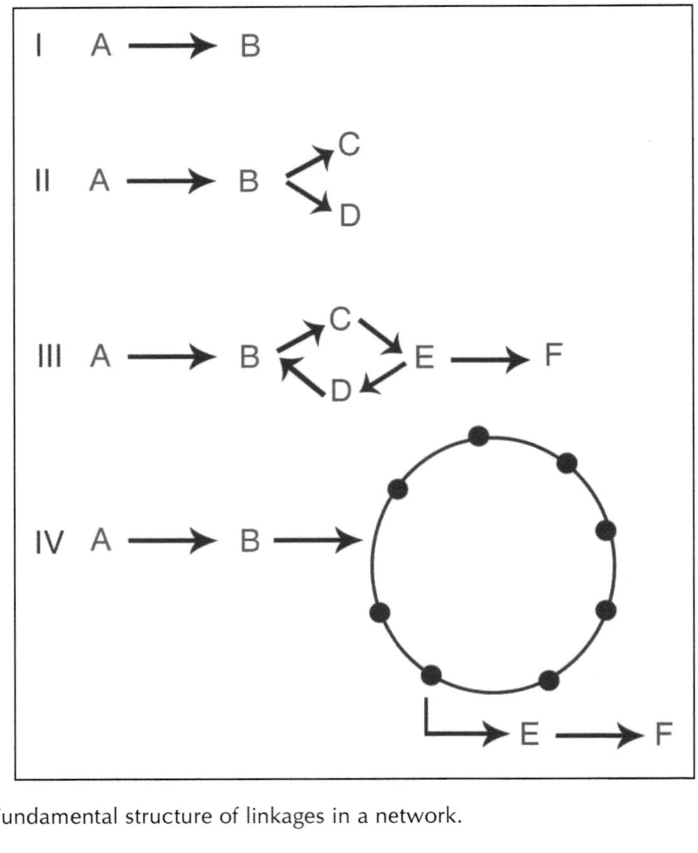


Figure 1. Fundamental structure of linkages in a network.

***(ii) BioJAKE***

Researchers at the National University of Singapore created the BioJAKE program for the visualization, creation and manipulation of metabolic pathways. It has been designed to provide a familiar and easy-to-use interface while allowing for the input and manipulation of metabolic data. It also provides a mechanism by which remote database queries can be stored and performed with respect to individual molecules within a pathway. This remote database access functionality is offered in addition to the local database creation, management and querying capability. The program has been developed in Java to provide platform independence and maximum extendibility.

***(iii) Electric Arc***

ElectricArc is a Perl and Tk-based diagram drawing tool. It is intended to be a general-purpose graph editor and as such, it pushes the application of graphs to the limits of generality. With varying degrees of convenience, ElectricArc can be used to design everything from abstract graphs to electronic circuits, database schema, computer networks and metabolic pathways. ElectricArc borrows most generally useful ideas from electronic CAD technology. It is based on two abstract graph objects, Node and Arc. The code consists of the two tools named symbol and net, the former being used to create the data and symbols for Nodes, while the latter serves the task of laying out the networks of Nodes by connecting them with Arcs.

***(iv) BioPath***

BioPath is a system for the exploration and automatic visualization of biochemical pathways. It was developed to obtain an electronic version of the *Boehringer Biochemical Pathways. BioPath* is linked to a database that contains reactions and a hierarchical clustering of reactions and reaction networks. It provides automatic generation of pathways from the database and their visualization.

***(v) Pathway Browser***

URL: http://www-pr.informatik.uni-tuebingen.de/?site=forschung/metabolic_paths/metabolic_paths

Pathway Browser is an application for the visualization of Metabolic Pathways. In order to run Pathway Browser, a JAVA Runtime Environment for JAVA 2 must be installed. It has following features: XML Input/Export Filters, automatic layout of diagram, advanced navigation features like zooming, overview, etc., printing capabilities, displaying the data at several levels of detail and showing user-defined data.

## *1.2 Metabolic Pathways*

The term pathway describes all biochemical transactions of a cell. Pathways may come in many flavours e.g., metabolic pathways, signaling and genetic networks and drug metabolism pathways. Essentially all of them represent a continuous flow of information. Some of the prominent maps, pathways and databases used for modeling purposes are:

### 1.2.1 IUBMB-Nicholson Minimaps

URL: http://www.iubmb-nicholson.org/

Donald Nicholson of the Department of Biochemistry and Molecular Biology, The University, Leeds, England has created the IUBMB-Nicholson minimaps. It supplements the 21 edition old Metabolic Pathway Charts produced over the past 40 years. A special feature of these maps is the incorporation of information on compartmentation, enzymes and regulation aspects by using coloured backgrounds. The pathways flow from a highlighted starting point to a highlighted ultimate product. The maps are available online in three versions: GIF, SVG and PDF.

### 1.2.2 Boehringer Mannheim Biochemical Pathways

URL: http://www.expasy.ch/cgi-bin/search-biochem-index

Boehringer Mannheim Biochemical Pathways are a standard wall chart on any laboratory workbench. It was created by Boehringer Mannheim researcher Dr. Gerhard Michal (now retired). It is comprehensive, updated and spans many organisms and pathways. Currently it is available on the ExPASy Molecular Biology server in both online and paper format.

### 1.2.3 Kyoto Encyclopedia of Genes and Genomes (KEGG)

URL: http://www.genome.ad.jp/kegg/

The KEGG (Kyoto Encyclopedia of Genes and Genomes) project was initiated in May 1995 under the Japanese Human Genome Program. The primary objective of KEGG is to computerize metabolic pathways, regulatory pathways and molecular assemblies. Additionally, KEGG maintains gene catalogs for all the organisms that have been sequenced and links each gene product to a component on the pathway. KEGG also organizes a database of all chemical compounds in living cells and links each compound to a pathway component.

KEGG consists of the following five types of data:

1. Pathway maps—represented by graphical diagrams
2. Ortholog group tables—represented by HTML tables
3. Molecular catalogs—represented by HTML tables or hierarchical texts
4. Genome maps—represented by Java graphics
5. Gene catalogs—represented by hierarchical texts

These data are linked with each other and with the existing databases through DBGET/LinkDB, an integrated database retrieval system that has been developed in-house.

### 1.2.4 What Is There (WIT)

After several years in service, the tool has been retired and superceded by Seed and PUMA2.

### 1.2.5 Enzyme and Metabolic Pathway (EMP)

This tool is no longer avilable online.

Contact: Evgeni (Zhenya) Selkov

Email: selkovsr@mcs.anl.gov

### 1.2.6 Biopathways Consortium

URL: http://www.biopathways.org/

The Mission of BioPathways Consortium, an open forum, is to develop technologies and open standards for representing, handling, accessing, analyzing and adding value to pathways and protein interaction information.

Some of its goals are: (1) Specify biochemical pathways and protein interactions. Apply this knowledge to genomics, functional genomics, comparative genomics and proteomics. (2) Bring together leaders in these areas from academia, pharmaceutical/biotech industry and database institutions. (3) Develop an online platform for exchange information regarding current and potential technologies.

### 1.2.7 EcoCyc

URL: http://ecocyc.org/

EcoCyc is an encyclopedia of *E. coli* genes and metabolism.

The EcoCyc database describes the genome, metabolic pathways and signal transduction pathways of *E. coli*. It describes each metabolic enzyme of *E. coli*, including its cofactors, activators, inhibitors and subunit structure. EcoCyc is a literature-derived database housing annotations of all *E. coli* genes, as well as the DNA sequence of each *E. coli* gene. EcoCyc describes all known pathways of *E. coli* metabolism. Each pathway is described in rich detail with external links to databases and biomedical literature. The Pathway Tools software provides query and visualization services for EcoCyc. The long-term goal of the project is to create a functional catalog of *E. coli* to facilitate its system-level understanding.

### 1.2.8 PathDB

This tool is no longer available online.
Contact: Jeffrey L. Blanchard
Email: blanchard@microbio.umass.edu

### 1.2.9 The University of Minnesota Biocatalysis/Biodegradation Database (UM-BBD)

URL: http://umbbd.ahc.umn.edu/

UM-BBD is a database storing microbial biocatalytic reactions and biodegradation pathways. The goal of the UM-BBD is to provide information on microbial enzyme-catalyzed reactions that are important for biotechnology. Additionally, UM-BBD is being used to teach enzymology online.

### 1.2.10 Metavista

URL: http://www.metabolic-explorer.com

METAVISTA supports three types of data input: proteomic profiling by 2D gel electrophoresis, metabolic profiling by NMR and/or mass spectroscopy, metabolic flux analysis by 13C stable isotope labeling and NMR and/or mass spectroscopy. METabolic EXplorer's bioinformatic tool, METAVISTA®, is dedicated to the storage, management and analysis of metabolic data resulting from METabolic EXplorer's platform and links it with genetic information of key reference organisms: E. coli, S. cerevisiae and A. thaliana. Its potential applications are: (a) identification and quantitation of metabolic pathway activities in vivo, (b) evaluation of the relative contributions of alternative pathways to product synthesis, (c) determination of the loss of carbon in competing pathways, (d) identification of limiting pathway stochiometries by metabolic network analysis, (e) establishment of a cause-effect relationship between genetic changes and metabolic response, (f) definition of new targets for metabolic engineering and (g) monitoring of pathway activity changes during the transition from growth to the production phase.

### 1.2.11 Metabolic Pathways in Biochemistry

URL: http://www.gwu.edu/%7Empb/index.html

The Metabolic Pathways of Biochemistry is an online reference of metabolism for students and scientists. This site is a teaching aid to represent graphically all major metabolic pathways, primarily those important to human biochemistry.

### 1.2.12 THCME Medical Biochemistry

URL: http://themedicalbiochemistrypage.org/

This site contains description of various metabolic and regulation pathways and serves as an excellent teach aid.

## *1.3 Regulatory Pathways*

### 1.3.1 KEGG Regulatory Pathways

URL: http://www.genome.jp/kegg/

Minoru Kanehisa and his group at Kyoto University (Japan) developed the KEGG database with government funding (see 1.2.3). It is free for academic and non-academic use.

### 1.3.2 BioCarta

URL: http://www.biocarta.com/

BioCarta (founded in April 2000) serves as an interactive web-based resource for life scientists, especially in the areas of gene function and proteomics. The site provides information on pathways involved in developmental biology, hematopoeisis, immunology, metabolism, neuroscience, adhesion, apoptosis, cell activation, cell cycle regulation, signaling and cytokines/chemokines. Biocarta is free to use.

### 1.3.3 Biomolecular Interaction Network Database (BIND)

This project has evolved into Bondplus database.

### 1.3.4 Signal Pathway Database, SPAD

URL: http://www.grt.kyushu-u.ac.jp/spad/

Researchers at Kyushu University (Japan) have developed the SPAD (Signaling PAthway Database) on a Sun workstation. The objective is to understand the overview of signaling transduction (ST) pathways. SPAD classifies ST into four categories based on extracellular signal molecules (growth factor, cytokine, hormone and stress) that initiate the intracellular signaling pathway. SPAD houses information on protein-protein interaction, protein-DNA interaction, DNA sequence information and also provides external links.

### 1.3.5 Cell Signaling Networks Database, CSNDB

URL: http://www.chem.ac.ru/Chemistry/Databases/CSNDB.en.html

The Cell Signaling Networks Database (CSNDB) is a data- and knowledge- base for signaling pathways of human cells. It compiles the information on biological molecules, sequences, structures, functions and biological reactions which transfer the cellular signals. Signaling pathways are compiled as binary relationships of biomolecules and represented by graphs drawn automatically.

### 1.3.6 Munich Information Centre for Protein Sequences, MIPS

URL: http://mips.gsf.de/proj/yeast/CYGD/db/index.html

The MIPS Comprehensive Yeast Genome Database (CYGD) aims to present information on the molecular structure and functional network of the entirely sequenced, well-studied model eukaryote, the budding yeast Saccharomyces cerevisiae. In addition the data of various projects on related yeasts are used for comparative analysis.

### 1.3.7 Wnt Signaling Pathway

URL: http://www.stanford.edu/group/nusselab/cgi-bin/wnt/

Wnt, an amalgam of the two founding members (int-1 in the mouse (now called Wnt-1) and wingless in Drosophila), is a family of highly conserved proteins that regulate cell-to-cell developmental interactions in Drosophila. This is an excellent site on Wnt signaling pathways developed by Stanford University researchers.

### 1.3.8 Transpath

Transpath is essentially a signal transduction browser. It is an information system on gene-regulatory pathways. It focuses on pathways involved in the regulation of transcription factors. Elements of the relevant signal transduction pathways like hormones, enzymes, complexes and transcription factors are stored together with information about their interaction. The TRANSPATH database is free for users from nonprofit organizations.

## *1.4 Transcription Factors*

### 1.4.1 TRANSFAC—Transcription Factor Database

URL: http://www.biobase-international.com/product/transcription-factor-binding-sites

TRANSFAC is a database on eukaryotic cis-acting regulatory DNA elements and trans-acting factors. It covers the whole range from yeast to human.

TRANSFAC started 1988 with a printed compilation (Nucleic Acids Res. 16: 1879-1902, 1988) and was transferred into computer-readable format in 1990 (BioTechForum—Advances in Molecular Genetics (J. Collins, A.J. Driesel, eds.) 4:95-108, 1991).

### 1.4.2 RegulonDB

URL: http://regulondb.ccg.unam.mx/

RegulonDB is a database on transcription regulation and operon organization for different organisms, especially *E.coli*. It describes regulatory signals of transcription initiation, promoters, regulatory binding sites of specific regulators, ribosome binding sites and terminators, as well as information on genes clustered in operons.

### 1.4.3 DBTBS

URL: http://dbtbs.hgc.jp/

DBTBS is a database of *B. subtilis* promoters and transcription factors.

### 1.4.4 SCPD

URL: http://rulai.cshl.edu/SCPD

SCPD is the promoter database of Saccharomyces cerevisiae. It contains information on the promoter regions of about 6000 genes and ORFs in yeast genome. It also provides information on genes with mapped regulatory regions.

## *1.5 Gene Expression*

### 1.5.1 GEO: Gene Expression Omnibus

URL: http://www.ncbi.nlm.nih.gov/geo

GEO is a gene expression/molecular abundance repository supporting MIAME compliant data submissions and a curated, online resource for gene expression data browsing, queries and retrieval.

### 1.5.2 NEXTDB

URL: http://nematode.lab.nig.ac.jp/

NEXTDB is the database to integrate all information from the Caenorhabditis elegans expression pattern project.

### 1.5.3 MAGEST

MAGEST supplies data of DNA sequences and expression patterns of ESTs from maternal mRNAs of the ascidian egg.

## *1.6 Enzyme Databases*

### 1.6.1 Brenda

URL: http://www.brenda-enzymes.info/

BRENDA is the main collection of enzyme functional data available to the scientific community. It is available free of charge for academic, nonprofit users. Currently there are 3500 enzymes in the database; the projected aim is to house information on 40,000 different enzymes from various organisms.

### 1.6.2 ExPASy

URL: http://www.expasy.ch/

ExPASy is an acronym for the Expert Protein Analysis System that analyses protein sequences and structures by browsing through SWISS-PROT, PROSITE, SWISS-2DPAGE, SWISS-3DIMAGE, ENZYME, CD40Lbase and SeqAnalRef as well as other cross-referenced databases (such as EMBL/GenBank/DDBJ, OMIM, Medline, FlyBase, ProDom, SGD, SubtiList, etc).

### 1.6.3 NC-IUBMB

URL: http://www.chem.qmw.ac.uk/iubmb/enzyme/

C-IUBMB stands for Nomenclature Committee of the International Union of Biochemistry and Molecular Biology and contains comprehensive information on enzyme nomenclature.

### 1.6.4 Ligand Chemical Database

URL: http://www.genome.jp/kegg/ligand.html

KEGG LIGAND consists of COMPOUND, DRUG, GLYCAN, REACTION, RPAIR and ENZYME databases.

## 1.7 Scientific Literature Search

### 1.7.1 PubMed

URL: http://www.ncbi.nlm.nih.gov/sites/entrez

PubMed, available via the NCBI Entrez retrieval system, was developed by the National Center for Biotechnology Information (NCBI) at the National Library of Medicine (NLM) located at the National Institutes of Health (NIH). Entrez is the text-based search and retrieval system used at NCBI for all major databases including PubMed, Nucleotide, Protein, Structures, Genome, Taxonomy, OMIM and many others. PubMed was designed to provide access to citations from biomedical literature. Subsequently, a linking feature, LinkOut, was added to provide access to full-text articles at journal web sites and other related web resources. PubMed also provides access and links to the other Entrez molecular biology databases. It is free to use and no membership is required.

### 1.7.2 Medline

URL: http://www.nlm.nih.gov/bsd/pmresources.html

Medline is a very comprehensive database of publications, conference reports and publications from 1966 onwards. The literature can be seamlessly integrated into reference managing tools like EndNote, ReferenceManager, ProCite, Papyrus and Bookends. BioMedNet also offers the scope for creating virtual journals hosted by Medline.

### 1.7.3 Scirus

URL: http://www.scirus.com

Scirus is a meta-search tool of Elsevier Science that enables users to locate data, university sites for reports, homepages and articles. It currently covers the web, ScienceDirect, BioMedNet, Beilstein on ChemWeb, Neuroscion, BioMed Central and patents from the USPTO. Scirus reads nontext files such as PDF, postscript and other formats. It currently covers more than 69 million science-related Web pages, abstracts and full-text publications from databases externally connected to it.

### 1.7.4 ScienceDirect

URL: http://www.sciencedirect.com

ScienceDirect offers an advanced web delivery system for biological information. It was first launched commercially in 1997 and presently stores two million full-text scientific papers and 1200 titles. Browsing is free, but downloading publications comes at a price.

### 1.7.5 CrossRef

URL: http://www.crossref.org

CrossRef is a nonprofit independent organization that provides seamless integration of different literature databases. To date, CrossRef has more than 6,127 journals with more than 4.6 million article records in the database. CrossRef plans to incorporate encyclopedias, textbooks, conference proceedings and other relevant literature in future. It is free to use.

# 2. Mathematical Representation

## *Introduction*

Experimental biology has reached a stage where it is safe to take off to the next level i.e., virtual biology. This new field requires a strong coupling of computational approaches with biological data. Though static representation of data through maps helps develop an overall perspective, dynamic modeling is what actually provides us with an environment to understand and maneuver cellular machinery in-silico.

## *Basic Concepts*

Mathematical modeling is an art of converting biology into numbers. At the root of mathematical representation lies the need for a clear operational description of a model. By definition, a model is an optimal mix of hypotheses, evidence and abstraction to explain a phenomenon. When constructing a model we also use terms like abstraction and mathematical equations.

Hypothesis is a tentative explanation for an observation, phenomenon or scientific problem that can be tested by further investigation. In order to explain an observation something needs to be taken as true for the purpose of argument or investigation.

Evidence describes information that helps in forming a conclusion or judgment. In the present context it refers to experimental data.

Abstraction is an act of filtering out the required information to focus on a specific property only. For example, categorizing cars based on the year of manufacture irrespective of the model would be an example of abstraction. In this process, we lose some detail and gain some. Since we somewhat incompletely understand biology now, we often end up describing the available part of the system instead of the whole. Furthermore, researchers from different areas of specialization may view the same cellular transactions differently. For example, metabolic engineers would focus more on control elements that regulate flux, physicist would look for atomic interactions that govern biology, neurobiologists would pay more attention to the electro-chemical signal processing than metabolic event modeling and biotechnologists would view it more as a serial assembly-line process than a parallel processing system. The bottom line is that in abstraction we gain some and lose some.

Before setting out on a modeling journey, a checklist of biological phenomena that call for mathematical representation is in order. Broadly speaking, the whole cell metabolism may be classified into enzymatic and non-enzymatic processes. Enzymatic processes cover most of the metabolic events while non-enzymatic processes include gene expression and regulation, signal transduction and diffusion. However, knowing the cell inventory is not enough. The point is how to improve its overall performance or to alter selective output of a given product.

The following events would be important to model a complete virtual cell:

1. DNA replication and repair
2. Transcription and its regulation
3. Translation
4. Energy metabolism
5. Cell division
6. Chromatin modeling
7. Signaling pathways
8. Membrane transport (ion channels, pump, nutrients)
9. Intracellular molecular trafficking
10. Cell membrane dynamics
11. Metabolic pathways

To achieve this objective, we not only require precise qualitative and quantitative data but also an appropriate mathematical representation of each event. For metabolic modeling the data input consists of kinetics of individual reactions and also effects of cofactors, pH and ions on the model. The key step in modeling is to choose an appropriate assumption. During metabolic pathway modeling, we come across a number of situations that demand individual attention. For example, a metabolic pathway may be a mix of forward and reverse reactions (uni, bi, ter) of ordered/random types. Furthermore, inhibitors that are part of the pathway (or maybe separate entities) may influence some reactions. At every step, therefore, we must carefully choose enzymatic equations that best describe the process. The mathematical basis of these equations can range from simple algebra and calculus to Laplace transforms. Kinetic modeling is greatly dependent on the accuracy of the data. It may be noteworthy to mention that good data is more of an exception than the rule!

Briefly, mathematical model building calls for skills in mathematics (calculus and linear algebra), numerical methods (scientific computing, etc.), modelling techniques (dimensionless groups, model reduction, etc.), systems science (dynamic simulation, control theory, system identification, etc.) and biophysics (biomechanics, transport phenomena, etc.). Differential equations have been widely used to represent biology numerically due to their ability to incorporate time-based variations. The main advantage is evaluation of the reaction rate with respect to time and the concentration of metabolites. However, differential equations may be less-than-ideal tools in modeling complex and nonlinear systems with feedback loops. Mathematical techniques e.g., linear regression, nonlinear regression and maximum likelihood estimation, are used to fit models to data (in a process called optimization).

Another situation arises when the model itself generates data. In this case the simulator is fed with partial data and asked to find missing pieces. Though computer simulations have enormous advantages, problems arise mostly due to numerical reasons—stiffness and parameter sensitivity. The main difference between model-to-data and data-to-model approaches is that in the former we start from substrate concentration, enzyme concentration and modifier concentrations to get a particular velocity curve, while in the latter, we fix kinetic constants and velocity of reaction values in the beginning. However, the difference between these two approaches sometimes blurs. Due to the paucity of good data, real life modeling often calls for manual data fitting approaches. It is common to assume values in order to match an expected output or hypothesis. The 'litmus-test' of course, is the degree of similarity between computer output and experimental data. Simulation not only represents a given phenomenon but also extrapolates behavior of a system, even in presence of a hypothetical condition such as a cell having multiple knockouts of vital genes!

## 3. Computer Simulation

Cell simulation engines are dynamic representations of entities. The essential job of a simulator is to depict behavior of a system over time and allow pulse analysis of entities. Whole cell simulation calls for discrete event and continuous-time simulations. The former simulation usually includes random number generators and are useful in simulating stochastic processes like signal transduction and gene regulation. In contrast, continuous-time simulations are based on differential equations.

### *3.1 Software Tools*

A number of promising tools are available for studying metabolic pathways. A cross section of some of the popular ones are:

#### 3.1.1 DBSolve

URL: http://en.bio-soft.net/other/DBsolve.html

DBSolve is an integrated development environment for metabolic, enzymatic and receptor-ligand binding simulation. DBSolve derives an ordinary differential equation (ODE) model from a stoichiometric matrix defining the complex enzymatic reaction or metabolic pathway and calculates the steady state solution along a parameter range using the original parameter continuation algorithm. The main part of DBSolve is a general-purpose fitting and optimisation procedure. For storing all the information about a dynamic model it uses a special platform-independent SLV format and contains information about the mathematical model; including the stoichiometric matrix of the process, enzyme/reaction and compound attributes and parameters for numerical methods.

#### 3.1.2 Gepasi

URL: http://www.gepasi.org/

Gepasi is a Microsoft Windows program that simulates the steady-state and time-course behaviour of reactions in several compartments of different volumes. The user supplies the program with information about the stoichiometric structure of the pathway, kinetics of each reaction, volumes of the compartments and initial concentration of all chemical species. The program then builds the differential equations that govern the behaviour of the system and solves them. Results can be imported into spreadsheets and also plotted in 2D and 3D graphs. Gepasi characterises the steady states that it finds using Metabolic Control Analysis and linear kinetic stability analysis.

#### 3.1.3 Jarnac

URL: http://sbw.kgi.edu/software/jarnac.htm

Jarnac is a language for describing and manipulating cellular system models and can be used to describe metabolic, signal transduction and gene networks, or any physical system which can be described in terms of a network and associated flows. Eventually Jarnac will replace SCAMP and may be considered Scamp II.

Dr. Herbert M Sauro's (author of Jarnac) other products include JDesigner and Linear Pathway Modeller.

### 3.1.4 Dynafit

URL: http://www.biokin.com/

BioKin, Ltd. manages and markets *DynaFit* for simulation of chemical and biochemical reactions. In addition it also provides *ViraFit* for statistical analysis of Hepatitis-C viral dynamic data, *BatchK* (client-server application) for determination of tight-binding enzyme inhibition constants and *PlateKi* which is equivalent to BatchK but runs as a standalone Microsoft Windows application.

### 3.1.5 ModelMaker

URL: http://www.modelkinetix.com/

ModelMaker allows you to model continuous and discontinuous functions, stiff systems and stochastic systems. It also provides you optimization, minimization, Monte Carlo and sensitivity analysis.

### 3.1.6 Metamodel

URL: http://bip.cnrs-mrs.fr/bip10/modeling.htm

MetaModel 3.0 is a DOS-based program that allows you to build simple models that contain up to 20 reactions (enzymes) and up to 30 metabolites and to define conservation constraints on the metabolite concentrations . It is a good teaching aid for simulating biochemical reactions.

### 3.1.7 DMSS

Discrete Metabolic Simulation System (DMSS) is a recent entrant that does not employ kinetic parameters, stoichometry matrices or flux coefficients. Instead, the rate of a reaction is modeled based on competing metabolite concentrations or metabolite affinities to enzymes including metabolite and enzyme concentrations.

### 3.1.8 E-Cell

URL: http://www.e-cell.org/ecell/

E-Cell System is a modeling and simulation environment. E-Cell with 127 genes was the first virtual cell created in 1995. The basic concepts and applications of E-Cell Technology are detailed in sections that follow.

### 3.1.9 Virtual Cell

URL: http://www.nrcam.uchc.edu/

Virtual Cell is a modeling tool for cell biological processes. It associates biochemical and electrophysiological data describing individual reactions with experimental microscopic image data describing their subcellular locations. An underlying mathematics framework develops numerical simulations and results can be analyzed as images. Access to the Virtual Cell modeling software is available via the internet using a Java-based interface. Distinct biological and mathematical frameworks are encompassed within a single graphical interface.

### 3.1.10 Cellware

URL: http://www.bii.a-star.edu.sg/achievements/applications/cellware/

The first grid-based modeling and simulation tool for the systems biology community. See the website for details.

## General Concepts on Whole Cell Modeling

### *Modeling Fundamentals*

A model is a closet replica of the phenomena under investigation. The reason why we build models is that they are easy to understand, controllable and can store and analyze large amounts of information. A well-built model has diagnostic and predictive abilities.

### *Why Model Cells?*

A cell by itself is a complete biochemical reactor that contains all the information one needs to understand life. It offers an ideal middle path between the extreme ends of atomic interactions and whole organs. By creating a whole cell model it is possible to travel in either direction. In addition, it can be engaged for jobs like cell cycle, physiology, spatial organization and cell-cell communication.

### *Strategy for Whole Cell Modeling*

Whole cell modeling is a data-driven science that uses two types of data: qualitative and quantitative. Qualitative modeling analyzes logical relationships among components, while quantitative modeling provides a snapshot of an actual amount of matter that flows from one step to the next, from one pathway to the next or from one network to the next. For productive modeling, both qualitative and quantitative modeling approaches are required.

1. Catalog all the substances that make up a cell.
2. Make a list of all the reactions, enzymes and effectors.
3. Map the entire cellular pathways: gene regulation, expression, metabolism etc.
4. Build a stoichometric matrix of all the reactions v/s substances (for qualitative modeling).
5. Add rate constants, concentration of substances, strength of inhibition (if any) (for kinetic modeling).
6. Assume appropriate mathematical representations for individual reactions.
7. Simulate reactions with suitable simulation software.
8. Diagnose the system with system-analysis software.
9. Perturb the system and correlate its behavior to an underlying genetic and/or biochemical phenomenon using a hypothesis generator.

### *Challenges*

1. To identify global gene regulatory switches and crosstalking metabolic pathways.
2. Currently, it is not possible to depict fluxes among pathways over a wide range of physiological conditions like pH or temperature. In addition to the computational constraints, the main bottleneck is lack of experimental data. Thus, in the absence of a demonstrated ability to overcome this barrier, the virtual cell will continue to remain "stiff".
3. True steady states never occur in real life. The best we can hope is to bring an experimentally observed steady state to a quasi-steady state of a cell.
4. Ignorance of complete cellular networks, poor choice of assumptions and mathematical errors.

## Conclusion

Whole Cell modeling is an emerging branch of biological research that aims at a systems level understanding of genetic or metabolic pathways by investigating structure and behavior of genes, proteins and metabolites. The principal aim of systems biology is to provide both a conceptual basis and working methodologies for the scientific explanation of biological phenomena. Frequently, it is the process of formal modeling rather than the mathematical model obtained that is the valuable outcome. The purpose of a conceptual framework is, therefore, to help explain unknown relationships, to make predictions and to help design experiments, suggesting which variables to measure and why. The field itself is new and many challenges need to be overcome before the research community can use it in parallel with wet-bench research tools.

# Chapter 2

# Foundations of E-Cell Simulation Environment Architecture

**Nathan Addy and Koichi Takahashi***

## Introduction

The thorough overview of the E-Cell Simulation Environment in this chapter provides a foundation for understanding the systems biology research that uses the E-Cell Simulation Environment presented within this book. To begin this inquiry, we open with the most general question possible: what is the E-Cell Simulation Environment? The answer is that the E-Cell Simulation Environment (commonly abbreviated E-Cell SE, or even SE) is a simulator of cellular systems models. It is the primary component of a three-program software platform, collectively called the E-Cell System, for creating, simulating and analyzing biological models. As the simulator in this larger environment, the E-Cell Simulation Environment takes user-defined abstract model descriptions, translates them into its own internal model format and calculates trajectories of those models through time, either by recording the results in a file for future analysis, or in real time where the model state can be viewed or modified by the user at any point during execution.

For any simulator, two of the most relevant questions are about the type of system the program models and the algorithms the program can use in performing the modeling. As stated above, the E-Cell System was created to model and simulate cellular systems, but this is not the complete story. The E-Cell System generally and the E-Cell Simulation Environment specifically are fundamentally generic modeling platforms. While they come specialized "out of the box" for cellular modeling, they can simulate any mathematical model. What does this mean? It means that whenever a system can be described formally as a set of variables interacting through mathematical relationships such as equations, relations and constraints, that model can be expressed (and then simulated) in a natural way as an E-Cell Simulation Environment model. E-Cell SE can simulate any mathematical model, no matter what types of mathematical relationships that model describes, or the combinations in which those relationships occur.

The following simple example illustrates how the E-Cell Simulation Environment is more generic than the average biochemical simulator. To model a biochemical system containing three chemical species—A, B and C, such that A and B react to form C with some observed rate—there are two (many more than two, actually) ways to proceed, depending upon the interpretation of the verb "react". You can define it using a differential equation that states the quantities involved convert from one to another at a rate proportional to the product of the concentrations of the reactants: a mass-action reaction. A second way to describing a "reaction" would be as a Gillespie Process, which states that A and B react to form C in atomic jumps corresponding to individual reaction events, where the times of those events are calculated by sampling exponential distributions that depend on the population numbers of A and B and whose action is to decrease the value of each of A and B by one and increase the value of C by one. These two models are distinct and

*Corresponding Author: Koichi Takahashi—Molecular Sciences Institute, 2168 Shattuck Avenue, 2nd floor, Berkeley, California 94704, USA. Email: ktakahashi@molsci.org

*E-Cell System: Basic Concepts and Applications*, edited by Satya Nanda Vel Arjunan, Pawan K. Dhar and Masaru Tomita. 

equally valid mathematical descriptions of the described physical system. While most biological simulators use either mass-action equations or Gillespie equations for describing systems (that is, they typically are built around a single type of algorithm), the E-Cell Simulation Environment can use either. Furthermore, what really makes the E-Cell Simulation Environment generic is its extensibility: any mathematical description of what the word "reacts" might mean can be translated into computer instructions and then used within E-Cell model files.*

To understand how E-Cell Simulation Environment works, this chapter examines how the E-Cell SE allows for any mathematical model to be expressed as an E-Cell model capable of being simulated and also the architecture used to make this possible.

Although the E-Cell Simulation Environment is a generic simulator, the E-Cell Simulation Environment comes packaged with many features, including a toolkit of algorithms commonly used in the field, that put the focus of the E-Cell Simulation Environment on cellular modeling and simulation.

The key to understanding how the generic core of the E-Cell Simulation Environment works is in the intersection between model syntax, model semantics and algorithm implementation. The basic idea is that within the E-Cell Simulation Environment, all processes that update variable values (these correspond to mathematical relationships within the model, for example, a single mass-action equation) are defined in terms of the same internal interface, called the Process interface. (An object possessing such an interface in the SE environment is called a Process. Whenever the word is capitalized, it refers to an algorithm that has this interface in E-Cell SE.) This interface supports reading variable values within the simulation environment followed by instantaneously updating either some variable values or some variable derivatives. Because any algorithm used for systems modeling can be described as a process that updates certain variable values and velocities given the state of other variables and variable velocities, the E-Cell Simulation Environment is able to treat all conceivable simulation algorithms uniformly, without a priori needing information as to their implementation. The result is that internally to the E-Cell Simulation Environment, models are represented as combinations of variables lists and abstract Processes lists that supply the relationships between those variables. While the E-Cell Simulation Environment treats all algorithms both abstractly and uniformly, when called upon to act (to "fire" in E-Cell SE terminology), each Process has its own individual implementation, which defines the exact behavior of that algorithm. By using different combinations of variables and Processes connecting those variables, users can construct E-Cell models that represent any physical system (or any mathematical model, depending on one's point of view), which can then be simulated in the Simulation Environment. The Process interface defined by E-Cell is the foundation for the entire E-Cell Simulation Environment and makes E-Cell SE both generic and extendible.

To illustrate how E-Cell SE uses the universal Process interface to simulate generic models, let us revisit the above example, with two species that combine into a third, represented using either mass-action equations or Gillespie equations. Because E-Cell SE views models through the lens of the Process interface, the models have an identical structure according to this view. Both possess a list of three variables, A, B and C, and both have one Process that reads and then updates the variable values. The difference in model behavior comes from the implementation of the two different Processes. In the mass-action based model, the Process reads the value of A and B, along with the always-defined E-Cell SE variable called volume. The Process uses this information to calculate the concentrations of A and B and then uses the product to calculate a velocity delta, which it adds to the variable C (recall that a mass-action equation representing the reaction A+B -> C is a differential equation of the form $d[C]/dt = k[A][B]$). In the Gillespie system model, the Process uses the volume, the values of A and B, along with a random number, to determine the time at which the values of A and B should decrement by one and the value of C increment by one.

While these two models have different simulation trajectories, the difference is entirely encapsulated within the algorithms' implementation, hidden from the E-Cell Simulation Environment behind identical interfaces. With this system, E-Cell SE only has to be concerned with defining variables, defining the universal Process interface and driving the two. Model builders can implement any algorithms, as long as they follow the rules of the E-Cell Process interface. Then, as they build models, they can do so using any combination of algorithms, simply by invoking them within model files using the names defined concomitant to their implementations. The way the E-Cell Simulation Environment treats algorithms uniformly allows all the semantics of models simulated by the E-Cell Simulation Environment to be defined by the model builders themselves.

The goal is that by combining model building with algorithm implementation, the modeling of any system within the E-Cell Simulation Environment will be as easy and as open ended as directly mathematically modeling the same system. The resultant model structure will ultimately be custom built to the user's needs and not according to the software capabilities.

Hopefully the reader is by now convinced of the veracity of E-Cell SE ability as a generic simulator. And now, with that perspective of the program covered, we move in the other direction and emphasize that the E-Cell Simulation Environment, as well as the E-Cell System, comes structured and organized as a biological simulator of cellular systems. In fact, virtually all literature discussing the E-Cell System discusses it almost exclusively as this type of simulator only. How can this be understood, given the effort just spent discussing how the core E-Cell Simulation Environment is a generic simulator? Although E-Cell SE is a fundametally generic platform, it was created as one part of an ongoing biological project to simulate whole-cell models on computers. Because of this, E-Cell is set up out of the box to support cellular modeling. Common algorithms used within this field are supplied already implemented for use within E-Cell models and need only be called within model files in order to be used within a model. Additionally, the organization of the E-Cell Simulation Environment application—which includes but is not limited to its generic kernel, the component that actually drives the simulation of models—has been developed with the needs of biologists in mind. Its default workflow is applicable to many nonbiological fields and can also be extended or modified as needed for those projects where it is inadequate, but the default configuration of the E-Cell System has been created with the needs of systems biologists and other cellular modelers in mind. This explains the dual generic/specialized nature of the E-Cell System: while the core engine of the E-Cell Simulation Environment is a completely generic and extendible system for simulating arbitrary models, it comes "pre-extended" for cellular and sub-cellular modeling.

## Background

At this point, we understand that the E-Cell Simulation Environment is a unique blend of generic and cellular simulation systems. We also have a basic understanding that this blend is possible because of the way the E-Cell Simulation Environment uniformly treats algorithms, which allows users to extend the Simulation Environment with any new algorithm they need to include in their models. Before we cover the architectural details used by the Simulation Environment to make this possible, knowing the background of the E-Cell project will help provide a better understanding of the forces that have forged the E-Cell System and the E-Cell Simulation Environment into the unique form they take today.

The origins of these programs began at Keio University in 1996, with the launch of a biological program called the E-Cell Project that aimed to reconstruct a whole cell in silico. For this project the organism *Mycoplasma genitalium*, which possesses the smallest known genome, was chosen as the target. One branch of the project consisted of initial work on a simulator that could simulate the whole cell models the project would produce. (This simulator would come to eventually develop into the current version of the E-Cell Simulation Environment, over a period of many years and several major software releases.) The initial work in engineering this program was to perform a meta-study of the field of biological modeling in order to establish a requirements analysis that would determine what features a simulator capable of running whole-cell models would have to possess.This investigation uncovered that, while the simulation of biological cells is similar in many respects to the simulation of many other types of complex systems, cellular systems typically have features that pose unique challenges to their simulation. The specific discovery was that in categorizing systems based on modeling requirements, there are at least three axes of complexity and cellular systems rank particularly high on two of them.

The first type of complexity the E-Cell Project observed was that cellular systems typically have high copy numbers of components, implying that the total number of interactions taking place within a cell during any given time interval is large. This type of complexity is common in the world of simulation. However, the second type of complexity observed within cellular systems by the E-Cell group was less often found in the world of complex systems. This type of complexity is ontological, which means that within most cellular systems the number of distinct interaction types that can be observed is large. Cellular processes including metabolism, signal transduction, gene expression, cytoskeletal dynamics and cytoplasmic streaming are all processes that cause interactions between intracellular components but otherwise differ fundamentally from one another in their behaviors, possessing different properties such as time scales, number of intracellular components affected, global effects on the cell, dynamics, etc.

Ontological complexity poses a challenge to programs that wish to simulate these systems. Because of the variety of intra- and extracellular behaviors, the current state of the art in cellular simulation is a rich ecosystem of algorithms, each representing some aspect of the processes that occur within cellular systems. Note that the alternative to this approach would be to attempt to produce a monolithic "universal" algorithm that would be able to model all these different processes by itself. However at the present time, no algorithm known to the field of cellular modeling can claim to be universal, in the sense that that it could be used to produce accurate simulations of all cellular systems in a timely fashion. For example, it is possible to build whole cell models consisting entirely of systems of mass action equations. While such a model potentially could be efficiently simulated, it probably would not be particularly accurate, because it likely would represent a gross oversimplification of the system. At the other extreme, it would also be possible to build whole cell models by modeling all cellular contents and interactions in terms of Brownian motion, collisions between three-dimensional objects and geometry. But while such a simulation might be very accurate, it would also be simply too large to simulate on any conceivable computer. Given the range of intracellular behaviors, it seems unlikely that a universal algorithm will ever be found; at minimum, such an algorithm does not currently exist. Therefore, to produce serious whole-cell models, the only realistic course is to focus on how to use large sets of algorithms in various combinations to create and simulate our models in order to allow different algorithms to be used where they are best suited.

Given the necessity of using many different algorithms to model whole-cell systems, the E-Cell group made yet another finding. It was observed that the behavior of cellular systems, on both the sub-system and whole-system levels, have highly nonlinear dynamics in all but the most trivial cases. The implication is that no matter which sub-systems of the cell are studied and no matter how well sub-system behaviors are individually understood, that knowledge will form an incomplete framework for understanding the whole system. Such investigations can be very useful in understanding the behavior of whole cells, but in the end cannot be completely explanatory. Some understanding of whole cell behavior can only come through considering the system as a whole. This property made it clear to the E-Cell Project that a strategy of using many different simulators to independently investigate different cellular subsystems would be doomed from the start to be incomplete. The ultimate conclusion reached was that to model and simulate cellular systems, a new type of generic simulator that could use arbitrary algorithms within the same model must be built. With that understanding, the concept of the E-Cell System was conceived.

With the bold goal of building a generic simulator set out during the first phase, work turned to implementation. How could arbitrary algorithms be used within the same simulation framework? This problem was solved by Koichi Takahashi[1] with the development of a computational scheme he called the meta-algorithm. The meta-algorithm provides the theoretical solution as to how a model using multiple algorithms can be simulated as a single unit to produce a trajectory of the whole system. The true importance of the meta-algorithm to the success of the E-Cell System can be expressed by noting that the entire core of the E-Cell Simulation Environment is hardly more than an implementation of the meta-algorithm.

The meta-algorithm works by classifying each potential simulation algorithm that can be mathematically defined into two types based on whether they are continuous (equations that represent continually changing quantities) or discrete (equations representing quantities that change at specific moments). For each algorithm in each of these groups, the meta-algorithm records which variables the algorithm reads as input and which it modifies as its output and uses this to calculate a dependency relation amongst the algorithms used within the model: one algorithm is dependent on another if it reads variables that the other modifies. The meta-algorithm then specifies the exact order in which the different algorithms should be used (these are called events) on an initial state as well as how much time should be advanced for each event in order to simulate the whole model.

The meta-algorithm framework provides the platform that resolves both concerns raised above: the need to use many different algorithms and in a combined form. Thus, this platform allows the building of cellular models using appropriate representations at each level of modeling. Put simply, the meta-algorithm makes a platform for generic modeling possible. Although a generic system like this is more difficult to implement and requires a more complicated architecture than a simple simulator that implements only one algorithm, it has many advantages that easily allow it to surpass any such concrete system. For instance, any model that can be run in any specific simulator can be run within E-Cell, because a model using only one formalism is a special case of a multi-algorithm model. A second advantage is that being able to use multiple algorithms encourages modelers to perform their craft in a very natural way: by mentally decomposing systems into sub-systems, modeling the sub-systems individually using appropriate algorithms and then specifying the coupling between the sub-systems to create a whole cell model. Not only is this a very natural and straightforward way to model large systems, but it also allows the sub-systems to be simulated individually with no additional work. This was the first major set of results produced by the E-Cell Project in the direction of whole cell modeling.

Other design considerations made by the E-Cell Project leading up to the construction of the E-Cell Simulation Environment came from the experience of E-Cell Project members as to how biological simulators are ultimately used by systems biology researchers in labs. "In silico" research is usually only one part of a complicated process of biological knowledge creation, involving wet lab experimentation, modeling, simulation and analysis. In these laboratory settings, biological models are built from experimental results and their purpose is to explain and extend those results. In these dynamic environments, each new piece of data and each limitation in the explanatory power of a model, is likely to propagate changes in the model. At the frontiers of biological research, a model representing "best understanding" could be under near constant revision. In addition, the simulation of models must be configurable to accommodate the range of approaches scientists might wish to use as a part of their research. These approaches might include scripting multiple simulation runs with varying inputs, running simulations on parallel or grid-based hardware and investigating models through a graphical user interface where each variable in the model can be looked at and modified at any moment in time. Another aspect of this configurability is that within labs simulators are often used as one link in a chain of software programs; any generic biological simulator must be configurable enough so that it can collect data from and send results to arbitrary data sources. This high level of configurability is critical for a simulator to be useful to a community of researchers, each with different needs.

## The E-Cell System

With an initial requirements analysis completed and a theoretical foundation for development laid out in the meta-algorithm, work began on building a specific software system for modeling whole-cell systems. As we now know, the result of this work was a suite of software, called the E-Cell System, which is a complete environment for the modeling, simulation and analysis of complex biological systems. (Fig. 1) The E-Cell System consists of three components: the E-Cell Modeling Environment, which allows for collaborative and distributed modeling of cellular systems, the E-Cell Simulation Environment, which runs simulations of models and the E-Cell Analysis

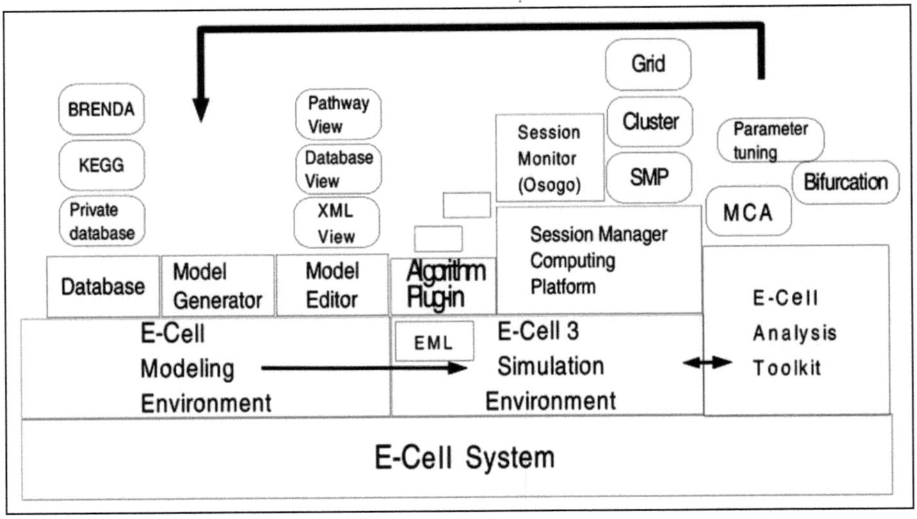


Figure 1. Overview of the E-Cell System. The E-Cell System consists of three components, the Modeling Environment, the Simulation Environment and the Analysis Toolkit.

Toolkit, which is composed of a set of scripts for mathematically analyzing the results of E-Cell Simulation Environment simulations.

The E-Cell Modeling Environment (also called E-Cell ME) is a computer environment for the modeling of cellular systems. As computer processing speeds increase, along with the quantities of available genomic and proteomic data for any given system, the average size of biological models is constantly increasing. Preparing models by hand is becoming increasingly difficult and will likely become impossible on average in the near future. In order to take advantage of faster computers and additional data, new automated methods of model production must be created, so that computers can be "taught" how to build models by humans, instead of humans doing all the work manually. The E-Cell Modeling Environment is an attempt to meet this need. The E-Cell Modeling Environment is built around the idea that model building occurs in several stages: data collection, data integration and initial editing of the model, which results in an initial approximation of a model of the system. This model is simulated and analysis of the results leads to additional model refinement. The E-Cell Modeling Environment provides tools that address each of these stages and has been created as a generic modeling environment, analogous to the way the E-Cell Simulation Environment is a generic simulation environment.

Once a model has been created using the Modeling Environment and simulated in the Simulation Environment, it must be analyzed either to refine the model, or to learn new facts about the behavior of the system being modeled. For this, the E-Cell System provides the E-Cell Analysis Toolkit, which consists of a series of mathematical scripts that analyze the behavior of a model. For tasks such as model refinement, the E-Cell Analysis Toolkit provides scripts for parameter tuning that help fit a model to some observed system output. For the analysis of already-tuned models, the E-Cell Analysis Toolkit provides scripts for bifurcation analysis, which analyze a model that might have several different behaviors depending on the initial conditions in order to provide boundary conditions on the state space such that different regions lead to one outcome versus the other.

These two programs, along with the E-Cell Simulation Environment, combine to form a complete platform for "in silico" biological research and provide a useful tool for biological researchers in the field.

## The Meta-Algorithm

The E-Cell Simulation Environment enables the simulation of models constructed using virtually any combination of continuous and discrete algorithms using a formalism called "the meta-algorithm", which is a framework in which various simulation algorithms can be run in concert. The importance of the meta-algorithm to E-Cell cannot be overstated. Because the implementation of the kernel of the Simulation Environment is primarily an implementation of the meta-algorithm, the architecture of the meta-algorithm forms a substantial subset of the architecture of the E-Cell Simulation Environment and thus bears our initial attention.The meta-algorithm originated in the field of discrete event simulation. One important insight obtained by this field is that all time-driven simulation algorithms can be classified into one of three categories based on how they update variable values: differential equations (equations that modify variables by changing their velocities), discrete time equations (equations that update variables by instantaneously and directly modifying their values) and discrete event equations (equations that represent quantities changed as the result of another event within the model occurring). Using this classification, discrete event simulation provides another result, given by Ziegler,[2] which states these three types of algorithms can be integrated in what is called a discrete-event world view (DEVS). In this formalism, a model state consists of a set of variables that is updated at discrete times along with a global event queue listing the state-changing events that are scheduled to occur and their times of occurrence.

Time advances in a discrete event system by taking the first event in the event queue, advancing global time to the moment of that event's occurrence and executing the event, which causes state changes to the model. The type of event, either discrete or continuous, results in either the model variable values being modified directly or in changes to variables within the model. Next, time advances from the occurrence of the first event to the next scheduled event by using the recorded variable velocities to integrate all model variables to the time of the next event. By alternately executing events and integrating state, a DEVS simulator can calculate the trajectory of the model through time by calculating a sequence of states, one for each time an event occurs. If the model state is needed between the occurrences of two events, the model state can always be integrated from the time of the previously occurring event to the time the state is needed. Thus the discrete-event world view describes one way to create a generic simulator.

The meta-algorithm, developed by Koichi Takahashi, is a concrete specification of a discrete-event world view system that has been implemented with efficiency in mind. The discussion of the meta-algorithm we present here will only be general, as a more detailed account is outside the scope of this text. See Takahashi, 2003, for the definitive treatment.

The meta-algorithm describes in detail how a model using multiple algorithms can be unified in a discrete-event world view framework. It is called a "meta"-algorithm because it is only a template for a simulator and only becomes a concrete algorithm when a particular model using a particular combination of algorithms is interpreted. The specification of the meta-algorithm begins by specifying the data structures used to represent a multi-algorithm model. The most fundamental data structure defined is an object called Model, which is defined as a set of Variable objects and a set of Stepper objects. A Variable is defined as a single named real value, such that the Model object has the property that its state at any given time is completely described by the state of its set of Variables.

A Stepper can be explained by describing it as a computational subunit of the Model object, representing some subset of the total set of interactions that occur within the Model. Each Stepper object consists of a set of Processes, which are objects encapsulating specific algorithms, an interruption method, a local Stepper time and a time step interval. Each event in the meta-algorithm framework consists of a single Stepper "stepping", a term that describes the process by which a Stepper uses its Processes to update the Model, notify other Steppers in the Model of the changes made and prepare itself for stepping again by rescheduling itself as an event.

Within these computational subunits, a Process is defined as an object that uses some subset of the current Model state as well as a time interval to update Variables in the Model to a new state. Processes are organized by the way in which they use Model's current state to modify that state by noting that for any Process in a Model, two sets of variables can be identified. The first is that Process' set of accessor variables, which are the variables used by that Process to read the environment in order to calculate the future state. The second are the mutator variables, which are the variables actually updated by this Process (note that a particular Variable might appear within both sets). Using the theorem from Discrete Simulation presented above, the meta-algorithm characterizes any Process as either continuous or discrete; it further states that individual Steppers can only drive a set consisting of one type of Process and calls these types Continuous Steppers, Discrete Time Steppers or Discrete Event Steppers.

At this point, the Model specified by the meta-algorithm globally looks like a set of real values, as well as a set of computational subunits, each of which represents continuous or discrete sets of behaviors that causes change within the model. Two more pieces of data are required. The first is a global time value (which is always equal to the minimum of the set of local times of the Steppers). The second is a binary relation on the Steppers, called the Stepper Dependency. This relation is defined in the following way: A pair of non-equal Steppers ($S_1$, $S_2$) is in the Stepper Dependency if Stepper $S_1$ contains a Process $P_i$ and Stepper $S_2$ contains a Process $P_j$ such that the intersection of the mutator variables of $P_i$ with the acccessor set of $P_j$ is nonnull, which means that two Steppers are related if the first modifies a value that the second needs to read. This is the data the meta-algorithm works on and with that covered, we can now move on to explaining how the meta-algorithm advances time and drives simulation.

For any system represented as a Model, the meta-algorithm specifies how time can be advanced. Like any system built using a discrete-event world view, time is advanced within the meta-algorithm as a series of discrete events, where events consist of individual Steppers "firing". Therefore, each iteration of the meta-algorithm consists of several parts: choosing the next Stepper to execute by comparing their local times, preparing the Model to run that event, "firing" that Stepper and then resolving the Model so that everything is ready to iterate again.

Each iteration begins with choosing the next Stepper to execute. Because each Stepper keeps a record of when it ought to step next, finding the next executing Stepper is quite simple: it is the Stepper with the smallest time of next firing.

The next step is to advance time in the Model to the time of the scheduled event. Because each event occurs at a discrete time, the interval between any two consecutive events is, in general, nonzero. And because each round of iteration can end leaving Variables with nonzero velocity, this means that the Model state at the time of the previously occurring event must be integrated to the present time, using some kind of extrapolation based on previously recorded variable velocity changes.

Next comes Stepper stepping, a process consisting of several parts: modifying global time, updating variable values within the model, preparing to run again in the future and notifying other Steppers of the changes made.

The first portion consists of the executing Stepper's step function being called. The step function may call one or more of the Processes owned by that Stepper, which, depending on whether the Stepper is of the continuous or the discrete variety, results in either discrete changes to the values of the Variables or changes to the Variable value velocities. This function also causes the time variables of the executing Stepper to be modified. First, the Stepper's local time is updated by adding the current step interval to the current local time; second, based on the Model state after Processes have been fired, a new time-step interval is chosen, preparing the Stepper for its next firing.

The second portion of the firing process consists of notifying all Steppers whose Processes access variables are modified by the firing Stepper to inform them of relevant changes to the model and update their future behavior accordingly, such as the next time they are scheduled to step. For this, the global Stepper Dependency is used. For an executing Stepper S, all pairs (S, D) are found and the interruption method for each such Stepper D is called. This allows Steppers that depend on the data modified by the executing event to examine those changes and update their next time of execution if needed. Once this is completed, Stepper firing is finished, leaving only the "in-between steps" of recording the model state and checking to see if simulation-end conditions have been met.

This is the meta-algorithm. It specifies how a generic simulator simulating any model can be efficiently implemented using a particular implementation of a discrete-event world view simulator. Conceptually, this meta-algorithm forms the foundation for the E-Cell Simulation Environment. In fact, the E-Cell Simulation Environment kernel is practically a direct implementation of the formalism specified above. Everything else is largely a product of software design, wrapping this generic simulator in clothing that makes it configurable and easy to use.

## The E-Cell SE Kernel

Now that we have an overview of the theoretical foundations of the E-Cell Simulation Environment, we can move on to its implementation, called Libecs, which is the name of the simulator kernel of the E-Cell Simulation Environment. This kernel is written entirely in standard ISO C++, and not only implements the meta-algorithm, but also provides the fundamental API to all the essential features of the core system, such as data logging and model object creation.

With regards to calculation, Libecs does three things. It defines the data structures which represent the state of the model, the data structures which represent the forces on the model and the functions that advance time by manipulating these two sets of data.

Data definition in the Libecs implementation begins with the definitions of four basic object classes, which form the parent classes for the different types of model components. Three of these types, called Variable, Process and Stepper, conceptually correspond to the identically named objects in the meta-algorithm (Fig. 2). The fourth, called System is new and acts as a type of set

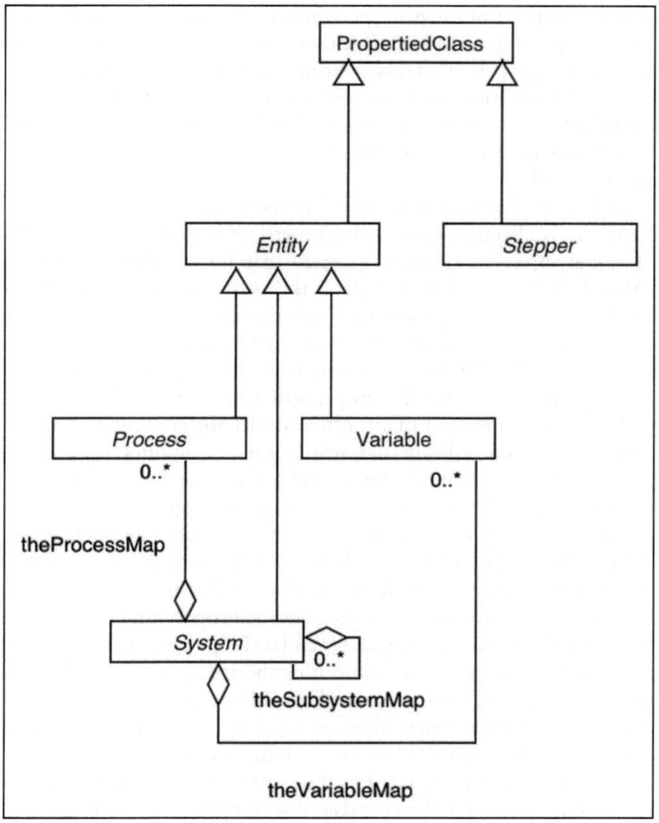


Figure 2. Overview of the fundamental classes of E-Cell.

that contains Variables as well as other Systems and serves the role of organizing all the state data within the model. To quickly discuss the roles of these objects, Variables represent the basic quantities of model state (the number of some specific chemical species, for example). Process objects represent individual mathematical relationships within the model (such as an equation that relates the values of two model Variables). Stepper objects define computational subunits of a model and control entire sets of Processes by activating the set as a group. That activation, which is called a "step" and is initiated by calling a Steppers's "step()" method, constitutes the atomic action in the discrete event system which Libecs implements. As mentioned above, Systems organize the Variables that make up the model state. In fact, the set of all Variables, as defined in the meta-algorithm, is represented in Libecs by a single System object, called the root system, that acts as the one and only container for state data by containing all other model Systems and Variables inside itself. By creating different combinations of these objects, Libecs can represent any model.

One more common feature of these types must be discussed. In this framework, which hopes to construct a representation of any generic model by creating combinations of arbitrarily defined Process, Variable and Stepper object types, an important requirement is a way of assigning to those different objects arbitrary properties of various types. For example, any Process that describes some type of reaction between different chemical species requires additional rate information beyond simply specifying reactants and products. Because we wish to be able to build arbitrary models using arbitrary components, Libecs defines a property API, so that arbitrary property names, paired with a mutable data value of a polymorphic type, can be added to an arbitrary object in the Model. Some properties come predefined for all objects. For instance, each Variable object has a "Value" property of either Real type or of Integer type, where it might represent population count. Each System has a "Size" property that is a real value that represents the volume of that compartment; every object has a "Name" property that takes a string. Furthermore, by using this interface, models simulated in the E-Cell Simulation Environment have the property that the collection of all object properties is equivalent to the model state (many classes defined by Libecs do have nonproperty, member data, but this all corresponds to data about the state of the simulator itself and not the state of the simulated model.)

In order to implement this kind of universal property interface within Libecs, each model object in the kernel derives from a class of type PropertiedClass, which acts as a generic interface to properties of model objects by containing a static map listing all the PropertySlots owned by objects in the Model. A PropertySlot (Fig. 3.) is the association of a PropertyName (a string) with a PropertyValue, which is a polymorphic object that can be of type Real, Integer, String or a List (which itself is a list of other polymorphic types, including other Lists). Because each specific property of each individual Model object is associated with a single PropertySlot object, the static map of all these PropertySlots, owned by PropertiedClass, is universal in E-Cell—each Model object can directly access any property of any other Model object as easily as any other.

The Libecs implementation of Properties, whose software architecture is shown in Figure 3, has several advantages. First, it allows the basic model objects defined in Libecs to represent any generic type of model object. Any arbitrary set of properties a specific model object might have can be stored as a set of PropertySlots within this interface, which is uniquely associated with that object. Second, this scheme allows for multiple types of different property values to be assigned (this is called polymorphic behavior) without sacrificing efficiency. Commonly, a client directly accesses a polymorphic property value, finding the desired PropertySlot using the PropertiedClass interface and then using the generic getProperty() and setProperty() methods of that PropertySlot to access the value. This type of access assumes nothing about the underlying data type and is on the order of performance of standard C++ polymorphism. However, when a particular property must be accessed repeatedly, as is the case where the logging components of the software have to repeatedly access the same PropertySlots in order to record their values through time, the PropertySlot interface can also be used to get a concrete interface, called a PropertySlotProxy, that knows the underlying type of the PropertySlot object and accesses it directly, bypassing polymorphic behavior. When a PropertySlotProxy is created and cached between multiple accesses of a particular

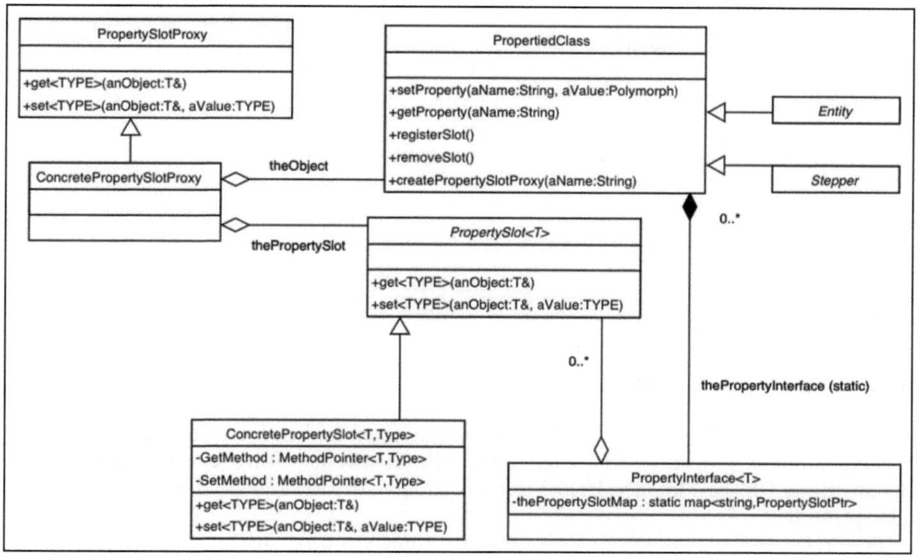


Figure 3. Object properties in E-Cell SE.

PropertySlot, it can be used to increase the speed to access that Property. Thus, this organization of all state data into different PropertySlots means that all that data is accessible at any time, even without knowing the type of data in advance. This organization also has the added advantage that when the client does know the type of data, this knowledge can be used to increase performance. With these advantages, the Property Interface is a very convenient organizational tool for all the data within an E-Cell Model.

If we understand the role of a Process object is to represent a specific algorithm within a model, then we can understand the role of the Stepper object is to a act as a computational subunit of the model because they contain and manage sets of Model Processes and act as an interface to coordinatethe execution of subsets of Processes within its set. Because of the distinction made in the field of discrete event simulation, Libecs divides Processes into two types: Continuous and Discrete. As you might expect, Continuous Processes represent differential equations, which describe how to simulate continuously changing quantities; Discrete Processes represent equations that describe discrete changes to the model state at specific times. Using these definitions as a foundation, Libecs defines four varieties of Steppers, which correspond to the four allowed ways that Processes can be grouped together within Libecs. These four types are DifferentialStepper, DiscreteTimeStepper, DiscreteEventStepper and PassiveStepper (Fig. 4).

A DifferentialStepper maintains a set of continuous Processes and acts as a unit for solving those differential equations: the individual Processes are the individual equations in the system and the DifferentialStepper is a program that actually solves that set of equations. The specific job of a DifferentialStepper is to act as the differential equation solver for its Processes by determining optimal times for recalculating trajectories so that recalculation of equations is performed as infrequently as possible while maintaining accuracy. A computational challenge in simulating trajectories of systems of differential equations comes when the set of differential equations contained by a DifferentialStepper is "stiff". A system of equations is said to be stiff when explicit numerical methods for that system become very inaccurate unless step sizes are small, oftentimes unacceptably so. In this case, implicit methods, which use past information as well as current state, become much more efficient (although under nonstiff conditions implicit methods are less effective). The Libecs implementation of the DifferentialStepper type performs adaptive switching between implicit and

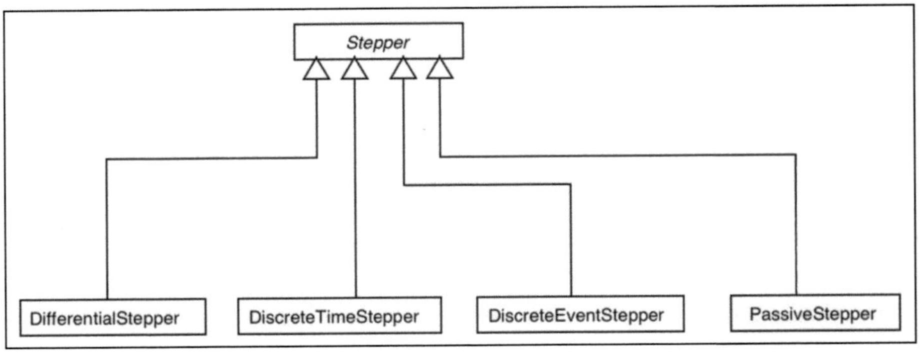


Figure 4. Stepper classes of E-Cell SE.

explicit methods between nonstiff and stiff regions, using an explicit Dormand-Prince algorithm (corresponding to a fourth-order Runge-Kutta with adaptive stepsizing) and an implicit Radau IIA algorithm (the best implicit Runge-Kutta equation currently known) in order to overcome these problems.

For driving discrete modeling, E-Cell provides three Steppers: DiscreteTime, DiscreteEvent and Passive. DiscreteTimeSteppers are used for algorithms that represent changes to the system that occur at discrete moments but where the actual time of "stepping" depends on the state of the system (an algorithm that calculates population changes by executing one reaction event after another, such as the Gillespie algorithm, is an example of this type of algorithm). DiscreteEvent Steppers are used for DiscreteProcesses where the Processes fire at intervals independent of Model state. Finally, PassiveSteppers control Processes that never spontaneously fire, where events happen only as a result of specific cues within the environment. These are the four types of Steppers that exist in the Libecs environment and correspondingly, these are the four types of events that can occur in E-Cell SE.

Last but not least, there is one other major component integral to the operation of the Libecs kernel, the LoggerBroker, which acts as an interface to all features of the kernel involving data logging. Using the LoggerBroker, Libecs can record the values of any or all of the PropertySlots in the Model during the course of simulation. The LoggerBroker object works by creating and managing collections of Logger objects, each of which is associated with a specific PropertySlot in the model (a PropertySlot, as you recall, is the combination of a PropertyName and PropertyValue belonging to a object in the Model). Immediately following the execution of each event during simulation runtime, the LoggerBroker executes its log() method, which records each of the PropertyValues associated with each of its Logger objects. The LoggerBroker interface provides several advantages to the E-Cell Simulation Environment. First, it provides a unified logging API that enables client access to logging capabilities either at the low Libecs level, or at the higher architectural levels that users use (we will later see how the E-Cell SE architecture wraps low level Libecs capabilities to higher level functions that can be easily used by human users). Having a single object in charge of this API also allows the logging process to be optimized in two ways. First, logged data is more efficiently stored in memory than might otherwise be possible, by internally having the LoggerBroker periodically move stored data between memory and the hard disc in order to optimize the handling of large data sets. Logger objects are also optimized for speed of access to PropertyValues by obtaining and caching a PropertyCacheProxy for that class, which allows for faster amortized accesses to the PropertyValue than through normal, polymorphic accesses.

Now that we are familiar with the individual objects contained within the kernel and understand how the fundamental simulation types can be combined to represent mathematical models, we can proceed to the process of how models are instantiated and simulated through time. When the kernel initializes, it begins by creating an object called a Model. The Model object contains,

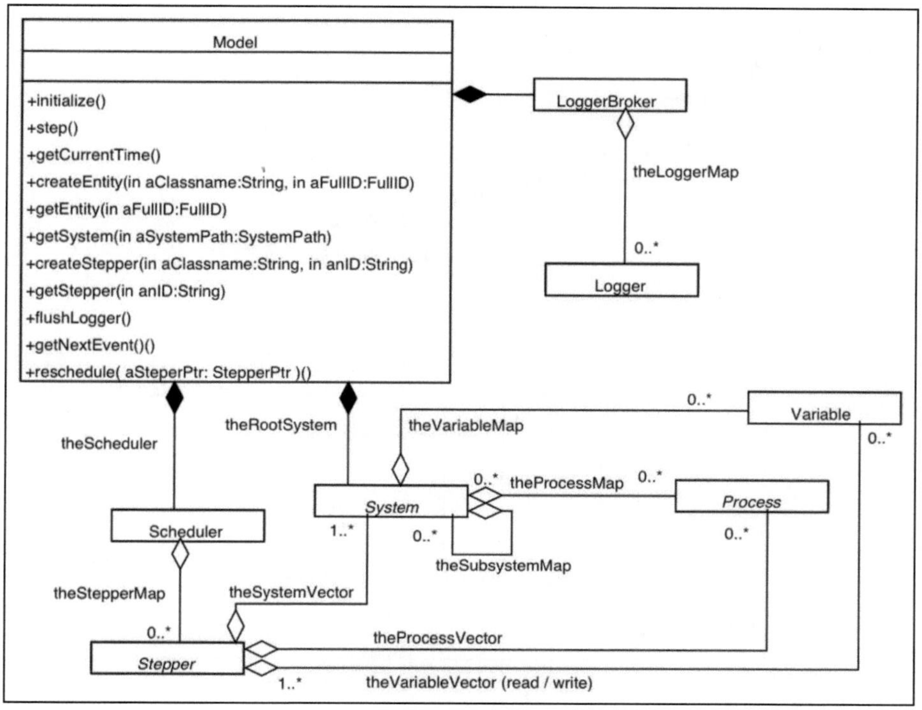


Figure 5. An overview of the class structure of the E-Cell SE kernel.

organizes and coordinates all the data and software components needed to represent a model and provides an interface to all the functionality of the E-Cell kernel: creating and setting up models in preparation for the running of a simulation, stepping the model and logging data through iterations of the meta-algorithm. The Model has three objects which help it to implement these tasks: a root System object, a Scheduler object and a LoggerBroker object. The root System object contains all Variables in the model as well as other Systems. The Scheduler object contains all the Steppers within the model and organizes the execution of Stepper events, which when called in order using their individual step() methods advances the state of the root System object through time. The LoggerBroker object logs object PropertyValues after each cycle of the meta-algorithm. This structure is shown in Figure 5. Please note that the Steppers are contained within the Scheduler and all the Processes in the model are contained within the different Steppers.

Once the Model class has been initialized, a model is instantiated within it by calling different factory methods for creating Variable, Process and Stepper objects within the Model, one at a time. These factory methods create the new objects either in the root System, in the Scheduler (if it is a Stepper) or in a Stepper (if it is a Process). Once each object has been individually added by Libecs to the Model class, a Model member function called initialize() is called, which prepares all additional data structures needed by the Model class. Most notably, both the Stepper Dependency and global time are set up during this stage, according to the specifications of the meta-algorithm. Likewise, one Event is created for each Stepper (each Event represents the simulation event consisting of the next stepping of its associated Stepper). These events are stored and maintained in an event queue owned by the Scheduler object and sorted by time of next planned stepping. Once the setup of all data structures is completed, advancement of time is ready to begin.

Implementation of the meta-algorithm (Fig. 6) is spread throughout the kernel. The entry point to the meta-algorithm is in Model's step() function, which executes one iteration of the

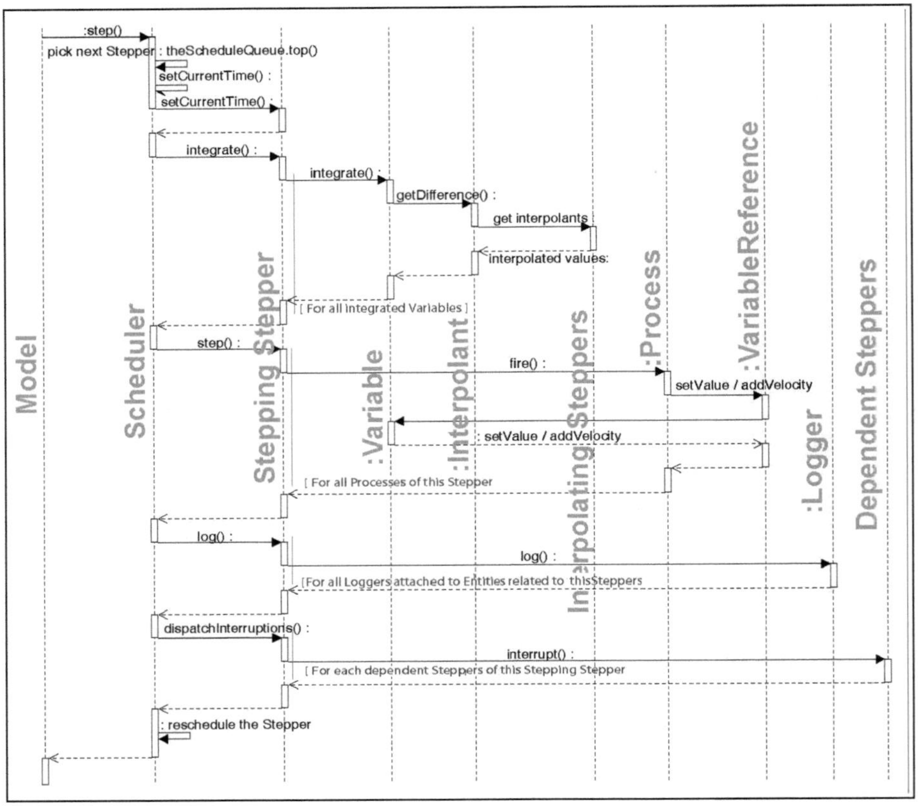


Figure 6. The time-advancement process in the E-Cell SE kernel.

meta-algorithm. Generally, this process consists of determining the time of the next occurring event and setting global time accordingly, integrating the model state to the new current time, stepping the scheduled Stepper by calling its step() method, which causes some Processes to be fired, logging the changes and using the StepperDependency to notify any dependent Steppers so they can reschedule themselves as well as modify any internal parameters as needed.

As mentioned, the first activity performed during a simulation cycle is a determination of the time of the next scheduled event. The Scheduler's event queue begins each step() cycle containing a list of executing events in order. Therefore, finding the time consists of inspecting the value of the scheduled execution time contained by the Event at the very top of the Event Queue.

The next step is to advance time by integrating all reference variables (the combined list of the variables each Process within that Stepper must read) associated with the about-to-be-executing Stepper. This is done by calling the integrate() method for each Variable in the executing Stepper's variable reference list, which uses recorded interpolants of that variable to extrapolate the future value at any specified time. The way this integration procedure works is related to the way in which velocity changes are recorded by Variables. Each Variable that is to be continuously modified is by definition a mutator reference for some Continuous Stepper registered with the kernel; each such Continuous Stepper contains an Interpolant class and during initialization each such Stepper registers an instance of the Interpolant class with each of its mutator reference Variables. When a Continuous Process needs to add a velocity change to a Variable, it does so by passing the changes through the Variable's Interpolant class, which translates velocity changes into interpolant values. When a Variable is called upon to integrate itself to a current time, it uses these interpolant values to calculate interpolant differences, summing over these differences to approximate the value of the Variable at the specified time. Thus, using its interpolant coefficients that are guaranteed to be up-to-date at each point of simulation, a Variable can give its value for any moment in time.

Once integration is completed, the scheduler executes the action of the Stepper, by calling its step() method, which fires some subset of the Processes associated with this Stepper. This step is general (it is implemented as a virtual method) and its exact behavior depends heavily on the type of Stepper. For example, in a DifferentialStepper, which contains Processes corresponding to differential equations, this method consists of calculating and updating velocities of variables through Interpolant classes, along with calculating approximate time steps for the next execution of the Stepper. However, in a DiscreteTimeStepper, this method consists simply of discretely updating the values of variables by firing the Processes within the Stepper.

Next comes logging, as the Stepper being stepped executes its log() method, which indicates to each logger associated with a PropertySlot of some Variable that Stepper references that it should record the value in that PropertySlot at the given time. This procedure is shown in Figure 7. The result is that each logger accesses its associated PropertySlot value through its PropertySlotProxy and inserts it into its PhysicalLogger object for recording.

Finally, using the time of next stepping calculated during its step() method, the Stepper is rescheduled in the Scheduler's event queue.

At this point, all state changes have been propagated into the model and time has been updated. The final activities of the meta-algorithm consist of resolving the model to incorporate the state changes during the current iteration by interrupting and rescheduling each Stepper that is dependent to the current one. This interruption process may change any implementation variables owned by the Stepper, most notably the next time of stepping. PassiveSteppers also fire their Processes here because they only execute after being interrupted by some occurrence. After being interrupted, each Stepper that updates its next firing time reschedules itself so that the Event Queue remains ordered by time as a post condition of Model's step method. At this point, an iteration of the meta-algorithm has been completed and the kernel is ready to advance time once again, choose the next Stepper to execute and so forth.

The major advantage to this architecture is due to the generic interfaces belonging to its fundamental classes. Specifically, because a Process class is only required to define initialize() and fire() methods, new Processes can be programmed and dynamically loaded by the Libecs kernel during runtime. As long as a modeling formalism can be encoded into an algorithm, it can be compiled as an E-Cell plug-in module and loaded into the E-Cell Simulation Environment.

## Interfaces to the Kernel

From a scientific programming perspective, Libecs is a complete implementation of a generic simulation platform. From the perspective of software engineering, it is not enough. Although the framework is extensible through the common algorithm interface provided by Libecs, it is cumbersome to invoke the core system library directly. Therefore, the kernel is wrapped in a Python interface layer to aid in programming, scripting and providing front ends to the kernel.

The Python interface layer API provides a thin interface to the kernel and is structured around a Session object. The Session object provides an interface for setting up models, running simulations and scripting sets of simulation runs. Methods provided by the Session API can be divided into five types. Entity and Stepper methods allow for individually creating or accessing these objects within a model. Logger methods allow for adding Loggers to a model, as well as saving the data recorded by those Loggers. Simulator methods allow for advancing time within a model, either by some fixed amount of time or by some number of steps. Finally, Session methods provide high-level functions for running the E-Cell Simulation Environment, most notably, methods for loading and saving models from E-Cell Model Language files (EML files). This Python API is covered in detail in the E-Cell Manual.[3]

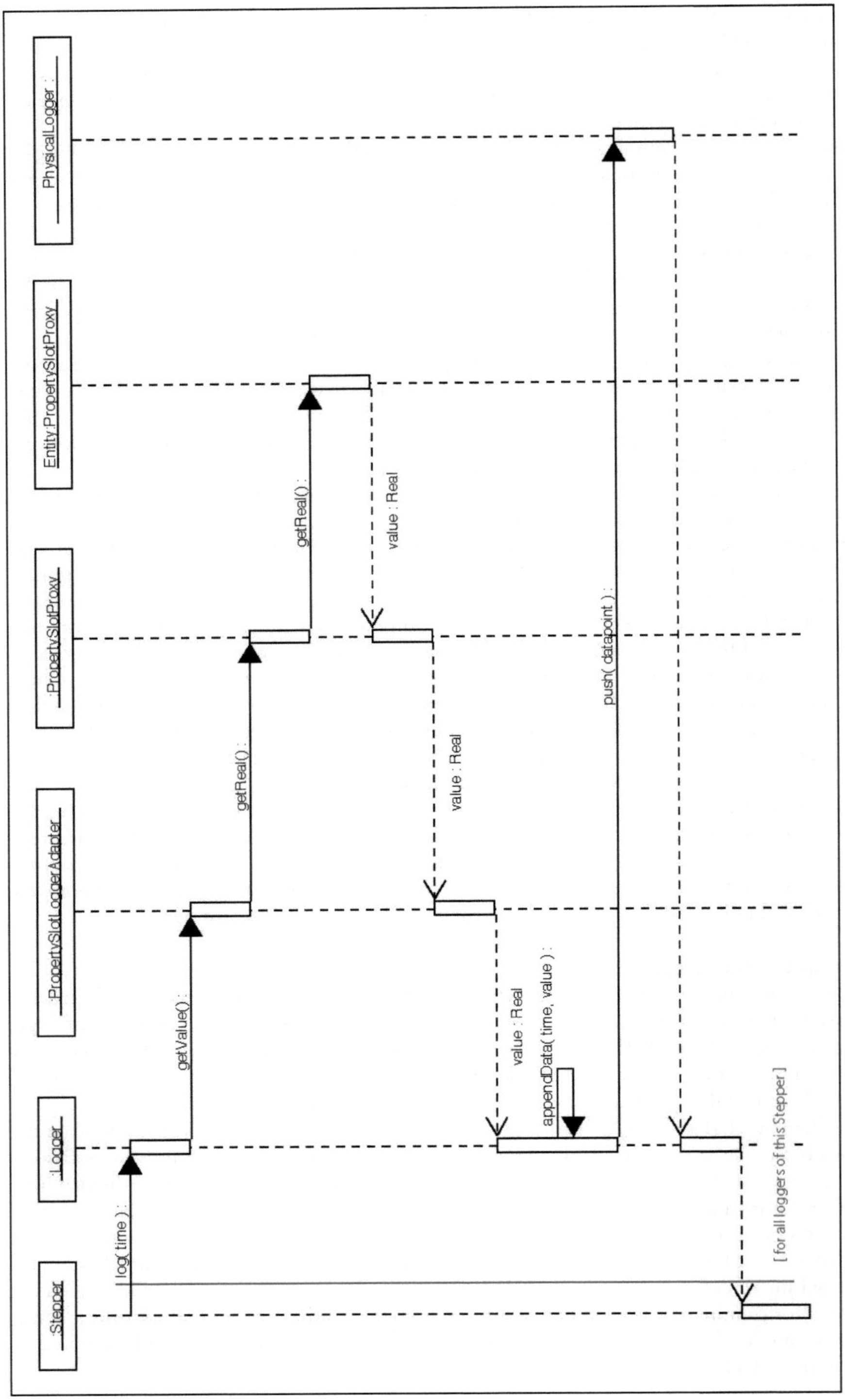


Figure 7. The logging process in the E-Cell SE kernel.

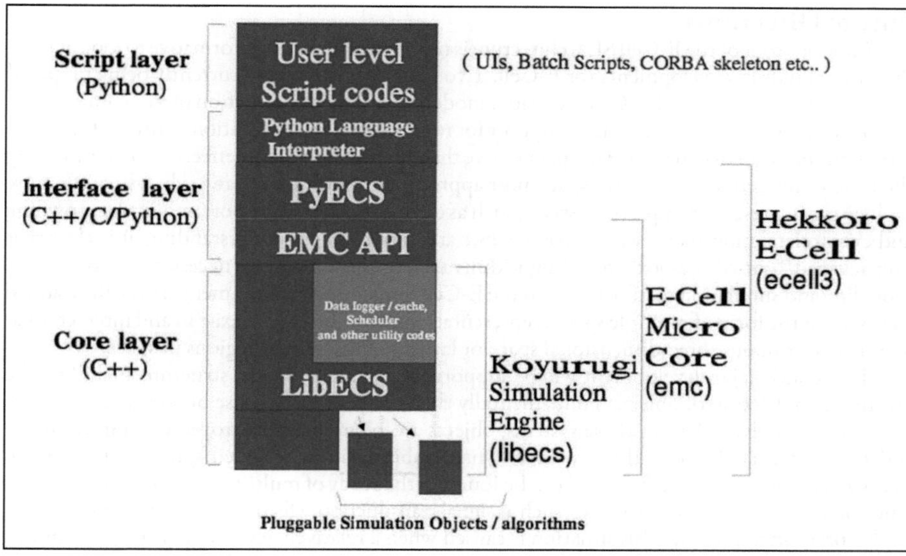


Figure 8. The architecture of the E-Cell Simulation Environment.

For E-Cell development, it is important to note that the Python interface layer does not directly wrap the kernel. Instead, a micro-core layer, called libemc, is built in C++ on top of the kernel, which contains many of the functions found in the Python interface. This layer is then wrapped in a Python interface and combined with other Python code known as PyEcell to produce the complete Python interface API upon which the front-ends to E-Cell are built. This layered architecture is presented in Figure 8.

Built on top of the Python API are three front ends provided by E-Cell: ecell3-session-monitor, ecell3-session and ecell3-session-manager.[3] Ecell3-session-monitor is a graphical user interface that is well suited for interactive model editing and running individual simulations. This is especially useful to researchers initially investigating the behavior of models as it provides numerous capabilities for investigating and analyzing the behavior of the model at any level. The behavior of individual components can be investigated individually or as a whole using a graphical interface. The second major front end component is the ecell3-session command, which provides a command line interface suitable for scripting and automating the processing of large models. This command line mode is an extension of a Python shell that directly reflects the Python session API. The final front-end is the ecell3-session-manager, which is designed for running multiple parallel sessions in either a grid or cluster environment. Ecell3-session-manager provides three classes, SessionManager, SessionProxy and SystemProxy.[4] Used in tandem, these provide a way for the E-Cell SE to be associated with a computing environment, whether that be a single computer, a grid or a cluster and then to automate the running of large numbers of similar models by creating jobs and farming them out to the execution environments registered with the system.While these tools have been designed to match common tasks users are faced with as they attempt to elucidate biological understanding from models, they are also an illustration of the extensible environment that the E-Cell Simulation Environment provides. E-Cell SE has been designed so that as much as possible users can modify or extend it according to their own needs. By wrapping the core simulation code in a programming API of an easily used programming language like Python, this goal is realized, providing nearly unlimited forms in which this software can be used.

## Future Directions

While our tour of the E-Cell SE architecture is nearly complete, it is informative to look at what the future holds in developments for E-Cell. Two major developments currently being prepared for the next major release of E-Cell are spatial modeling and the introduction of a dynamic model structure. Currently, there is no direct support for representing spatial location within E-Cell. One goal of the project is to encourage the perspective that models can be most effectively made by using the tools of reductionism and using the most appropriate algorithm for any sub-system. Because biologists can present examples of systems, such as diffusion, active transport, molecular crowding and cytoskeletal movement, where spatial views are important for understanding, it is clear that prepackaged, "out-of-the-box" spatial algorithms and representations are necessary in a biological modeling and simulation platform such as the E-Cell Simulation Environment. This will be added to E-Cell in the form of multiple spatial representations that objects can exist in and interact, such as either continuous three-dimensional space or lattices of discretised regions in space.

The second major development will be support for a dynamic model structure, including the creation and deletion of objects. Fundamentally this is important because biological systems are dynamic themselves. Within these systems, objects are created and destroyed constantly and in order to appropriately model these systems, dynamic abilities must be added. One specific example of how such a feature might be useful can be found in the study of multi-protein complexes. In the study of many intra-cellular processes, such as signal transduction, a feature known as combinatorial explosion is often present. This situation is caused when a relatively few numbers of proteins can combine in regular ways, producing situations where the number of complexes that can potentially be created is enormous, far greater than that which can ever be sensibly enumerated. Because of this, dynamic model structure must be provided so that these species no longer need to be a priori enumerated and can simply be dynamically created and added to a dynamic model during runtime, along with procedures for informing the rest of the model of the new changes.

An E-Cell System incorporating these features is currently under development. These processes will be critical to the biological modeling and simulation that must take place in order to make the most accurate models of complex systems possible.

## Conclusion

Development of the E-Cell Simulation Environment has been motivated by the belief that large-scale complex models can best be created and understood by composing models written with arbitrary algorithms. E-Cell supports this with a meta-algorithm incorporating a unique plug-in architecture that allows new algorithms to be written and seamlessly integrated into the E-Cell Simulation Environment. Secondary considerations for the design of E-Cell include a belief that this software should be extensible and customizable for users. While the E-Cell Simulation Environment provides in its default distribution several programs users should find quite useful, it will always be possible to write new interfaces that allow for simulation using the E-Cell SE. In this way, E-Cell SE can be a simulator that is relevant far into the future. As new algorithms are developed, they can easily be incorporated into E-Cell SE. As new workflows become needed, E-Cell SE can be molded to fit the required niche. In this way, we expect this generic platform to prove increasingly relevant, providing all the power and flexibility needed to users even as their ambitions only grow.

## References

1. Takahashi K. "Multi-Algorithm and Multi-Timescale Cell Biology Simulation", PhD thesis, Keio University, 2004.
2. Ziegler BP, Kim TG, Praenhofer H. "Theory of Modeling and Simulation: Integrating Discrete Event and Continuous Complex Dynamic Systems" (2nd edition). San Diego, London: Academic.
3. Takahashi K, Addy N. "E-Cell Simulation Environment Version 3.1.105 User's Manual", <http://www.e-cell.org/software/documentation/ecell3-users-manual.pdf>, 2006, Accessed 2006.
4. Sugimoto M, Takahashi K, Kitayama T et al. Distributed Cell Biology Simulations with E-Cell System. In: Konagaya A, Satou K., eds. Lecture Notes in Computer Science, Berlin: Springer-Verlag, 2005:20-31.

# CHAPTER 3

# Distributed Cell Biology Simulations with the E-Cell System

**Masahiro Sugimoto***

## Abstract

Analytical techniques in computational cell biology such as kinetic parameter estimation, Metabolic Control Analysis (MCA) and bifurcation analysis require large numbers of repetitive simulation runs with different input parameters. The requirements for significant computational resources imposed by those analytical methods have led to an increasing interest in the use of parallel and distributed computing technologies.

We developed a Python-scripting environment that can execute the above mathematical analyses. Also, where possible, it automatically and transparently parallelizes them on either (1) stand-alone PCs, (2) shared-memory multiprocessor (SMP) servers, (3) cluster systems, or (4) a computational grid infrastructure. We named this environment E-Cell Session Manager (ESM). It involves user-friendly flat application program interfaces (APIs) for scripting and a pure object-oriented programming environment for sophisticated implementation of a user's analysis.

In this chapter, fundamental concepts related to the design and the ESM architecture are introduced. We also describe an estimation of the parameters with some script examples executed on ESM.

## Introduction

Computer simulations are often used to understand complex biological mechanisms, reproducing dynamic behavior in cells, organs and individuals. Simulation models are important for simultaneously understanding the complex processing of biological phenomena and for revealing their mechanisms in vivo. To establish an in silico model to capture biological behavior, qualitative structural information concerning cellular elements including gene networks, metabolic pathways and cascades of signal transductions, along with parameters of reaction rates characterizing the dynamics of the model must be provided precisely and in sufficient detail. Quantitative parameters available from literature or public databases deteriorate the credibility of such constructed models because they often show noise and are measured under different conditions. Recently, a number of high-throughput measurement devices to perform time-course quantitative studies have been developed; these have been aimed at accumulating sufficient and accurate data that can be used for cell simulations.[1] Thus, development of sophisticated parameter estimation methods to determine parameters unavailable from observable data and to build quantitative models are required.

Estimation of parameters for large-scale models requires high-performance computing facilities because a number of simulation runs must be repeated using different parameters to produce models that represent specific time-courses. Generic parameter estimation approaches based on

*Masahiro Sugimoto—Institute for Advanced Biosciences, Keio University, Tsuruoka, Yamagata, 997–0017, Japan and Department of Bioinformatics, Mitsubishi Space Software Co. Ltd., Amagasaki, Hyogo, 661-0001, Japan. Email: msugi@sfc.keio.ac.jp

*E-Cell System: Basic Concepts and Applications*, edited by Satya Nanda Vel Arjunan, Pawan K. Dhar and Masaru Tomita. 

global optimizations such as genetic algorithm iterate independent simulations, which can be executed on coarse-grained parallel environments, e.g., cluster machines and grid infrastructures. A number of cell simulators implementing parameter estimation functions with parallel computing have been developed. Systems Biology Workbench (SBW) is an extensible and general framework that includes a biological simulation engine and parameter optimization modules.[2] Grid Cellware is an integrated simulation environment implementing the adaptive Swarm algorithm for parameter estimation.[3] OBIYagns is a parameter estimation system based on an epigone genetic algorithm called distance independent diversity control (DIDC) and has a Web-based graphical interface.[4] These systems exploit clusters or grid infrastructures to distribute simulation runs to reduce the total calculation time.

After constructing the structure and parameters needed in a simulation model, they need to be evaluated by comparing them with known biological data. At this stage, the validity of the model is investigated; this includes the ability to reproduce inter/intra cellular behaviors or its quantitative properties including sensitivity or stability of parameters and analyses using Metabolic Control Analysis (MCA), bifurcation analysis. These analyses can be parallelized at a coarse-grained level because they also repeat independent simulations with different parameters. Typical in silico experiments can also be parallelized in the same way such as over/under-activate a/some intercellular substrate(s) to virtually simulate gene knockout or overexpression and the cultivation of cells with different intracellular conditions such as pH or temperature to maximize/minimize concentrations of cellular products. Since many simulation applications in computational cell biology require repetitive runs of simulation sessions with different models and boundary parameters, distributed computation schemes are highly suitable for such applications.

Here, we discuss a scheme for job-level parallelism, or distributed computing. There is already some middleware software available for the assignment of jobs to distributed environments, e.g., Portable Batch System (PBS, http://www.pbs.org/), Load Sharing Facility (LSF, http://www.platform.com/), Sun Grid Engine (SGE, http://wwws.sun.com/software/gridware/) at the cluster level and Globus toolkit[5] at the grid level. While these low-level infrastructures are extremely powerful, they are not compatible with each other, nor are they readily accessible to an average computational biologist. On the other hand, higher-level parallelization systems with a Web-based user interface such as OBIYagns may help computer neophytes. Though these systems provide editable workflow functions such as myGrid[6] and ProGenGrid[7], they lack programming flexibility to implement a user's analysis algorithm for various research purposes.

In this chapter, we describe the architecture and the design of a distributed computing module of E-Cell3, called E-Cell Session Manager (ESM).[8] ESM was developed to produce higher-level APIs to provide users with a scripting environment and to transparently distribute multiple E-Cell sessions on stand-alone PC, SMP, cluster and grid environments. We also introduce parameter estimation scripts built on ESM as an example.

## Design of ESM

### *Architecture of ESM*

Figure1 shows the architecture of ESM. It is composed of three layers: (1) a class library for cell simulation (libecs) and its C++ API (libemc), (2) a Python language wrapper of libemc, PyEcs and pyecell which is the interface connecting the bottom and top layers and (3) a library of various front-end and utility modules written in Python. The pyecell library defines an object class called Session representing a single run of the simulator. ESM provides APIs for Python scripting and instantiates many Session objects.

The Class diagram of ESM is depicted in Figure 2. The Session Manager class provides the user with a flat API to create and run simulation sessions. The Session Manager class holds a System Proxy object as its attribute. System Proxy conceals the difference of distributed environments and communicates to the computer operating system or to the low-level middleware of the computing environment on which ESM is running (Fig. 3). Session Proxy executes a task in PC and SMP

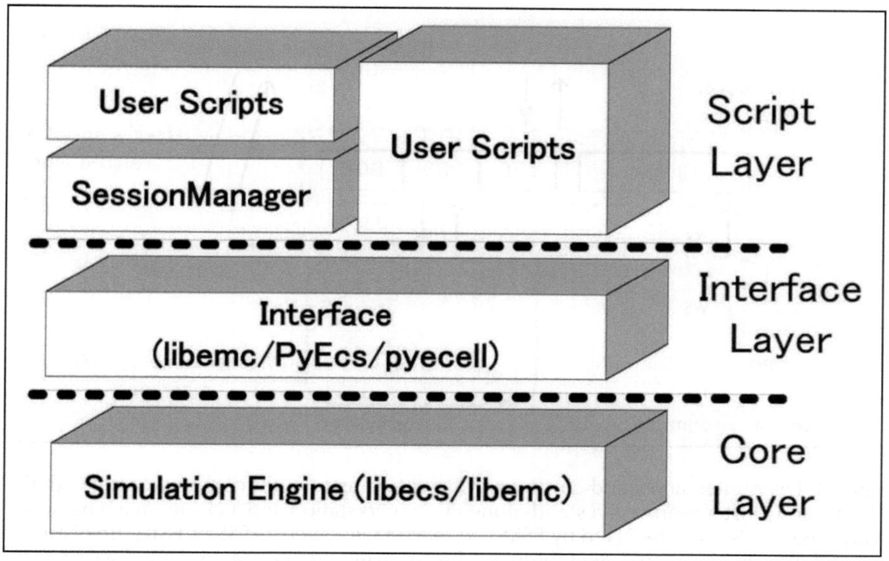


Figure 1. ESM architecture. The bottom layer includes a class library for cell simulation (libecs) and its C++ API (libemc). The top layer represents python front-end utilities such as ESM, GUI and analytical tools. The middle layer (libemc, PyEcs and pyecell) is the interface connecting the bottom and top layers.

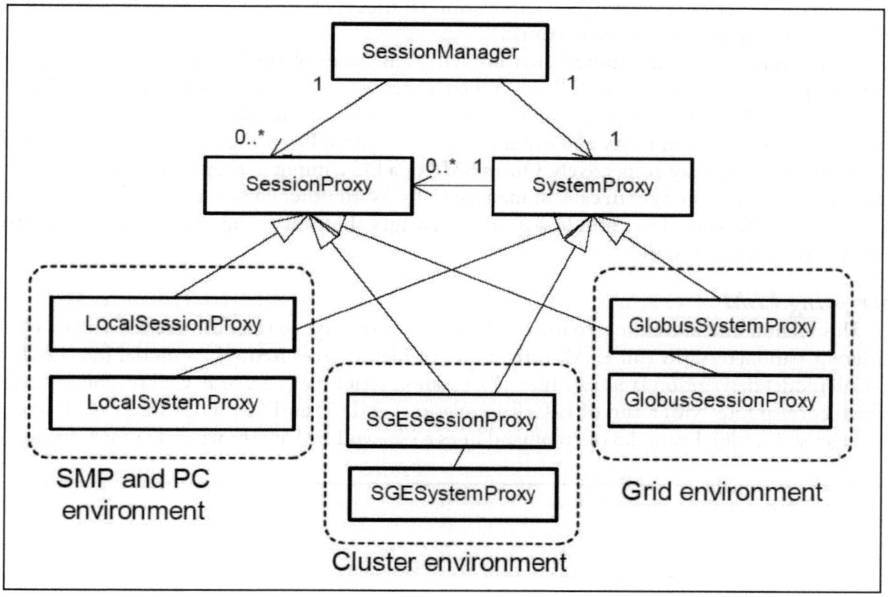


Figure 2. Class diagram of ESM. The Session Manager class provides flat APIs for user scripting. System Proxy is a proxy of a computing environment. Each object of Session Proxy corresponds to a process or a job. Reproduced from reference 8 with kind permission of Springer Science+Business Media.

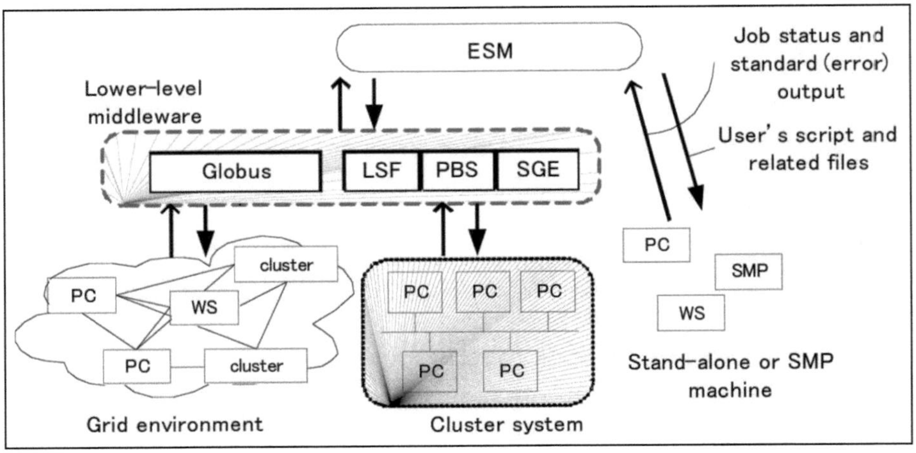


Figure 3. Distributed and stand-alone environment infrastructures communicating with ESM. PC, WS and cluster represent a stand-alone PC, a workstation and a cluster machine, respectively. The user's script received by ESM and related files, such as ESS or EML, are distributed to a grid or a cluster environment through a lower-level middleware. In a stand-alone or SMP machine, jobs are directly generated by ESM. The job dispatch and collection of the results are actually done by the subclass of System Proxy with Session Proxy.

environments or processes a job on cluster and grid environments and holds the status of the process or job (waiting, running, recoverable error, unrecoverable error or finished). Unrecoverable data are unrepeatable errors including job submission failures such as end of file (EOF) error due to instantaneous breakdown of the network.

To accommodate a distributed environment, subclasses of the Session Proxy and System Proxy objects are exemplified as follows. When a user uses a cluster machine on which the Sun Grid Engine (SGE) parallel batch middleware is installed, the Session Manager class generates instances of SGE Session Proxy and instances of SGE System Proxy that are subclasses of Session Proxy and System Proxy, respectively. On an SMP or a PC computer, they spawn processes in the local computer and use system calls to manage tasks. With other environments, these subclasses contact with the lower-level middleware that manages the computing environment to control jobs and so obtain job status.

## *Scripting ESM*

This section introduces how to use ESM and an ESM script to run multiple E-Cell tasks with different parameters. To run ESM, three types of files are required: (1) a model file (EML or E-Cell model description language file), (2) a session script file (ESS or E-Cell session script file which corresponds with a run of E-Cell simulation) and (3) an ESM script file (E-Cell session manager script file). Examples of command lines to spawn ESM are shown in Figure 4. Examples

```
% ecell3-session-manager --environment=Local ems.py                        (1)
% ecell3-session-manager --environment=SGE --concurrency=30 ems.py        (2)
% ecell3-session-manager --environment=Globus2 --concurrency=100 ems.py  (3)
```

Figure 4. Command line examples for running ESM. The '—environment=' and '—concurrency=' command-line arguments specify the computing environment and the concurrency of the distributed jobs, respectively. The last argument, 'ems.py', is an ESM script file for describing the ESM procedure, see Figure 5 for details of 'ems.py'. Reproduced from reference 8 with kind permission of Springer Science+Business Media.

```
MODEL_FILE='model.eml'
ESS_FILE='runsession.py'

# (2) Register jobs.
aJobIDList = []
for VALUE_OF_S in range(0,100):
        aParameterDict={'MODEL_FILE':MODEL_FILE, 'VALUE_OF_S':VALUE_OF_S}
        #           registerEcellSession(the script, parameters, files that the ESS uses)
        aJobID =    registerEcellSession(ESS_FILE, aParameterDict, [MODEL_FILE,])
        aJobIDList.append(aJobID)  # Memorize the job IDs in aJobIDList

# (3) Run the registered jobs.
run()

# (4) Examine the results.
for aJobID in aJobIDList:       # Print the output of each job.
        print getStdout(aJobID)
```

Figure 5. A sample ESM script. This script runs the session script 'runsession.py' 100 times by changing the parameter 'VALUE_OF_S' from 0 to 100. In the resister step (2), an ESS file 'runsession.py' is registered with the parameters ESS_FILE and VALUE_OF_S. The characters of MODEL_FILE and VALUE_OF_S in ESS are replaced for the values of MODEL_FILE and VALUE_OF_S, respectively. In step (3), all registered ESS files are executed. Step (4) simply prints out the standard output of all executed jobs. Reproduced from reference 8 with kind permission of Springer Science+Business Media.

```
loadModel( MODEL_FILE )                   # Load the model.

S = createEntityStub( 'Variable:/:S' )  # Create a stub object of
                                          # the simulator variable 'Variable:/:S'
S['Value'] = VALUE_OF_S                   # Set the value VALUE_OF_S given by the
                                          # ESM script in Fig.5 to the variable.

run( 200 )                                # Run the simulation for 200 seconds.

message( S['Value'] )                     # Print the value of 'Variable:/:S'.
```

Figure 6. A sample E-Cell session script (ESS). This script runs a simulation model for 200 seconds and outputs the value of the variable 'Variable:/:S' in the model after the simulation. The initial value of the variable is changed to the value of 'VALUE_OF_S' given by the ESM script in Figure 5. Reproduced from reference 8 with kind permission of Springer Science+Business Media.

of an ESM script file and an ESS file used in the script are shown in Figures 5 and 6, respectively. Details of an example ESM script are below.

## Setting System Parameters

The computing environment and concurrency needs to be set when running ESM. The computing parameters specify what types of facilities are to be used. The concurrency parameter specifies the maximum number of CPUs that ESM uses simultaneously. When no concurrency parameter is specified, a default value is used, e.g., 1 CPU is used on a stand-alone PC or numbers of all available queues on a cluster machine are used. These parameters are given as command-line arguments to the 'ecell3-session-manager' command, which runs an ESM indicated by the user. Alternatively, the user can specify the computing environment, named setEnvironment (environment) and setConcurrency (concurrency) in an ESM script. Other execution environmental conditions should be specified here, on top of the ESM scripts. For example, ESM generates intermediate files under a working directory, specified by setTmpRootDir(directory), during its calculation. These files are removed when the procedure reaches the end of the ESM scripts. Saving the setTmpDirRemoval (deleteflag) method with false arguments avoids deletion of these files and is useful for debugging ESM or ESS scripts.

**Registering Jobs**

The registerEcellSession method in an ESM script registers an E-Cell job. It accepts three arguments: (1) the E-Cell session script (ESS) to be executed, (2) the optional parameters given to the job and (3) the input files to the script (at least a model file) that must be available to the ESS upon execution. In the example in Figure 5, 100 copies of the session script 'runsession.py' have been registered with the model file 'model.eml'. An optional parameter to the script, 'VALUE_OF_S' is also given to each session in the range 0, 1, ..., 100. When a job is registered, a Session Proxy is instantiated and the registerEcellSession method returns a unique ID.

**Running the Application**

When the run method is called, registered jobs start to execute or are submitted to the lower-level middleware. During this step, System Proxy transfers the ESS file and all other related files to the execution environment. System Proxy communicates with the computer operating system or lower-level middleware at regular intervals to track the process and job status and to update the status of Session Proxy itself. Until all jobs and processes are either 'finished' normally or are stopped in 'unrecoverable error' states, the run method is repeated. Job execution in this method is parallelized, if possible.

**Examining the Results**

After running ESS, scripts such as that shown in Figure 5 print the results of the executed ESS to the screen; getStdout (aJobID) returns the standard output of the job specified by a job ID.

## Parameter Estimation on ESM

This section introduces parameter estimation for an example application scripting program built on ESM architecture. This program incorporates a genetic algorithm—an evolutionary algorithm—to identify a global minimum of given fitness functions, avoiding local minima. A brief overview of a genetic algorithm is as follows. First, individuals in arbitrary numbers are generated with searching parameter sets whose values are randomly distributed within the search space. Second, each individual is independently evaluated with the user-defined fitness function. A square-error function between given and simulation-predicted trajectories is often used as the fitness function. Third, individuals are proliferated or wiped-out from the group of individuals according to their fitness values. Fourth, individuals are crossed over. Fifth, each individual is mutated. These procedures are repeated unless individuals with a sufficient fitness value are found.

A detailed implementation of the genetic algorithm on ESM is described here. The first step of initialization includes parsing a file specifying the parameter estimation process (e.g., Fig. 7) and setting up working conditions, e.g., preparing a temporary working directory with setTmpRootDir (directory) and setting concurrency with setConcurrency (concurrency). Moreover, individual instances need to be tested with random parameters. The genetic algorithm itself is also initialized according to the specified values in the [GA] section of the setting file. In addition, the other parameters are parsed here for the following procedures.

```
Fundamental]
[Seed]
RANDOM SEED                          = 0

[GA]
MAX GENERATION                       = 4
POPULATION                           = 10
FINISH CONDITION                     = 0.005

[Input file or directory]
ESS FILE                             = runsession.py

EML KEY                              = _EML_
EML FILES                            = simple.eml
```

Figure 7. An example of part of a setup file for a step in a process of parameter estimation built on ESS. The format of this file simply follows 'items = value'. The value of 'RANDOM SEED' represents the initializing value for a random function used in a genetic algorithm. 'MAX GENERATION' and 'POPULATION' mean the maximum number of generations and the number population, respectively. The genetic algorithm stops when the best fitness value becomes less than or equal to the threshold by 'FINISH CONDITION'. The value of 'ESS FILE' is the ESS file in which the procedure to evaluate an individual and to calculate fitness value is written. The value of 'EML KEY' is used to specify an EML file in the ESS file. The value of 'EML KEY' in the ESS file will be replaced to the value of 'EML FILES' when the procedure is executed.

In the second step of the evaluation, E-Cell sessions with different searching parameters are registered using registerEcellSession (essfile, argument, extrafiles) methods; 'essfile' and 'extrafiles' represent an ESS file which includes search parameters and a list of training-time course data files to be used by the fitness function, respectively. Next, the call run method is simply applied to execute the registered ESS files (Fig. 8). Procedures described in an ESS run a simulation with given parameters and evaluate fitness values defined in the ESS. When all spawned sessions finish in success, all calculated fitness values are converged. Furthermore, the third step of selection, the fourth step of crossover and the fifth step of mutation follow and then go back to the second step of the evaluation.

On a stand-alone PC, the parameter estimation works as a simple genetic algorithm that executes all ESS scripts in sequence. In grid or cluster environments, it behaves as a master-slave parallel GA, where the master process works on a master node and the calculation of fitness values (procedures written in ESS) is evaluated concurrently in a slave process distributed in parallel computational resources.

## Discussion

We have evaluated ESM by implementing simple iterations of E-Cell sessions and a genetic algorithm on ESM. The procedure we described works transparently in both stand-alone and distributed computational environments. An ESM script is helpful for users who might not be familiar with programming parallel environments. It enables these users to implement analysis of algorithms and to easily parallelize them. All scripts can be written in the Python language utilizing ESM's user-friendly API methods. Indeed, the architecture of ESM is so generic that it can execute ordinary scripts, such as Python, Perl and Shell by the registerJobSession method rather than registerEcellSession.

In homogeneous parallel computing environments such as shared-memory machines or PC clusters, it is relatively easy to schedule jobs to minimize the total amount of processing time. On the other hand, heterogeneous environments such as PC grids require more sophisticated

```
from ecell.ECDDataFile import *
import os

# simulation
DURATION = 1000
START_TIME = 0
INTERVAL = 10

# parameters to be logged.
VARIABLE_LIST_FOR_LOGGER = [ 'Variable:/:S:Value', 'Variable:/:P:Value' ]

# (1) load an eml file
loadModel( _EML_ )

# (2) set parameters
anEntity = createEntityStub( 'Process:/:E' )
anEntity.setProperty( 'KmS', _KmS_ )
anEntity.setProperty( 'KcF', _KcF_ )

# (3) create logger stubs
aLoggerList = []
for i in range( len(VARIABLE_LIST_FOR_LOGGER) ):
    aLogger = createLoggerStub( VARIABLE_LIST_FOR_LOGGER[i] )
    aLogger.create()
    aLoggerList.append( aLogger )

# (4) run simulation
run( DURATION )

# (5) reading of training time-course (omitted)
# (6) saving predicted time-course (omitted)
# (7) calculation of the difference between training and prediction
#       simulated time-courses (omitted)

# (8) writing of the value of fitness function to 'result.dat'
open('result.dat','w').write(str(aDifferenceBetweenTheTimeCourses))
```

Figure 8. An example ESS (E-Cell session script file) for parameter estimation. Step 1) a model file is loaded; Step 2) KmS and KcF are set to values given by ESM to the model; Step 3) logger stubs are prepared for the model's time-courses; Step 4) simulation is executed; Step 5) given time-course data is read; Step 6) the simulated time-courses are saved to files; Step 7) simulated and given time-courses are compared to evaluate the model; and Step 8) the fitness value is placed into a file as a result.

scheduling because the topology of remote computation nodes and the network speed between them is generally unpredictably. Such environments deteriorate the parallelization performance of programs requiring synchronous timing of parallelized sessions such as the master-slave genetic algorithm. As an example to resolve this problem, Island-type genetic algorithms may reduce these adverse affects by reducing synchronous transactions among remote calculation nodes and are suitable for heterogeneous and coarse parallel environments. The implementation of such algorithms accommodating a heterogeneous environment is something we have set down for future work.

Medium scaled infrastructures including coarse-distributed computational resources where multiple PC-clusters are connected by grid technology are common network architectures. The current run method in an ESM script simply distributes all registered jobs, which means that job scheduling depends on lower layer middleware. Although submission in the grid version of ESS with cluster options is one solution to efficiently utilize such middleware, users must have detailed knowledge of the features of distributed environments to utilize them. In the future, we will investigate implementation of alternative methods with a sophisticated scheduling scheme.

We have also developed various kinds of other analytical scripts that run on ESM: a sensitivity analysis toolkit based on MCA and a bifurcation analysis toolkit that is used to estimate the stability of nonlinear models. We still need to design a scheduling scheme suitable for the algorithms commonly used in biological systems.

## Conclusion

We developed a distributed computing module for the E-Cell System that we named the E-Cell Session Manager (ESM). This software is a higher-level job distribution middleware providing a Python-scripting environment to transparently run simulation runs on any type of stand-alone, cluster or grid computing environments. An EMS script, a script language of ESM and parameter estimation built on ESM is included in the E-Cell Simulation Environment Version 3 package. This package can be downloaded from http://www.e-cell.org/.

## References


1. Voit EO, Marino S, Lall R, Challenges for the identification of biological systems from in vivo time series data. In Silico Biology 2005; 5(2):83-92.
2. Sauro HM, Hucka M, Finney A et al. Next generation simulation tools: the Systems Biology Workbench and BioSPICE integration. OMICS 2003; 7(4):355-372.
3. Dhar PK, Meng TC, Somani S et al. Grid cellware: the first grid-enabled tool for modelling and simulating cellular processes. Bioinformatics 2005; 21(7):1284-1287.
4. Kimura S, Kawasaki T, Hatakeyama M et al. OBIYagns: a grid-based biochemical simulator with a parameter estimator. Bioinformatics 2004; 20(10):1646-1648.
5. Foster I, Kesselman C. Globus: A metacomputing infrastructure toolkit. Int. J. Supercomput. Appl 1997; 11(3); 115-128
6. Stevens RD, Robinson AJ, Goble CA. $^{my}$Grid: personalised bioinformatics on the information grid. Bioinformatics 2003; 19:302-304.
7. Aloisio G, Cafaro M, Fiore S et al. ProGenGrid: a grid-enabled platform for bioinformatics. Stud Health Technol Inform 2005; 112:113-126.
8. Sugimoto M, Takahashi K, Kitayama T et al. Distributed cell biology simulations with E-Cell System Lecture Notes in Computer Science, Berlin, Springer-Verlag 2005; 3370:20-31.

# Chapter 4

# A Guide to Modeling Reaction-Diffusion of Molecules with the E-Cell System

**Satya Nanda Vel Arjunan***

## Abstract

The E-Cell System is an advanced platform intended for mathematical modeling and simulation of well-stirred biochemical systems. We have recently implemented the Spatiocyte method as a set of plug in modules to the E-Cell System, allowing simulations of complicated multicompartment dynamical processes with inhomogeneous molecular distributions. With Spatiocyte, the diffusion and reaction of each molecule can be handled individually at the microscopic scale. Here we describe the basic theory of the method and provide the installation and usage guides of the Spatiocyte modules. Where possible, model examples are also given to quickly familiarize the reader with spatiotemporal model building and simulation.

## Introduction

The E-Cell System version 3 can model and simulate both deterministic and stochastic biochemical processes.[1] Simulated molecules are assumed to be dimensionless and homogeneously distributed in a compartment. Some processes such as cell signaling and cytokinesis, however, depend on cellular geometry and spatially localized molecules to carry out their functions. To reproduce such processes using spatially resolved models in silico, we have developed a lattice-based stochastic reaction-diffuson (RD) simulation method, called Spatiocyte,[2] and implemented it as a set of plug in modules to the E-Cell System.[3] Spatiocyte allows molecular diffusion and reaction to take place between different compartments: for example, a volume molecule in the cytoplasm can diffuse and react with a surface molecule on the plasma membrane. Since molecules are represented as spheres with dimensions, it can also reproduce anomalous diffusion of molecules in a crowded compartment.[4,5] Using Spatiocyte simulated microscopy visualization feature, simulation results of spatiotemporal localization of molecules can be evaluated by directly comparing them with experimentally obtained fluorescent microscopy images.

The theory and algorithm of the Spatiocyte method are provided in Arjunan and Tomita (2010)[2] while the implementation details are described in Arjunan and Tomita (2009).[3] In this chapter, we provide a guide on how to build spatiotemporal RD models using Spatiocyte modules. We begin with the basic theory of the method and proceed with the installation procedures. The properties of each module are outlined in the subsequent section. Some example models are given to familiarize the reader with the common model structures while describing the modules. We conclude this chapter by outlining the planned future directions of Spatiocyte development.

*RIKEN Quantitative Biology Center, Furuedai, Suita, Osaka, Japan.
Email: satya@riken.jp

*E-Cell System: Basic Concepts and Applications*, edited by Satya Nanda Vel Arjunan, Pawan K. Dhar and Masaru Tomita. 

## Spatiocyte Method

In this section, we summarize the underlying features of the Spatiocyte method that are necessary to build an RD model. For a more detailed description of the method we direct the reader to a previous article.[2]

The Spatiocyte method discretizes the space into a hexagonal close-packed (HCP) lattice of regular sphere voxels with radius $r_v$. Each voxel has 12 adjoining neighbors. To represent a surface compartment such as a cell or a nuclear membrane, all empty voxels of the compartment are occupied with immobile lipid molecules. The method also allows molecules to be simulated at microscopic and compartmental spatial scales simultaneously. In the former, each molecule is discrete and treated individually. For example, each diffusing molecule at the microscopic scale is moved independently by a *DiffusionProcess* from a source voxel to a target neighbor voxel after a given diffusion step interval. Immobile molecules are also simulated at the microscopic scale. Conversely at the compartmental scale, molecules are assumed to be homogeneously distributed (HD) and thus, the concentration information of each HD species is sufficient without explicit diffusion movements. Depending on the simulated spatial scale and the mobility of the reacting species, molecules can undergo either diffusion-influenced or diffusion-decoupled reactions.

All second-order reactions comprising two diffusing reactants, or a diffusing and an immobile reactant are diffusion-influenced, and are therefore, executed by the *DiffusionInfluencedReactionProcess*. The remaining reactions, which include all zeroth- and first-order reactions, and second-order reactions that involve two adjoining immobile reactants or at least one HD reactant, can be decoupled from diffusion. These diffusion-decoupled reactions are performed by the *SpatiocyteNextReactionProcess*.

We proceed with the execution of *DiffusionInfluencedReactionProcess* for a reaction $j$. Following our discretized scheme[2] of the Collins and Kimball RD approach,[6] when a diffusing molecule collides with a reactant pair of $j$ at the target voxel, they react with probability

$$p_j = \begin{cases} \frac{k_{AB}}{6\sqrt{2}(D_A+D_B)r_v}, & A_v + B_v \xrightarrow{k_{AB}} \text{product(s)}, \\ \frac{k_{AA}}{6\sqrt{2}D_A r_v}, & A_v + A_v \xrightarrow{k_{AA}} \text{product(s)}, \\ \frac{\gamma k_{AB}}{D_A+D_B}, & A_s + B_s \xrightarrow{k_{AB}} \text{product(s)}, \\ \frac{\gamma k_{AA}}{D_A}, & A_s + A_s \xrightarrow{k_{AA}} \text{product(s)}, \\ \frac{\sqrt{2}k_{AB}}{3D_A r_v}, & A_v + B_s \xrightarrow{k_{AB}} \text{product(s)}, \\ \frac{24 k_S r_v}{(6+3\sqrt{3}+2\sqrt{6})D_A}, & A_v(+L_s) \xrightarrow{k_S} \text{product(s)}, \end{cases}$$

where the constant $\gamma = \frac{(2\sqrt{2}+4\sqrt{3}+3\sqrt{6}+\sqrt{22})^2}{72(6\sqrt{2}+4\sqrt{3}+3\sqrt{6})}$, $L$ is the lipid species, $k$ is the intrinsic reaction rate of $j$, $D$ is the diffusion coefficient, while the species subscripts $v$ and $s$ denote volume and surface species respectively.

The *DiffusionProcess* handles the voxel-to-voxel random walk of diffusing molecules and the collisions that take place between each walk. The latter is necessary when a diffusing species participates in a strongly diffusion-limited reaction and the time slice between each walk is too large for an accurate value of $p_j$. Given $t_s$ is the current simulation time, the next time a molecule of a diffusing species $i$ with a diffusion coefficient $D_i$ can be moved to a randomly selected neighbor voxel is

$$t_d^i = t_s + \frac{\alpha_i {r_v}^2}{D_i}$$

where in the HCP lattice, the constant $\alpha_i = \frac{2}{3}$ if it is a volume species or $\alpha_i = \left(\frac{2\sqrt{2}+4\sqrt{3}+3\sqrt{6}+\sqrt{22}}{6\sqrt{2}+4\sqrt{3}+3\sqrt{6}}\right)^2$

if it belongs to a surface compartment. However, if $i$ participates in a diffusion-limited reaction, a reactive collision may take place at time slices smaller than the walk interval $\frac{\alpha_i r_v^2}{D_i}$, causing $p_j > 1$. To ensure $p_j \leq 1$, we reduce the *DiffusionProcess* interval such that its next execution time becomes

$$t_d^i = \begin{cases} t_s + \frac{\alpha_i r_v^2}{D_i}, & \rho_i \leq P_i, \\ t_s + \frac{\alpha_i r_v^2 P_i}{D_i \rho_i}, & \rho_i > P_i. \end{cases}$$

Here $P_i$ is an arbitrarily set reaction probability limit (default value is unity) such that $0 \leq P_i \leq 1$, and $\rho_i = \max\{p_1, \ldots, p_J\}$ where $J$ is the total number of diffusion-influenced reactions participated by the species $i$. At each process interval, the molecule can collide as usual with a neighbor reactant pair and react with a scaled probability of $p_j P_i / \rho_i$. In the diffusion-limited case, $\rho_i > P_i$ and because of the reduced interval, the walk probability becomes less than unity to $P_i / \rho_i$.

Reactions that can be decoupled from diffusion such as zeroth- first-order reactions, and second-order reactions that involve two adjoining immobile reactants or at least one HD reactant, are event-driven by the *SpatiocyteNextReactionProcess*. The reaction product can be made up of one or two molecules, which can be either HD or nonHD molecules. The *SpatiocyteNextReactionProcess* is an adapted implementation of the Next Reaction (NR) method,[7] which itself is a variation of the Gillespie algorithm.[8,9]

In the process, the reaction propensity (unit $s^{-1}$) is calculated from the rate coefficient according to

$$a_\mu = \begin{cases} k_A A\#, & A \xrightarrow{k_A} \text{product(s)}, \\ \frac{k_S}{V} A\# S, & A \xrightarrow{k_S} \text{product(s)}, \\ \frac{k_{AB}}{V} A\# B\#, & A + B \xrightarrow{k_{AB}} \text{product(s)}, \\ \frac{k_{AA}}{V} A\#(A\# - 1), & A + A \xrightarrow{k_{AA}} \text{product(s)}. \end{cases}$$

Here, $S$ and $V$ are area and volume of the reaction compartment respectively, while $k_S$ (unit $ms^{-1}$) is the surface-average adsorption rate of an HD volume species $A$. In the second-order reactions, $V$ is replaced with $S$ if both reactants are in a surface compartment. The next reaction time of a randomly selected molecule in a first order reaction or a pair of molecules in a second-order reaction is given by

$$t_r^\mu = t_s - \frac{\ln u_r}{a_\mu},$$

with $u_r$ a uniformly distributed random number in the range (0,1).

If a reaction has a nonHD product, the new molecule will replace a nonHD reactant in the product compartment. Otherwise if the reaction only involves HD reactants or if the product belongs to a different compartment, the new nonHD molecule will be placed in a random vacant voxel of the product compartment. The placement of a second nonHD product also follows the same procedure. For intercompartmental reactions, a nonHD product will occupy a vacant voxel adjoining both compartments.

Dynamic localization patterns of simulated molecules can be directly compared with experimentally obtained fluorescence microscopy images and videos using the *MicroscopyTrackingProcess* and the *SpatiocyteVisualizer*. Together, these modules simulate the microphotography process by recording the trajectory of simulated molecules over the camera exposure time and displaying their spatially localized densities. The *MicroscopyTrackingProcess* records the number of times the molecules of a species occupy each voxel at diffusion step intervals over the exposure time. The *SpatiocyteVisualizer* then displays the species color at each voxel with intensity and opacity levels that are directly proportional the voxel occupancy frequency. Colors from different species occupying the same voxel are blended to mimic colocalization patterns observed in multiple-labeling experiments.

## Installing and Running Spatiocyte

The Spatiocyte source code is distributed as open source software under the GNU General Public License and is available at GitHub. At the time of writing, the Spatiocyte modules of the E-Cell System have been tested to run on Linux systems. Spatiocyte does not yet support other operating systems. Here we describe the installation procedures on a Ubuntu Linux system.

On a freshly installed Ubuntu Linux, E-Cell System version 3 and Spatiocyte require several additional packages:

```
$ sudo apt-get install automake libtool g++ libgsl0-dev python-numpy python-ply
libboost-python-dev libgtkmm-2.4-dev libgtkglextmm-x11-1.2-dev libhdf5-serial-dev
git valgrind
```

The general installation procedure of the E-Cell System version 3 is as follows:

```
$ cd
$ mkdir wrk
$ cd wrk
$ git clone https://github.com/ecell/ecell3.git
$ cd ecell3
$ ./autogen.sh
$ ./configure --prefix=$HOME/root
$ make -j3 (or just make, if there is only one CPU core available)
$ make install (files will be installed in the $HOME/root directory)
$ gedit ~/.bashrc (other editors such as emacs or vim can also be used here)
```

The following lines, which specify the environment variables of the E-Cell System should be appended to the .bashrc file:

```
  export PATH=$HOME/root/bin:$PATH
  export LD_LIBRARY_PATH=$HOME/root/lib:$LD_LIBRARY_PATH:.
  export PYTHONPATH=$HOME/root/lib/python:$HOME/root/lib/python2.7/site-
packages:$PYTHONPATH
  export ECELL3_DM_PATH=$HOME
```

In the line 3 above, the Python version number '2.7' should be updated if it is different in the installed system. Next, we load the new environment variables:

```
$ source -/.bashrc
$ ecell3-session-monitor (try opening it, the window shown in Figure 1 should appear, and then close it)
We can now attempt to run a simple model in the E-Cell Model (EM) language,
simple.em:
$ cd $HOME/wrk/ecell3/doc/samples/simple/
$ ecell3-em2eml simple.em
$ ecell3-session-monitor
```

Using `ecell3-em2eml`, the model file `simple.em` was converted into `simple.eml` in Extensible Markup Language (XML) format. The `simple.eml` file can now be loaded from the File menu of the E-Cell Session Monitor or the File open button (see Fig. 1). Try running the simulation by clicking on the Start button.

The steps to install E-Cell3-Spatiocyte are as follows:

```
$ cd $HOME/wrk
$ git clone git://github.com/ecell/ecell3-spatiocyte.git
$ cd ecell3-spatiocyte
$ make -j3 (or just make, if there is only one CPU core available)
```

The E-Cell3-Spatiocyte package includes the MinDE model (see Fig. 2) reported in Arjunan and Tomita (2010).[2] We can now attempt to run the model with the following steps:

```
$ cd $HOME/wrk/ecell3-spatiocyte/
$ ecell3-em2eml 2010.arjunan.syst.synth.biol.wt.em
$ ecell3-session-monitor
```

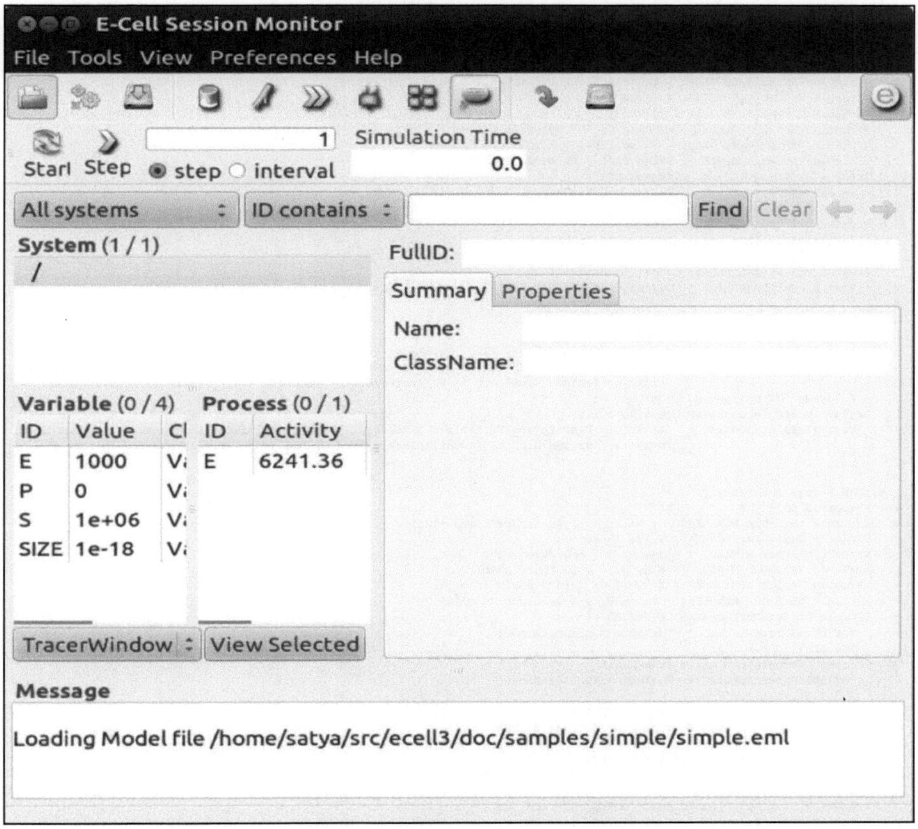


Figure 1. The E-Cell session monitor.

Load the model `2010.arjunan.syst.synth.biol.wt.eml` and try running the simulation for 90 seconds.

We can also run Spatioctye models using command line interface of the E-Cell System:

```
$ ecell3-session -f 2010.arjunan.syst.synth.biol.wt.em
<2010.arjunan.syst.synth.biol.wt.eml, t = 0>>> run(90)
<2010.arjunan.syst.synth.biol.wt.eml, t = 90>>> exit()
```

Models that are created using the Python script can be run as,

```
$ ecell3-session 2012.arjunan.chapter.neuron.py
```

When running a Spatiocyte model with the *VisualizationLogProcess* module enabled, the three-dimensional positional information of a logged molecule species will be stored in `visualLog0.dat` (default file name). The molecules can be viewed in a separate visualizer window even while the simulation is still running. To view them, we can run *SpatiocyteVisualizer* by issuing

```
$ ./spatiocyte
```

The visualizer will load the `visualLog0.dat` file by default and display the molecules at every log interval (see Fig. 3). The keyboard shortcuts that are available for the visualizer are listed in the *SpatiocyteVisualizer* module section.

```
Stepper SpatiocyteStepper(SS) { VoxelRadius 1e-8; } # m
System System(/) {
  StepperID SS;
  Variable Variable(GEOMETRY) { Value 3; } # rod shaped compartment
  Variable Variable(LENGTHX) { Value 4.5e-6; } # m
  Variable Variable(LENGTHY) { Value 1e-6; } # m
  Variable Variable(VACANT) { Value 0; }
  Variable Variable(MinDatp) { Value 0; } # molecule number
  Variable Variable(MinDadp) { Value 1300; } # molecule number
  Variable Variable(MinEE) { Value 0; } # molecule number
  Process DiffusionProcess(diffuseMinD) {
    VariableReferenceList [_ Variable:/:MinDatp] [_ Variable:/:MinDadp];
    D 16e-12; } # m^2/s
  Process DiffusionProcess(diffuseMinE) {
    VariableReferenceList [_ Variable:/:MinEE];
    D 10e-12; } # m^2/s
  Process VisualizationLogProcess(visualize) {
    VariableReferenceList [_ Variable:/Surface:MinEE] [_ Variable:/Surface:MinDEE] [_ Variable:/Surface:MinDEED]
                          [_ Variable:/Surface:MinD];
    LogInterval 0.5; } # s
  Process MicroscopyTrackingProcess(track) {
    VariableReferenceList [_ Variable:/Surface:MinEE 2] [_ Variable:/Surface:MinDEE 3] [_ Variable:/Surface:MinDEED 4]
                          [_ Variable:/Surface:MinD 1] [_ Variable:/Surface:MinEE -2] [_ Variable:/Surface:MinDEED -2]
                          [_ Variable:/Surface:MinEE -1] [_ Variable:/Surface:MinDEED -4] [_ Variable:/Surface:MinD -1];
    FileName "microscopyLog0.dat"; }
  Process MoleculePopulateProcess(populate) {
    VariableReferenceList [_ Variable:/:MinDatp] [_ Variable:/:MinDadp] [_ Variable:/:MinEE] [_ Variable:/Surface:MinD]
                          [_ Variable:/Surface:MinDEE] [_ Variable:/Surface:MinDEED] [_ Variable:/Surface:MinEE]; }
}

System System(/Surface) {
  StepperID SS;
  Variable Variable(DIMENSION) { Value 2; } # surface compartment
  Variable Variable(VACANT) { Value 0; }
  Variable Variable(MinD) { Value 0; } # molecule number
  Variable Variable(MinEE) { Value 0; } # molecule number
  Variable Variable(MinDEE) { Value 700; } # molecule number
  Variable Variable(MinDEED) { Value 0; } # molecule number
  Process DiffusionProcess(diffuseMinD) {
    VariableReferenceList [_ Variable:/Surface:MinD];
    D 0.02e-12; } # m^2/s
  Process DiffusionProcess(diffuseMinEE) {
    VariableReferenceList [_ Variable:/Surface:MinEE];
    D 0.02e-12; } # m^2/s
  Process DiffusionProcess(diffuseMinDEE) {
    VariableReferenceList [_ Variable:/Surface:MinDEE];
    D 0.02e-12; } # m^2/s
  Process DiffusionProcess(diffuseMinDEED) {
     VariableReferenceList [_ Variable:/Surface:MinDEED];
    D 0.02e-12; } # m^2/s
  Process DiffusionInfluencedReactionProcess(reaction1) {
    VariableReferenceList [_ Variable:/Surface:VACANT -1] [_ Variable:/:MinDatp -1] [_ Variable:/Surface:MinD 1];
    k 2.2e-8; } # m/s
  Process DiffusionInfluencedReactionProcess(reaction2) {
    VariableReferenceList [_ Variable:/Surface:MinD -1] [_ Variable:/:MinDatp -1] [_ Variable:/Surface:MinD 1]
                          [_ Variable:/Surface:MinD 1];
    k 3e-20; } # m^3/s
  Process DiffusionInfluencedReactionProcess(reaction3) {
    VariableReferenceList [_ Variable:/Surface:MinD -1] [_ Variable:/:MinEE -1] [_ Variable:/Surface:MinDEE 1];
    k 5e-19; } # m^3/s
  Process SpatiocyteNextReactionProcess(reaction4) {
    VariableReferenceList [_ Variable:/Surface:MinDEE -1] [_ Variable:/Surface:MinEE 1] [_ Variable:/:MinDadp 1];
    k 1; } # s^{-1}
  Process SpatiocyteNextReactionProcess(reaction5) {
    VariableReferenceList [_ Variable:/:MinDadp -1] [_ Variable:/:MinDatp 1];
    k 5; } # s^{-1}
  Process DiffusionInfluencedReactionProcess(reaction6) {
    VariableReferenceList [_ Variable:/Surface:MinDEE -1] [_ Variable:/Surface:MinD -1] [_ Variable:/Surface:MinDEED 1];
    k 5e-15; } # m^2/s
  Process SpatiocyteNextReactionProcess(reaction7) {
    VariableReferenceList [_ Variable:/Surface:MinDEED -1] [_ Variable:/Surface:MinDEE 1] [_ Variable:/:MinDadp 1];
    k 1; } # s^{-1}
  Process SpatiocyteNextReactionProcess(reaction8) {
    VariableReferenceList [_ Variable:/Surface:MinEE -1] [_ Variable:/:MinEE 1];
    k 0.83; } # s^{-1}
}
```

Figure 2. E-Cell Model (EM) description file for the MinDE model. The file is available in the Spatiocyte source package as 2010.arjunan.syst.synth.biol.wt.em.

If the program fails and crashes when loading or running a model, we can get some debugging information using the Valgrind tool:

```
$ valgrind —tool = memcheck —num-callers = 40 —leak-check = full python $HOME/
root/bin/ecell3-session -f modelFileName.eml
```

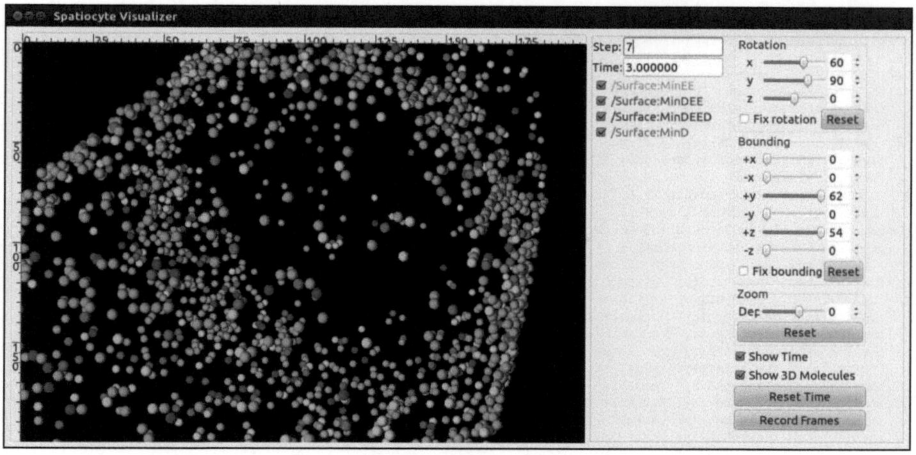


Figure 3. The *SpatiocyteVisualizer* displaying simulated membrane-bound proteins of the MinDE model.

## Spatiocyte Modules

In Spatiocyte modules, the unit of numeric values is given in meters, seconds, radians and molecule numbers. A Spatiocyte model file created using the E-Cell Model (EM) language is shown in Figure 2. The file contains the wildtype *Escherichia coli* MinDE cytokinesis regulation model that was reported in Arjunan and Tomita (2010).[2] A schematic representation of the model is given in Figure 4. Python script examples to build models with more complex compartments are provided in Figures 5 and 6. Figures 7 and 8 illustrate 3D visualizations of the resulting models.

### *Compartment*

Compartments are defined hierarchically and follow the format used by the E-Cell System version 3 (see the E-Cell Simulation Environment Version 3 User's Manual for details). Each sub-compartment within a parent compartment is created according to the alphabetical order of the compartment names. Predefined *Variables* that specify the *Compartment* properties include DIMENSION, GEOMETRY, LENGTHX, LENGTHY, LENGTHZ, ORIGINX, ORIGINY, ORIGINZ, ROTATEX, ROTATEY, ROTATEZ, XYPLANE, XZPLANE, YZPLANE, VACANT, DIFFUSIVE and REACTIVE. Examples of these variable definitions can be seen in Figures 2 (lines 4-7 and 33-34), 5 (lines 5-8, 17-24, 31-32, 41-49 and 52-54) and 6 (lines 46-49, 59-60, 63-69 and 71-72).

Molecule species within a *Compartment* are also defined as a *Variable*. The *Value* property of each species stipulates the molecule number during initialization. All species by default are nonHD. Examples of nonHD species definitions can be seen in Figures 2 (lines 8-10 and 35-38), 5 (line

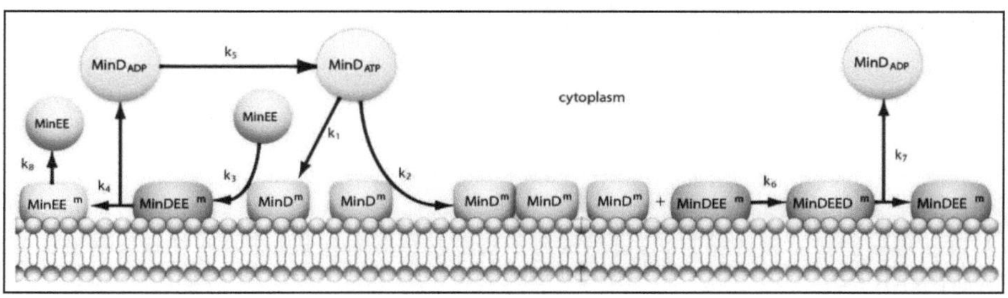


Figure 4. A schematic representation of the MinDE model.

```
1 # Example of python scripting to create a neuron with 5 minor processes
2 theSimulator.createStepper('SpatiocyteStepper', 'SS').VoxelRadius = 10e-8
3 # Create the root container compartment using the default Cuboid geometry:
4 theSimulator.rootSystem.StepperID = 'SS'
5 theSimulator.createEntity('Variable', 'Variable:/:LENGTHX').Value = 61e-6
6 theSimulator.createEntity('Variable', 'Variable:/:LENGTHY').Value = 25e-6
7 theSimulator.createEntity('Variable', 'Variable:/:LENGTHZ').Value = 5.5e-6
8 theSimulator.createEntity('Variable', 'Variable:/:VACANT')
9 logger = theSimulator.createEntity('VisualizationLogProcess', 'Process:/:logger')
10 logger.LogInterval = 1
11 logger.VariableReferenceList = [['_', 'Variable:/Soma/Membrane:VACANT'], ['_', 'Variable:/Soma:K']]
12 logger.VariableReferenceList = [['_', 'Variable:/Dendrite%d/Membrane:VACANT' %i] for i in range(5)]
13 populator = theSimulator.createEntity('MoleculePopulateProcess', 'Process:/:populate')
14 populator.VariableReferenceList = [['_', 'Variable:/Soma:K']]
15 # Create the Soma compartment of the Neuron:
16 theSimulator.createEntity('System', 'System:/:Soma').StepperID = 'SS'
17 theSimulator.createEntity('Variable', 'Variable:/Soma:GEOMETRY').Value = 1
18 theSimulator.createEntity('Variable', 'Variable:/Soma:LENGTHX').Value = 10e-6
19 theSimulator.createEntity('Variable', 'Variable:/Soma:LENGTHY').Value = 10e-6
20 theSimulator.createEntity('Variable', 'Variable:/Soma:LENGTHZ').Value = 6.5e-6
21 theSimulator.createEntity('Variable', 'Variable:/Soma:ORIGINX').Value = -0.48
22 theSimulator.createEntity('Variable', 'Variable:/Soma:ORIGINY').Value = -0.2
23 theSimulator.createEntity('Variable', 'Variable:/Soma:ORIGINZ').Value = -0.6
24 theSimulator.createEntity('Variable', 'Variable:/Soma:VACANT')
25 theSimulator.createEntity('Variable', 'Variable:/Soma:K').Value = 1000
26 diffuser = theSimulator.createEntity('DiffusionProcess', 'Process:/Soma:diffuseK')
27 diffuser.VariableReferenceList = [['_', 'Variable:.:K']]
28 diffuser.D = 0.2e-12
29 # Create the Soma membrane:
30 theSimulator.createEntity('System', 'System:/Soma:Membrane').StepperID = 'SS'
31 theSimulator.createEntity('Variable', 'Variable:/Soma/Membrane:DIMENSION').Value = 2
32 theSimulator.createEntity('Variable', 'Variable:/Soma/Membrane:VACANT')
33 # Parameters of Dendrites/Minor Processes:
34 dendritesLengthX = [40e-6, 10e-6, 10e-6, 10e-6, 10e-6]
35 dendritesOriginX = [0.32, -0.78, -0.48, -0.3, -0.66]
36 dendritesOriginY = [-0.2, -0.2, 0.52, -0.65, -0.65]
37 dendritesRotateZ = [0, 0, 1.57, 0.78, -0.78]
38 for i in range(5):
39   # Create the Dendrite:
40   theSimulator.createEntity('System', 'System:/:Dendrite%d' %i).StepperID = 'SS'
41   theSimulator.createEntity('Variable', 'Variable:/Dendrite%d:GEOMETRY' %i).Value = 3
42   theSimulator.createEntity('Variable', 'Variable:/Dendrite%d:LENGTHX' %i).Value = dendritesLengthX[i]
43   theSimulator.createEntity('Variable', 'Variable:/Dendrite%d:LENGTHY' %i).Value = 1.5e-6
44   theSimulator.createEntity('Variable', 'Variable:/Dendrite%d:ORIGINX' %i).Value = dendritesOriginX[i]
45   theSimulator.createEntity('Variable', 'Variable:/Dendrite%d:ORIGINY' %i).Value = dendritesOriginY[i]
46   theSimulator.createEntity('Variable', 'Variable:/Dendrite%d:ORIGINZ' %i).Value = -0.6
47   theSimulator.createEntity('Variable', 'Variable:/Dendrite%d:ROTATEZ' %i).Value = dendritesRotateZ[i]
48   theSimulator.createEntity('Variable', 'Variable:/Dendrite%d:VACANT' %i)
49   theSimulator.createEntity('Variable', 'Variable:/Dendrite%d:DIFFUSIVE' %i).Name = '/:Soma'
50   # Create the Dendrite membrane:
51   theSimulator.createEntity('System', 'System:/Dendrite%d:Membrane' %i).StepperID = 'SS'
52   theSimulator.createEntity('Variable', 'Variable:/Dendrite%d/Membrane:DIMENSION' %i).Value = 2
53   theSimulator.createEntity('Variable', 'Variable:/Dendrite%d/Membrane:VACANT' %i)
54   theSimulator.createEntity('Variable', 'Variable:/Dendrite%d/Membrane:DIFFUSIVE' %i).Name = '/Soma:Membrane'
55 run(100)
```

Figure 5. A Python script to create a neuron-shaped model. The file is available in the Spatiocyte source package as 2012.arjunan.chapter.neuron.py.

25) and 6 (line 50). To define a HD species, the *Name* property of the *Variable* should be set to "HD" as shown in the EM and Python examples below:

```
Variable Variable(A) {
      Value 100;
      Name "HD"; }
```

```
A = theSimulator.createEntity('Variable', 'Variable:.:A')
A.Value = 100
A.Name = "HD"
```

## DIMENSION

The DIMENSION variable defines the spatial dimension of the compartment, whether it is a line ('1'), surface ('2') or a volume ('3') type. At the time of writing, the line compartment type is still in

```
import math
import random
minDist = 75e-9
dendriteRadius = 0.75e-6
dendriteLength = 10e-6
lengths = [8.4e-6, 6.3e-6, 4.2e-6, 2.1e-6, 1e-6]
lengthFreqs = [7, 10, 11, 21, 108]
mtOriginX = []
mtOriginZ = []
mtOriginY = []
expandedLengths = []

def isSpacedOut(x, y, z, length):
  for i in range(len(expandedLengths)-1):
    maxOriX = mtOriginX[i]*dendriteLength/2 + expandedLengths[i]/2
    minOriX = mtOriginX[i]*dendriteLength/2 - expandedLengths[i]/2
    maxX = x*dendriteLength/2 + length/2
    minX = x*dendriteLength/2 - length/2
    y2 = math.pow((y-mtOriginY[i])*dendriteRadius, 2)
    z2 = math.pow((z-mtOriginZ[i])*dendriteRadius, 2)
    if((minX <= maxOriX or maxX >= minOriX) and math.sqrt(y2+z2) < minDist):
      return False
    elif(minX > maxOriX and math.sqrt(y2+z2+math.pow(minX-maxOriX, 2)) < minDist):
      return False
    elif(maxX < minOriX and math.sqrt(y2+z2+math.pow(maxX-minOriX, 2)) < minDist):
      return False
  return True

for i in range(len(lengthFreqs)):
  maxX = (dendriteLength-lengths[i])/dendriteLength
  for j in range(int(lengthFreqs[i])):
    expandedLengths.append(lengths[i])
    x = random.uniform(-maxX, maxX)
    y = random.uniform(-0.95, 0.95)
    z = random.uniform(-0.95, 0.95)
    while(y*y+z*z > 0.9 or not isSpacedOut(x, y, z, lengths[i])):
      x = random.uniform(-maxX, maxX)
      y = random.uniform(-0.95, 0.95)
      z = random.uniform(-0.95, 0.95)
    mtOriginX.append(x)
    mtOriginY.append(y)
    mtOriginZ.append(z)

theSimulator.createStepper('SpatiocyteStepper', 'SS').VoxelRadius = 0.8e-8
theSimulator.rootSystem.StepperID = 'SS'
theSimulator.createEntity('Variable', 'Variable:/:GEOMETRY').Value = 3
theSimulator.createEntity('Variable', 'Variable:/:LENGTHX').Value = dendriteLength
theSimulator.createEntity('Variable', 'Variable:/:LENGTHY').Value = dendriteRadius*2
theSimulator.createEntity('Variable', 'Variable:/:VACANT')
theSimulator.createEntity('Variable', 'Variable:/:K').Value = 100
diffuser = theSimulator.createEntity('DiffusionProcess', 'Process:/:diffuseK')
diffuser.VariableReferenceList = [['_', 'Variable:/:K']]
diffuser.D = 0.2e-12
visualLogger = theSimulator.createEntity('VisualizationLogProcess', 'Process:/:visualLogger')
visualLogger.LogInterval = 1
visualLogger.VariableReferenceList = [['_', 'Variable:/Membrane:VACANT'], ['_', 'Variable:/:K']]
theSimulator.createEntity('MoleculePopulateProcess', 'Process:/:populate').VariableReferenceList = [['_', 'Variable:/:K']]
theSimulator.createEntity('System', 'System:/:Membrane').StepperID = 'SS'
theSimulator.createEntity('Variable', 'Variable:/Membrane:DIMENSION').Value = 2
theSimulator.createEntity('Variable', 'Variable:/Membrane:VACANT')
for i in range(len(expandedLengths)):
  theSimulator.createEntity('System', 'System:/:Microtubule%d' %i).StepperID = 'SS'
  theSimulator.createEntity('Variable', 'Variable:/Microtubule%d:GEOMETRY' %i).Value = 2
  theSimulator.createEntity('Variable', 'Variable:/Microtubule%d:LENGTHX' %i).Value = expandedLengths[i]
  theSimulator.createEntity('Variable', 'Variable:/Microtubule%d:LENGTHY' %i).Value = 6e-9
  theSimulator.createEntity('Variable', 'Variable:/Microtubule%d:ORIGINX' %i).Value = mtOriginX[i]
  theSimulator.createEntity('Variable', 'Variable:/Microtubule%d:ORIGINY' %i).Value = mtOriginY[i]
  theSimulator.createEntity('Variable', 'Variable:/Microtubule%d:ORIGINZ' %i).Value = mtOriginZ[i]
  theSimulator.createEntity('Variable', 'Variable:/Microtubule%d:VACANT' %i)
  theSimulator.createEntity('System', 'System:/Microtubule%d:Membrane' %i).StepperID = 'SS'
  theSimulator.createEntity('Variable', 'Variable:/Microtubule%d/Membrane:DIMENSION' %i).Value = 2
  theSimulator.createEntity('Variable', 'Variable:/Microtubule%d/Membrane:VACANT' %i)
  visualLogger.VariableReferenceList = [['_', 'Variable:/Microtubule%d/Membrane:VACANT' %i]]
run(100)
```

Figure 6. A Python script to create a compartment with randomly distributed microtubules. The file is available in the Spatiocyte source package as 2012.arjunan.chapter.microtubules.py.

development. A surface compartment encloses its parent volume compartment, and as a result, it cannot be defined independently without a volume compartment to enclose with. A surface compartment does not have any child volume or surface compartment. The root compartment should always be defined as a volume compartment. Since the default DIMENSION value is '3', a volume compartment can be defined without the DIMENSION variable. A volume compartment can also use the predefined variables GEOMETRY, LENGTHX, LENGTHY, LENGTHZ, ORIGINX, ORIGINY, ORIGINZ,

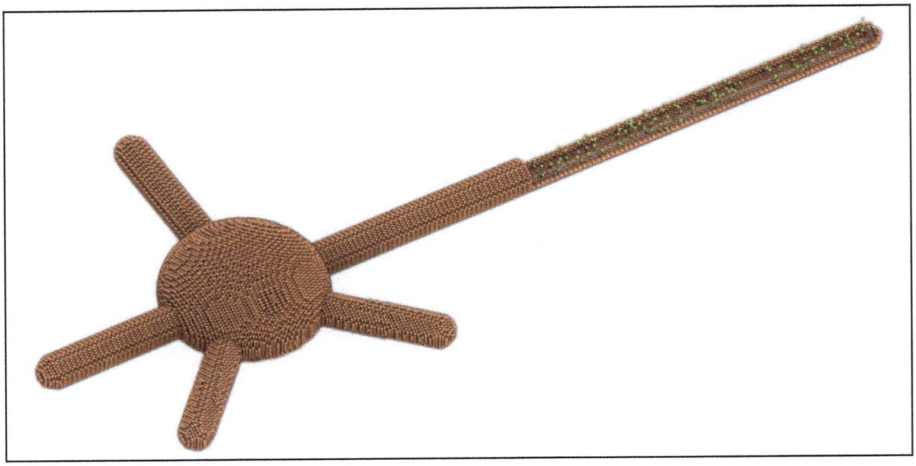

Figure 7. A neuron-shaped compartment created from a combination of rod and ellipsoid compartment geometries. The model is created from the Python script shown in Figure 5.

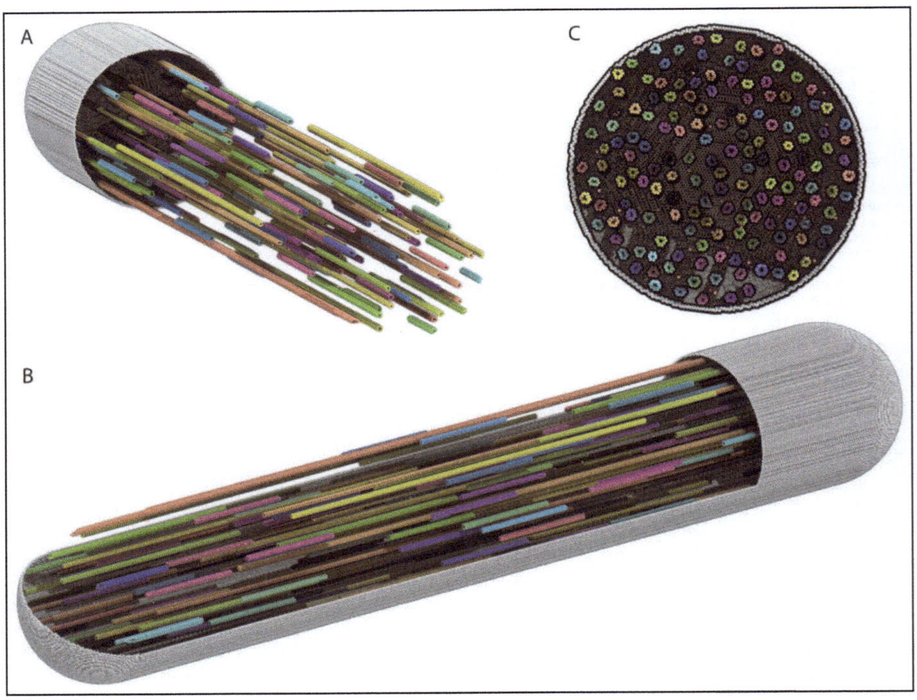


Figure 8. A rod compartment containing randomly distributed microtubules built from cylinder compartments. The model is created from the Python script shown in Figure 6. The steps to create each of the displayed panels in *SpatiocyteVisualizer* are as follows: (A) (i) select all species (i.e., the default configuration), (ii) decrease the +x range to the desired level, (iii) deselect the membrane.VACANT species, (iv) increase the +x range to the maximum level, and (v) select the membrane.VACANT species; (B) the same steps as in (A) and increase -y range to the desired level; and (C) the same steps as in (A) and rotate to the desired angle.

ROTATEX, ROTATEY, ROTATEZ, XYPLANE, XZPLANE, YZPLANE, DIFFUSIVE and VACANT, whereas a surface compartment only requires the DIMENSION and VACANT variables and inherits the remaining relevant properties from its parent compartment. In addition, surface compartments can also define the DIFFUSIVE and REACTIVE variables. See Figures 2 (line 33), 5 (lines 31 and 52) and 6 (lines 59 and 71) for examples of the DIMENSION variable definition.

**GEOMETRY**

The GEOMETRY variable of a volume compartment specifies one of the six supported geometric primitives: cuboid ('0'), ellipsoid ('1'), cylinder ('2'), rod ('3'), torus ('4') and pyramid ('5'). More complex forms can be constructed using a combination of these primitives. Figures 4 and 6 illustrate the construction of a neuron-shaped model using a combination of ellipsoid and rod compartments. Compartments without the GEOMETRY definition is set to the cuboid form since the default value is '0'. For examples of GEOMETRY definition see Figures 2 (line 4), 5 (lines 17 and 41) and 6 (lines 46 and 63).

**LENGTH[X, Y, Z]**

The three variables LENGTH[X, Y, Z] can specify the compartment lengths in the directions of [x, y, z]-axes, respectively. The cuboid, ellipsoid and pyramid compartments use all three variables. If all three lengths are equal, a cube or a sphere compartment can be created with a cuboid or an ellipsoid geometry, respectively. For the pyramid compartment, LENGTH[X, Y, Z] stipulate its base length, height and base width, respectively. For a cylinder compartment, LENGTHX defines the cylinder length, while its diameter is given by LENGTHY. In the case of a rod compartment, LENGTHX indicates the length from the tip of one pole to the other while LENGTHY defines its diameter. For a torus, its larger diameter (from the torus center to the edge) is given by LENGTHX, whereas LENGTHY determines the tube diameter. LENGTH[X, Y, Z] definitions examples are given in Figures 2 (lines 5-6), 5 (lines 5-7, 18-20, and 42-43) and 6 (lines 47-48 and 64-65).

**[XY, XZ, YZ]PLANE**

When a volume compartment has the cuboid geometry, the boundary type or the presence of the [xy, xz, yz]-plane surfaces enclosing the compartment can be specified using [XY, XZ, YZ]PLANE variables. The boundary type can be reflective ('0'), periodic ('1') or semi-periodic ('2'). A semi-periodic boundary allows nonHD molecules to move unidirectionally from one boundary to the other. When a surface compartment is defined to enclose the cuboid compartment, we can remove one or both faces of the cuboid in a given [XY, XZ, YZ]PLANE. To remove the surface on the upper or the lower face of the cuboid in a plane, we can set the variable to '3' or '4', respectively, whereas to remove both faces we can set it to '5'. If the variable is not defined, the boundary type is set to the default reflective ('0') type. Examples in EM and Python to remove both of the cuboid XYPLANE faces are given below:

```
Variable Variable(XYPLANE) { Value 5; }

theSimulator.createEntity('Variable', 'Variable:.:XYPLANE').Value = 5
```

**ORIGIN[X, Y, Z]**

A child volume compartment can be placed at any location within a parent compartment using the variables ORIGIN[X, Y, Z]. The variables define the origin (center) coordinates of the child compartment relative to its parent center point. The variable values '−1' and '1' correspond to the normalized lowest and the highest points of the parent compartment in a given axis, respectively. Since the default value of these variables is '0', the child compartment will be placed at the center of its parent if they are not defined. Figures 5 (lines 21-24 and 44-46) and 6 (lines 66-68) give some examples of the ORIGIN[X, Y, Z] variables definition.

**ROTATE[X, Y, Z]**

A compartment can be rotated along the [x, y, z]-axis with the origin at the compartment center using the ROTATE[X, Y, Z] variables respectively. The unit of the variables is in radians. If there are multiple rotation definitions, they follow the [x, y, z]-axis rotation order. Compartments are not rotated if the variables are not defined since their default value is '0'. An example of compartment rotation definition is given in Figure 5 (line 47).

### VACANT

Every compartment must have a VACANT variable that represents the 'species' of empty voxels within the compartment. The VACANT voxels of a surface compartment are analogous to the lipid molecules mentioned in the Spatiocyte Method section and in Arjunan and Tomita (2010).[2] Examples of the VACANT variable definition are shown in Figures 2 (lines 7 and 34), 5 (lines 8, 24, 32, 48 and 53) and 6 (lines 49, 60, 69 and 72). The variable can be used to define sink (e.g., A -> VACANT) and membrane binding reactions (e.g., $B_V$ + $VACANT_S$ -> $B_S$) of non-HD species, as shown in the EM and Python examples below:

**First-Order Sink Reaction, A → Ø**

```
Process SpatiocyteNextReactionProcess(sink) {
      VariableReferenceList [_ Variable:/:A -1]
                            [_ Variable:/:VACANT 1];
      k 0.3; }
```

**Second-Order Surface-Adsorption Reaction, $B_v$ + Surface.VACANT → $B_s$**

```
Process DiffusionInfluencedReactionProcess(bind) {
      VariableReferenceList [_ Variable:/:B -1]
                            [_ Variable:/Surface:VACANT -1]
                            [_ Variable:/Surface:B 1];
      k 2e-8; }
```

**First-Order Sink Reaction, A → Ø**

```
sinker = theSimulator.createEntity('SpatiocyteNextReactionProcess',
'Process:/:sink')
sinker.VariableReferenceList = [['_', 'Variable:/:A', '-1']]
sinker.VariableReferenceList = [['_', 'Variable:/:VACANT', '1']]
sinker.k = 0.3
```

**Second-Order Surface-Adsorption Reaction, $B_v$ + Surface.VACANT → $B_s$**

```
binder = theSimulator.createEntity('DiffusionInfluencedReactionProcess',
'Process:/:bind')
binder.VariableReferenceList = [['_', 'Variable:/:B', '-1']]
binder.VariableReferenceList = [['_', 'Variable:/Surface:VACANT', '-1']]
binder.VariableReferenceList = [['_', 'Variable:/Surface:B', '1']]
binder.k = 2e-8
```

For a volume compartment, the *Value* of the VACANT variable determines if the compartment has a higher occupancy priority when it intersects with a peer compartment. Figure 9 displays

***Table 1. Combinations of volume and surface VACANT values and their corresponding intersected peer compartment forms. In all cases X is an integer and the DIFFUSIVE variable is not set***

| Green Sphere Compartment | | White Sphere Compartment | | Intersection |
|---|---|---|---|---|
| Volume VACANT.Value | Surface VACANT.Value | Volume VACANT.Value | Surface VACANT.Value | Form in Figure 9 |
| X | 0 | X | 0 | A |
| X | nonzero | X | nonzero | B |
| X | 0 | X | nonzero | C |
| <X | 0 | X | 0 | D |
| <X | 0 | X | nonzero | E |
| <X | nonzero | X | nonzero | F |

cross-sections of various intersection forms of two spherical peer compartments with different volume and surface VACANT values (listed in Table 1). In the case of a surface compartment, the VACANT variable determines if it fully encloses a parent compartment that has an intersection. A nonzero value indicates that the parent will be fully enclosed even at the location of intersection. Otherwise if the value is '0', the surface will be open at the intersecting region. Figure 10 shows four possible

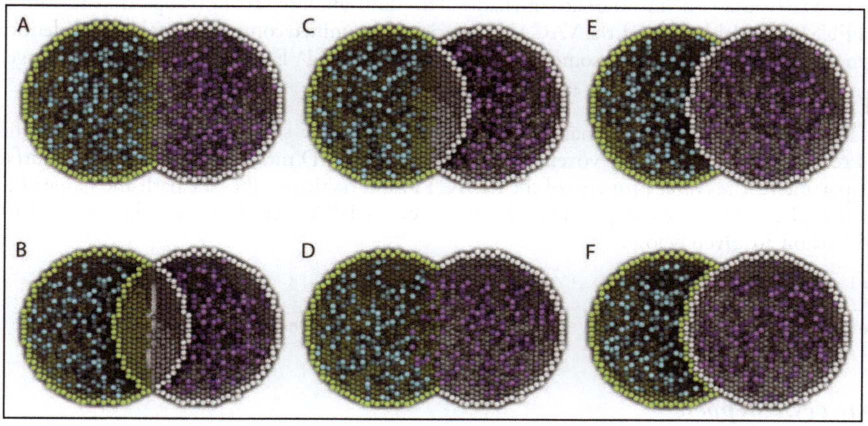


Figure 9. Cross-sections of two intersected peer compartments. Two sphere compartments in green and white are intersecting in space. Turquoise and purple molecules belong to the green and white compartments respectively. See text of the VACANT variable and Table 1 for a detailed description of the intersections. The EM file to create the intersections is available in the Spatiocyte source package as 2012.arjunan.chapter.peer.em.

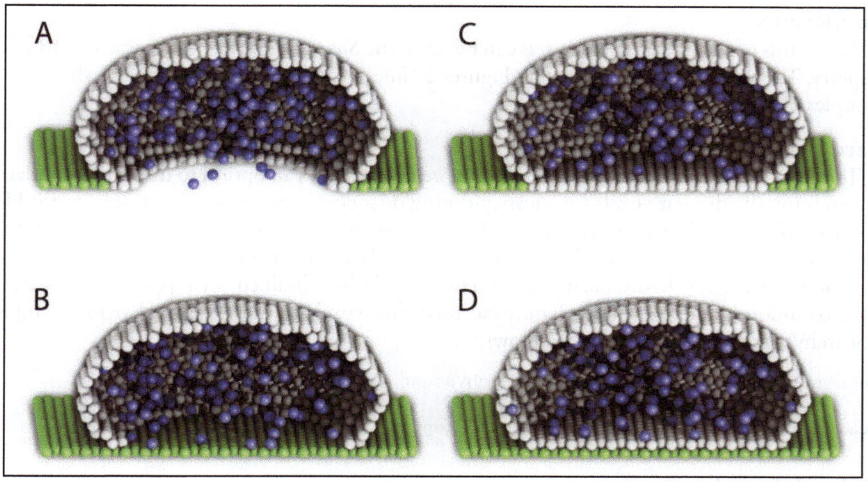


Figure 10. Cross-sections of intersected root and child compartments. The VACANT surface voxels of the cuboid root compartment are shown in green while those of the ellipsoid child compartment are in white. The blue molecules belong to the child volume compartment. (A) root surface.VACANT = 0 and child surface.VACANT = 0, (B) root surface.VACANT = 1 and child surface.VACANT = 0, (C) root surface.VACANT = 0 and child surface.VACANT = 1, and (D) root surface.VACANT = 1 and child surface.VACANT = 1. The EM file to create the intersections is available in the Spatiocyte source package as 2012.arjunan.chapter.root.em.

enclosure forms when a compartment intersects with a root compartment. Figure 7 illustrates the intersection of various compartments to create a unified neuron-shaped compartment.

**DIFFUSIVE**

To unify intersecting compartments, the DIFFUSIVE variable can be specified. It enables nonHD molecules to diffuse into and from an intersecting compartment. The *Name* property of the DIFFUSIVE variable defines the path and name of the diffusible intersecting compartment. With the DIFFUSIVE variable defined, the VACANT species of the unified compartments become identical. Figure 5 (lines 49 and 54) gives some examples of the DIFFUSIVE variable definition and usage.

**REACTIVE**

The REACTIVE variable enables nonHD molecules in a surface compartment to collide and react with the VACANT voxels (i.e., lipids) and nonHD molecules in an adjacent surface compartment. The *Name* property of the REACTIVE variable specifies the path and name of the reactive adjacent surface compartment. Examples of the REACTIVE variable definition in EM and Python are given below:

```
Variable Variable(REACTIVE) { Name "/Cell:Surface"; }

theSimulator.createEntity('Variable', 'Variable:/Surface:REACTIVE').Name = "/
Cell:Surface"
```

## *SpatiocyteStepper*

The *SpatiocyteStepper* is the only stepper used by Spatiocyte in the E-Cell System and must be defined to run all simulations. It advances the simulation in an event-driven manner. Initialization examples of the *SpatiocyteStepper* are shown in Figures 2 (line 1), 5 (line 2) and 6 (line 44). In each compartment, the StepperID must be set to the *SpatiocyteStepper* ID. Examples of *SpatiocyteStepper* ID definition in compartments are given in Figures 2 (lines 3 and 32), 5 (lines 4, 16, 30, 40 and 51) and 6 (lines 45, 58, 62 and 70).

**VoxelRadius**

The radius of the HCP lattice voxels can be set in the *SpatiocyteStepper* using the VoxelRadius property. The default radius is 10e-9 m. Figures 2 (line 1), 5 (line 2) and 6 (line 44) show some examples of the VoxelRadius initialization.

**SearchVacant**

The SearchVacant property of the *SpatiocyteStepper* provides an option to direct the simulator to search for all adjacent voxels for vacancy during dissociation reactions that result in nonHD product molecules. The reaction can only take place if there is an available target vacant voxel. This option is useful when evaluating the effects of a crowded compartment. The value of SearchVacant by default is true ('1'). To disable it, we can set it to '0'. When disabled, an adjacent target voxel is selected randomly and the reaction is only executed if the voxel is vacant. EM and Python examples of SearchVacant initialization are as follows:

```
Stepper SpatiocyteStepper(SS) { SearchVacant 0; }

theSimulator.createStepper('SpatiocyteStepper', 'SS').SearchVacant = 0
```

## *MoleculePopulateProcess*

The initial positions of all nonHD species with nonzero initial molecule numbers must be specified with the *MoleculePopulateProcess*. The molecules can be either uniformly or normally distributed within the compartment. By default, without any *MoleculePopulateProcess* parameter definition, molecules are uniformly distributed over the entire compartment. Otherwise if the GaussianSigma is set to a nonzero value, the compartment will be populated according to the Gaussian distribution. *MoleculePopulateProcess* definitions can be seen in Figures 2 (lines 26-28), 5 (lines 13-14) and 6

```
# Example of python scripting to populate molecules at the poles of a rod compartment
theSimulator.createStepper('SpatiocyteStepper', 'SS').VoxelRadius = 8e-8
# Create the root container compartment using the rod geometry:
theSimulator.rootSystem.StepperID = 'SS'
theSimulator.createEntity('Variable', 'Variable:/:GEOMETRY').Value = 3
theSimulator.createEntity('Variable', 'Variable:/:LENGTHX').Value = 10e-6
theSimulator.createEntity('Variable', 'Variable:/:LENGTHY').Value = 2e-6
theSimulator.createEntity('Variable', 'Variable:/:VACANT')
logger = theSimulator.createEntity('VisualizationLogProcess', 'Process:/:logger')
logger.LogInterval = 1
logger.VariableReferenceList = [['_', 'Variable:/Surface:A'], ['_', 'Variable:/Surface:B']]
populator = theSimulator.createEntity('MoleculePopulateProcess', 'Process:/:populateLeft')
populator.VariableReferenceList = [['_', 'Variable:/Surface:A']]
populator.OriginX = -1
populator.UniformRadiusX = 0.5
populator = theSimulator.createEntity('MoleculePopulateProcess', 'Process:/:populateRight')
populator.VariableReferenceList = [['_', 'Variable:/Surface:B']]
populator.OriginX = 1
populator.UniformRadiusX = 0.5
# Create the surface compartment:
theSimulator.createEntity('System', 'System:/:Surface').StepperID = 'SS'
theSimulator.createEntity('Variable', 'Variable:/Surface:DIMENSION').Value = 2
theSimulator.createEntity('Variable', 'Variable:/Surface:VACANT')
theSimulator.createEntity('Variable', 'Variable:/Surface:A').Value = 500
theSimulator.createEntity('Variable', 'Variable:/Surface:B').Value = 500
run(100)
```

Figure 11. A Python script to populate molecules at the poles of a rod surface compartment. The file is available in the Spatiocyte source package as 2012.arjunan.chapter.populate.py.

(line 57). A Python example showing two different species populated at the poles of a rod surface compartment is also listed in Figure 11 with the corresponding output in Figure 12.

### Origin[X, Y, Z]

Origin[X, Y, Z] is the origin point relative to the compartment center point for a species population. The molecules may have a uniform or a Gaussian distribution from this point. The range of the point along each axis covering the entire compartment is [−1, 1]. Therefore, the origin is at the center of the compartment if Origin[X, Y, Z] is fixed to [0, 0, 0], the default set of values.

### GaussianSigma[X, Y, Z]

GaussianSigma[X, Y, Z] stipulates the sigma value for a Gaussian distributed population from the origin in [x, y, z]-axis, respectively.

### UniformRadius[X, Y, Z]

The uniformly distributed normalized population radius from the origin point in [x, y, z]-axis is given by the UniformRadius[X, Y, Z] parameter. Since the default values of UniformRadius[X, Y, Z] and Origin[X, Y, Z] are [1, 1, 1] and [0, 0, 0], respectively, the molecules are spread uniformly within the entire compartment when the parameters are not defined.

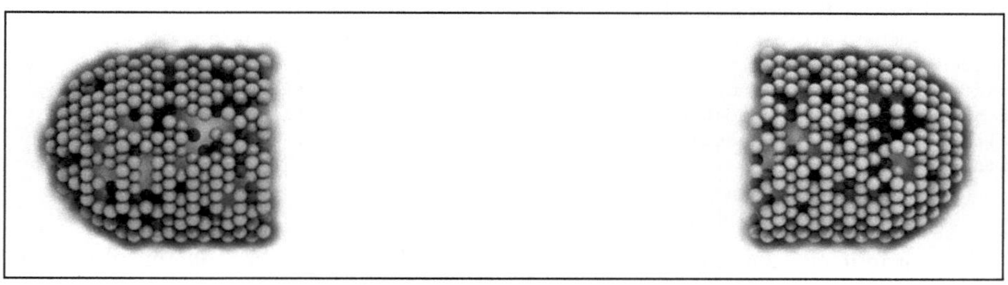

Figure 12. Visualization of molecules populated at the poles of a rod surface compartment. The model is created from the Python script shown in Figure 11.

**ResetTime**

To place the molecules at a certain interval after the simulation has started, we can use the ResetTime parameter. This parameter is useful when the positions of a molecule species need to be actively altered after a simulation interval.

## *DiffusionProcess*

The *DiffusionProcess* handles the voxel-to-voxel random walk of diffusing molecules and the collisions that take place between each walk. Examples of the *DiffusionProcess* usage are shown in Figures 2 (lines 11-16 and 39-50), 5 (lines 26-28) and 6 (lines 51-53).

**D**

In the *DiffusionProcess*, the diffusion coefficient of the molecule species is set with *D*, which has the unit $m^2s^{-1}$. The default value is 0 $m^2s^{-1}$.

**P**

*P* is an arbitrarily set reaction probability limit of the diffusing species, within the range [0, 1]. The default value is '1', which is sufficient to produce accurate simulations. We can set it to a smaller value to perform reaction-diffusion processes at smaller intervals.

## *PeriodicBoundaryDiffusionProcess*

We can use the *PeriodicBoundaryDiffusionProcess* in place of the *DiffusionProcess* when a molecule species needs to be diffused across periodic two-dimensional surface edges. The surface compartment must be enclosing a cuboid parent compartment. The process overcomes the limitation of setting [XY, XZ, YZ]PLANE of the *Compartment* variable to periodic, which only supports periodic volume edges. It inherits the diffusion coefficient, D and the reaction probability limit, P from the *DiffusionProcess*. Examples of *PeriodicBoundaryDiffusionProcess* in EM and Python are as follows:

```
Process PeriodicBoundaryDiffusionProcess(diffuse) {
     VariableReferenceList [_ Variable:/Surface:A];
     D 0.2e-12; }

diffuser = theSimulator.createEntity('PeriodicBoundaryDiffusionProcess',
'Process:/:diffuse')
diffuser.VariableReferenceList = [['_', 'Variable:/Surface:A']]
diffuser.D = 0.2e-12
```

## *DiffusionInfluencedReactionProcess*

The *DiffusionInfluencedReactionProcess* is used to execute all second-order reactions comprising two diffusing reactants, or a diffusing and an immobile reactant that are diffusion-influenced. Figure 2 (lines 51-60 and lines 67-69) shows several usage examples of *DiffusionInfluencedReactionProcess*. A python example of the process definition is provided below:

**Second-Order Reaction A + B → C**

```
binder = theSimulator.createEntity('DiffusionInfluencedReactionProcess',
'Process:/:associate')
binder.VariableReferenceList = [['_', 'Variable:/:A', '-1']]
binder.VariableReferenceList = [['_', 'Variable:/:B', '-1']]
binder.VariableReferenceList = [['_', 'Variable:/:C', '1']]
binder.p = 0.5
```

**k**

The intrinsic rate constant of the diffusion-influenced reaction is set to *k*. The relationship between the intrinsic rate constant with the macroscopic rate constant $k_{on}$ is given by $1/k_{on} = 1/k + 1/k_d$, where $k_d = 4\pi DR$ is the maximally diffusion-limited reaction rate, *D* is the diffusion coefficient and *R* is the contact radius. The units of *k* for various reaction types are given in Table 2.

***Table 2. Units of the rate constant,* k *in* DiffusionInfluencedReactionProcess *and* SpatiocyteNextReactionProcess**

| Reactant 1 | Reactant 2 | *k* (units) |
|---|---|---|
| Volume Molecule | Volume Molecule | $m^3s^{-1}$ |
| Surface Molecule | Surface Molecule | $m^2s^{-1}$ |
| Volume Molecule | Surface Molecule | $m^3s^{-1}$ |
| Volume Molecule | Surface.VACANT | $ms^{-1}$ |

**p**

The absolute reactive collision probability of the reaction is given by *p*. This process requires either the value of *k* or *p*.

### *SpatiocyteNextReactionProcess*

The *SpatiocyteNextReactionProcess* is used to execute all reactions that can be decoupled from diffusion such as zeroth- and first-order reactions, and second-order reactions that involve two adjoining immobile reactants or at least one HD reactant. Each reaction is performed according to the Next Reaction method.[7] Unlike in the *DiffusionInfluencedReactionProcess*, the membrane-adsorption reaction where a HD species binds to the membrane is represented as a first-order reaction (see example below). EM examples of the *SpatiocyteNextReactionProcess* are given in Figure 2 (lines 61-66 and 70-75), while Python examples of zeroth- and first-order (surface-adsorption) reactions are given below:

**Zeroth-Order Reaction, Ø → A**

```
zero = theSimulator.createEntity('SpatiocyteNextReactionProcess',
'Process:/:create')
zero.VariableReferenceList = [['_', 'Variable:/:A', '-1']]
zero.k = 0.01
```

**First-Order Surface-Adsorption Reaction, $A_v \rightarrow A_s$**

```
uni = theSimulator.createEntity('SpatiocyteNextReactionProcess',
'Process:/:dissociate')
uni.VariableReferenceList = [['_', 'Variable:/:A', '-1']]
uni.VariableReferenceList = [['_', 'Variable:/Surfact:A', '1']]
uni.k = 0.01
```

**k**

The rate constant of the event-driven reaction. For second-order reactions, the units are listed in Table 2. For all first-order reactions, the unit is in $s^{-1}$.

### *VisualizationLogProcess*

We can use the *VisualizationLogProcess* to log the coordinates of nonHD species at a specified periodic interval. The *SpatiocyteVisualizer* can load the log file to display the molecules in 3D. Figures 2 (lines 17-20), 5 (lines 9-12) and 6 (lines 54-56 and 73) show some examples of *VisualizationLogProcess* usage.

**FileName**

FileName is the name of the binary log file. The default name is 'visualLog0.dat', which is also the default file name loaded by *SpatiocyteVisualizer*.

**LogInterval**

The interval for logging the coordinates is determined by LogInterval. The default value is '0', which means that the interval would be set to the smallest diffusion or collision interval of the logged nonHD species. If LogInterval > 0, the log interval will be set to the specified value. The unit of LogInterval is in seconds.

### *MicroscopyTrackingProcess*

The *MicroscopyTrackingProcess* mimics the fluorescent microphotography process by logging the trajectory of nonHD molecules averaged over a specified camera exposure time. It inherits the FileName and LogInterval properties from the *VisualizationLogProcess*. After each LogInterval, the number of times a voxel is occupied by a molecule species is counted. At the end of a given ExposureTime, the frequency is averaged over the total number of intervals and logged. Figure 2 (lines 21-25) shows an example of the MicroscopyTrackingProcess definition. A Python example is given below:

```
tracker = theSimulator.createEntity('MicroscopyTrackingProcess',
'Process:/:track)
tracker.VariableReferenceList = [['_', 'Variable:/Surface:MinEE', '2']]
tracker.VariableReferenceList = [['_', 'Variable:/Surface:MinDEE', '3']]
tracker.VariableReferenceList = [['_', 'Variable:/Surface:MinE', '-2']]
tracker.VariableReferenceList = [['_', 'Variable:/Surface:MinDE', '-2']]
tracker.VariableReferenceList = [['_', 'Variable:/Surface:MinE', '-1']]
tracker.FileName = "microscopyLog0.dat"
```

*MicroscopyTrackingProcess* enables representation of different fluorescent colored subunits within a complex according to the coefficient assigned to each *variable*. In the Python example above, the coefficient of the first variable MinEE is 2, representing two subunits of MinE within the complex MinEE. Similarly for MinDEE, the three subunits (one MinD and two MinE's) are represented by the coefficient 3. Each unique variable with a negative coefficient is assigned a different color during visualization. The first negative variable, MinE, has a coefficient of –2, which means that two subunits from the first positive variable, MinEE, are assigned a unique color of MinE. The second negative variable MinDE also has a coefficient of –2, specifying that two subunits of the second positive variable, MinDEE, is assigned the color of MinDE. The third negative variable MinE has a coefficient of –1, corresponding to the color of the remaining one MinE subunit of the second positive variable MinDEE.

#### ExposureTime

The simulated camera exposure time is specified by ExposureTime. The default value is 0.5 s.

#### MeanCount

MeanCount is the maximum number of voxel occupancy frequency before it is averaged. The default value is '0', which indicates that the specified LogInterval or the smallest collision or diffusion interval should be used. In this case, the MeanCount will be ExposureTime/LogInterval. Otherwise if MeanCount > 0, the LogInterval is set to ExposureTime/MeanCount.

### *IteratingLogProcess*

The *IteratingLogProcess* executes multiple simulation runs with different random seeds and logs the averaged physical values of molecules, such as their displacement or survival probability, over the total runs. The values are logged in a file using the comma-separated values (csv) format. By default the process logs the number of available molecules of recorded species at the specified interval periodically.

#### LogDuration

LogDuration is the total duration of a simulation run (i.e., an iteration).

#### LogInterval

LogInterval is the interval for logging physical values of molecules within an iteration.

#### Iterations

The number of simulation runs before the logged values are averaged and saved in the log file is specified by the Iterations parameter.

**FileName**

The file name of the log file is given by FileName. The default file name is "Log.csv".

**SaveInterval**

When running many iterations, it is useful to save the logged data in a backup file for quick analysis, or to avoid restarting the runs because of some unexpected failures (e.g., power failure). To this end, a backup file of the logged values can be saved at the iteration intervals given by Iterations/SaveInterval. The default value of SaveInterval is '0', which indicates that a backup file will not be saved.

**Survival**

The Survival parameter can be set to '1' to log the survival probability of a molecule species. The default value of the parameter is '0'.

**Displacement**

Set the Displacement to '1' to log the displacement of a molecule species. The default value of Displacement is '0'.

**Diffusion**

If the Diffusion parameter is set to '1', the apparent diffusion coefficient of a molecule species will be logged. The default Diffusion value is '0'.

***SpatiocyteVisualizer***

The *SpatiocyteVisualizer* can be started by executing ./spatiocyte in the Spatiocyte directory. Figure 3 illustrates the *SpatiocyteVisualizer* interface, whereas its features and keyboard shortcuts are listed in Table 3. To change the color of a species, right mouse click on the species and select a desired color. The visualizer can display each species within a specified range in each axis using the bounding feature. Figure 8 displays the output after specifying a set of ranges for the cell membrane.

***Table 3.*** **SpatiocyteVisualizer** ***features and keyboard shortcuts***

| Feature | Keyboard Shortcut(s) |
|---|---|
| Play Forward | Right arrow |
| Play Backward | Left arrow |
| Step Forward | Up arrow or Enter |
| Step Backward | Down arrow or Shift+Enter |
| Pause/Play | Space |
| Zoom In | Ctrl++ or Ctrl+ = or Page Up |
| Zoom Out | Ctrl+- or Page Down |
| Reset View | Ctrl+0 or Home |
| Rotate along x-axis clockwise | Ctrl+Up Arrow |
| Rotate along x-axis counter-clockwise | Ctrl+Down Arrow |
| Rotate along y-axis clockwise | Ctrl+Right Arrow |
| Rotate along y-axis counter-clockwise | Ctrl+Left Arrow |
| Rotate along z-axis clockwise | z |
| Rotate along z-axis counter-clockwise | Z |
| Translate Up | Shift+Up Arrow |
| Translate Down | Shift+Down Arrow |
| Translate Right | Shift+Right Arrow |
| Translate Left | Shift+Left Arrow |
| Save current frame as a PNG image | s |
| Start/Stop recording PNG frames | S |

Each displayed frame can be saved into the Portable Network Graphics (PNG) image format. A quick way to create a movie from the saved images is to use the ffmpeg program:

```
$ ffmpeg -i image%07d.png -sameq out.mp4
```

## Conclusion

Building computational models of biochemical processes is usually a demanding task, especially for experimental biologists without modeling experience. This chapter aims to provide a guide on how one can quickly build and simulate spatially resolved biochemical models with the available Spatiocyte modules. We started with the basic theory of the Spatiocyte method and continued with the installation and simulation procedures. The various modules available to Spatiocyte users were also explained with accompanying model examples.

We plan to continuously develop and improve the Spatiocyte software and user experience. The contents of this guide will also therefore, evolve with the addition of new features and enhancements. The latest version of this guide will be available along with the Spatiocyte source code, which at the time of writing, is hosted at GitHub. The Spatiocyte website, http://spatiocyte.org also contains the latest information about the Spatiocyte method and software.

In future, we would like to introduce the ability of subunits to polymerize on the membrane and in the cytoplasm. A polymerization strategy using the HCP lattice was proposed recently.[10] Diffusion of compartments, and molecules with different shapes and sizes are also in the future development plan. Parallel implementation of the Spatiocyte method to run on multi-core architectures and graphics processing units is also being considered. We are also currently working on introducing compartments with complex surface geometries. Spatiocyte users are encouraged to submit feature requests and bug reports, while independent developers can submit their own algorithm modules, code improvements and bug fixes.

## References


1. Takahashi K, Kaizu K, Hu B et al. A multi-algorithm, multi-timescale method for cell simulation. Bioinformatics 2004; 20(4):538-546.
2. Arjunan SNV, Tomita M. A new multicompartmental reaction-diffusion modeling method links transient membrane attachment of E. coli MinE to E-ring formation. Syst Synth Biol 2010; 4(1):35-53.
3. Arjunan SNV, Tomita M. Modeling reaction-diffusion of molecules on surface and in volume spaces with the E-Cell System. IJCSIS 2009; 3(1):211-216.
4. Dix JA, Verkman AS. Crowding effects on diffusion in solutions and cells. Annu Rev Biophys 2008; 37:247-263.
5. Hall D, Hoshino M. Effects of macromolecular crowding on intracellular diffusion from a single particle perspective. Biophys Rev 2010; 2(1):39-53.
6. Collins FC, Kimball GE. Diffusion-controlled reaction rates. J Colloid Sci 1949; 4(4):425-437.
7. Gibson M, Bruck J. Efficient exact stochastic simulation of chemical systems with many species and many channels. J Phys Chem A 2000; 104(9):1876-1889.
8. Gillespie DT. A general method for numerically simulating the stochastic time evolution of coupled chemical reactions. J Comput Phys 1976; 22(4):403-434.
9. Gillespie DT. Exact stochastic simulation of coupled chemical reactions. J Phys Chem 1977; 81(25):2340-2361.
10. Arjunan SNV. Modeling three-dimensional spatial regulation of bacterial cell division. PhD Thesis, Keio University 2009.

# Part 2
# Applications

# Chapter 5

# A Model Library of Bacterial Chemotaxis on E-Cell System

**Yuri Matsuzaki***

## Introduction

Bacterial organisms like *Escherichia coli* have developed mechanisms to detect and direct cell movement toward substrate when starved. Such behavior is known as chemotaxis (15 for recent review).

Some nutrition (amino acids, sugar, etc.) can be sensed by the chemotaxis signal transduction system (Fig. 1). When the concentration of attractants increases, a signal is transmitted from the chemoreceptors to flagellar motor which influences the random walk of the bacterium. The fraction of time spent in run gets longer as the signal is transmitted, permitting the cells to be close to the nutrition rich environment for a longer period of time.

There are two modes of swimming behavior that are controlled by flagellar motor rotation: counter clockwise rotation, which causes the cell to 'run' and clockwise rotation, which makes the cell 'tumble' more frequently. In a nonstimulated environment, cells run four times longer than tumbling. Attractants like aspartate (Asp) shorten the tumbling time to increase a smooth run and lead cells to be in a more favorable environment.

The signal molecule that transmits the chemical signal to the flagellar motor is CheY protein. The phosphorylated form of CheY can interact with the flagellar motor protein FliM and make the motor rotate clockwise.[14] Under a nonstimulated environment, large fraction of CheA, which forms a complex with CheW and the receptor protein (Tar, for Asp), are in active form and undergo autophosphorylation of this histidine kinase.[7] CheA then transfers its phosphate to methyl esterase CheB or response regulator CheY. In exposure to attractants, the receptor complex tends to be in an inactive form, which in consequence decreases the phosphorylation level of CheY and then changes the switching of the flagellar motors to make cells tumble less.[4]

After stimulation, cells gradually adapt to the stimulus. This is a result of feedback by the receptor methylation caused by methyltransferase CheR and methyl esterase CheB. Methylation level of the Tar receptor is known to be enhanced by ligand binding and the methylated receptors recover its activity even in the sustained existence of attractants.

A number of models has been proposed to explain how a chemotaxis system controls this swimming behavior quantitatively, because this system is qualitatively one of the best understood signal transduction system in the field of molecular biology. This system shows two remarkable properties, high gain of signals and precise adaptation. Explanations of how these properties are achieved should be given using quantitative data and analysis. Most biochemical data needed to construct models can be retrieved from papers published from 1970s to now, which enables us to construct and simulate models and analyze this system quantitatively.

However, each modeling study employs different formulisms and simulation algorithms, so comparisons of their performance is a nontrivial problem. To study the characteristics of each of

*Yuri Matsuzaki—Institute for Advanced Biosciences, Keio University, Japan.
Email: yuri@sfc.keio.ac.jp

*E-Cell System: Basic Concepts and Applications*, edited by Satya Nanda Vel Arjunan, Pawan K. Dhar and Masaru Tomita. 

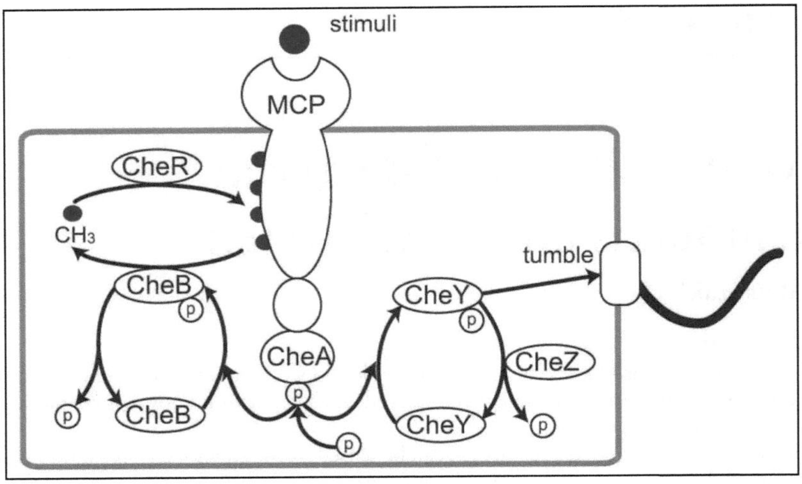


Figure 1. Signaling pathway of chemotaxis. A kinase CheA phosphorylates itself and transfers the phosphate to CheB or CheY. The state of the chemoreceptor modification controls the efficiency of CheA phosphorylation and consequently the CheY phosphorylation level. Receptors take active or inactive form; active receptor complex undergo autophosphorylation of CheA. It can be methylated by CheR. Inactive receptor complex can be demethylated by phosphorylated form of CheB.

these models and to compare their behavior, it would be helpful to be able to execute simulations on a single platform. The E-Cell Simulation Environment Version 3 (E-Cell 3) provides a flexible framework in which both deterministic and stochastic algorithms can be used to simulate models with either continuous or discrete variables. Our main goal is to test E-Cell's multi algorithm capabilities with a well-characterized system. To demonstrate the utility of this framework, we have constructed a model library of *E. coli* chemotaxis that allows comparative analysis of previously published models. It thus would be interesting when we try to analyze and get new insight on biological problems to compare models which have different assumptions and see which characteristics of each model bring the difference in representations of these models.

In this chapter, we introduce basic assumptions and profiles of the imported models and make clear the difference between reference models and imported E-Cell models. We have the following three models on E-Cell 3 thus far: (i) a minimal deterministic model of adaptation, based on Bray et al[5] in which receptors have only a single methylation site, (ii) a more detailed, deterministic model in which the receptor has four methylation sites, as proposed by Mello and Tu[8] and (iii) a stochastic model which explicitly represents the kinetics of all reactions present in (ii), based on Morton-Firth and Bray.[10]

These models are available at the following URL:

http://www.e-cell.org/

## Models and Methods

Initial amount of substances, kinetic equation and kinetic parameters are taken from the original models and published papers. All these data are shown in our website.[16]

### *Shared Assumptions*

The implemented models share two assumptions; a two-state model of receptor activation[1] and a robust adaptation mechanism[2,9] (Fig. 2). Based on two-state model, chemoreceptors are in equilibrium between two conformations (S: swimming/T: tumbling). S receptors are called inactive receptors, for CheA activity in complex with S receptor is low. On the other hand, T receptors are called active receptors. Attractants bind to T receptors and shift equilibrium between S/T to

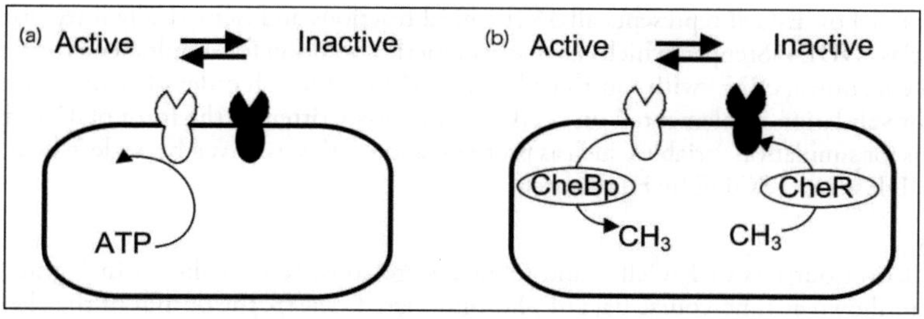


Figure 2. Two-state model and robust perfect adaptation mechanism. a) Two-state model. The receptor complex forms either active or inactive conformation. Receptor complex in active conformation promotes CheA autophosphorylation. b) Robust perfect adaptation mechanism. Methyltransferase CheR only binds to the inactive form of the receptor complex, while methyl esterase CheB in phosphorylated form can only bind to the active form.

increase S receptors. Simultaneously, S receptors accept methylation. Methylation causes receptors to more favorably shift to T form, although kinetic rates of methylation and demethylation are small compared to the effect induced by attractants. Barkai and Leibler[2] and Morton-Firth and Bray[9] suggested conditions to gain robust perfect adaptation that assume receptor methylation changes depending on activity of the receptor, thus CheR only bind receptors in inactive conformation while CheB only bind receptors in active conformation.

## *Canonical Adaptation Model (Loosely Based on Bray et al, 1993)*

### Methods

Model (i) employs the simplest mechanism for adaptation, loosely based on the reference.[5] The reference model has the following features: (i) assumes the existence of only Tar receptors and does not incorporate effects from four other chemoreceptors (Tap, Trg, Tsr, Aer) that the Che protein can interact with, (ii) simplifies receptor methylation states in only two forms (methylated/not methylated), which denotes that the chemoreceptor has only two methylation sites (Fig. 3).

As E-Cell 3 was still in early development at the time we developed the model library, we needed to clarify the accuracy of the numerical integration of E-Cell system. For this purpose, we implemented the same model to GNU Octave and compared the results brought by the two software programs.

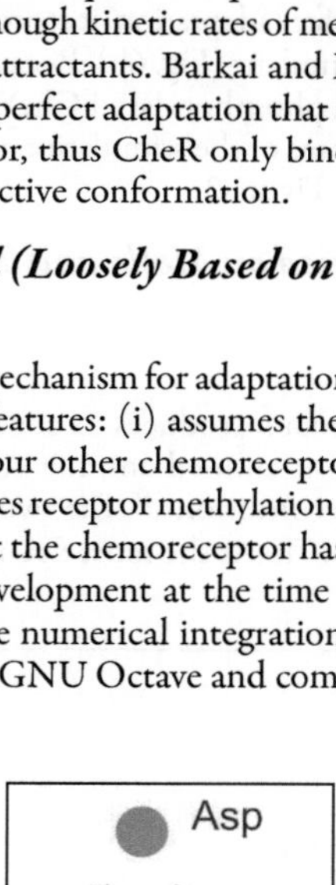


Figure 3. Binding states of the Tar complex in model (i). 'm' represents the methyl group, 'p' represents the phosphate group. Asp, m, p can bind to the Tar complex with a distinct binding site for each. The Tar complex can form eight different binding states in this model.

The model on E-Cell represents all 36 chemical reactions and numerically integrates by the Stepper class ODE45Stepper, which calculates numerical solution for simultaneous ordinary differential equations (ODE) with fourth order of precision and fifth order of error control.[13] The model for validation implemented on GNU Octave was written in the form of 12 differential equations for simulation variables, such as proteins, and ODE was solved by lsode, which is based on the ODE solver LSODE by Hindmarch.

**Results**

Simulation outputs of E-Cell 3 and Octave were consistent as shown in Figure 5a. The results are shown as time-course data of phosphorylated CheYp, the output of the chemotaxis signal transduction system, which interacts directly to a flagellar motor. Simulation results are shown in Figure 5b. Attractants were induced at 2000 seconds when the system has reached steady state and then removed 2000 seconds after the stimulation when the cell adapted to the stimulation. The model can partially adapt to the stimulus. The Adaptation errors were under 3%, which do not meet perfect adaptation criterion.[2] The Adaptation error shows a strong correlation with the magnitude of the stimulation (Fig. 6a). It enhances exponentially depending on the induced Asp concentration.

Though the model didn't show perfect adaptation, it reproduced the dependence of adaptation time to the magnitude of induced stimulant (Fig. 6b). Because this model didn't adapt perfectly, time spent to recover half of reduced phosphorylated CheY is plotted to show adaptation time. It shows sigmoid curve to the logarithms of the stimulation magnitudes, which is consistent with experimental data published in ref. 3, Figure 2.

## *Perfect Adaptation Model (Based on Mello and Tu, 2003 and Morton-Firth and Bray, 1999)*

**Methods**

Mello and Tu[6] proposed a model that introduces six conditions derived in an analytical study of the perfect adaptation. They also examined another model that is biologically consistent but moderately violates two of these conditions.[10] The two models adapt almost equally exact, with adaptation error lower than 1%. This is the most detailed deterministic model that can be

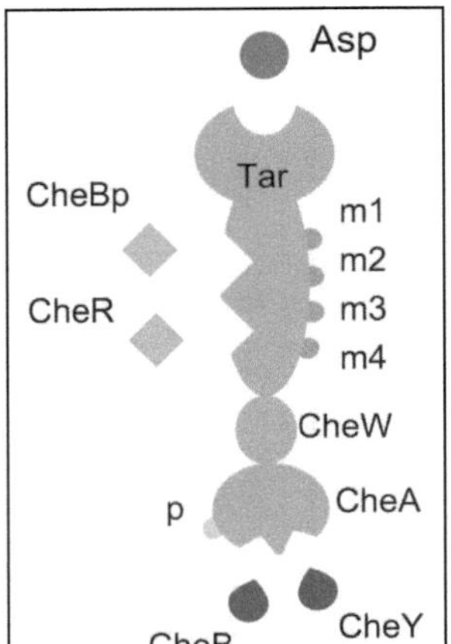


Figure 4. Binding states of the Tar complex in model (ii) and (iii). 'm1', 'm2', 'm3', and 'm4' represent the methyl group, 'p' represents the phosphate group. CheBp and CheR exclusively bind to NWETF motif of Tar, while CheB and CheY compete to bind to the $P_2$ domain of CheA. The Tar complex can form 180 different binding states in this model.

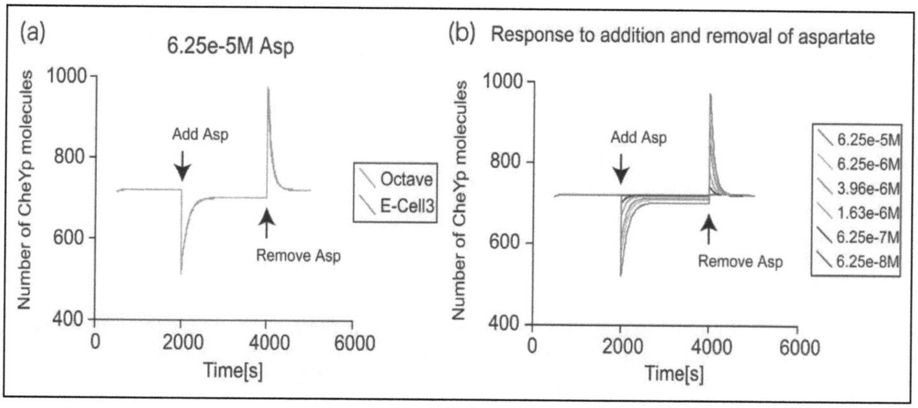


Figure 5. Simulation results of model (i). a) Comparison of simulation results by GNU Octave and E-Cell 3. The number of phosphorylated CheY molecules in response to the addition and removal of 0.625*10^-5 M Asp are shown. b) The response of CheYp molecules to the addition and removal of six magnitudes of Asp.

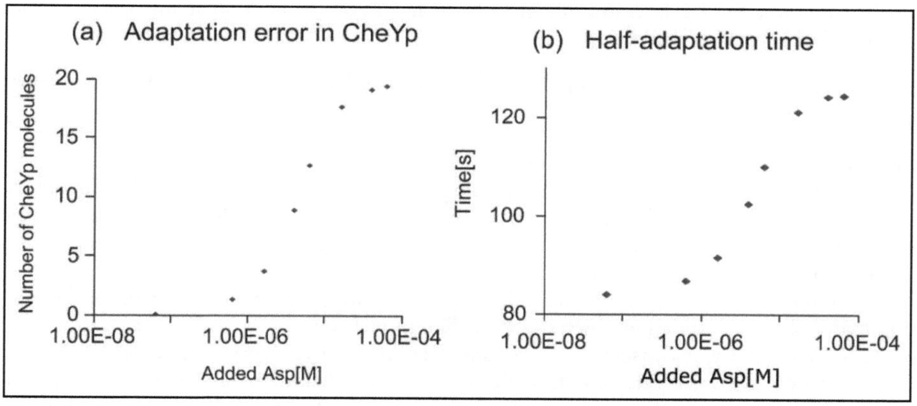


Figure 6. a) Adaptation error observed in model (i). Difference of CheYp molecules before and after adaptation. b) Adaptation time in model (i). Half adaptation times are plotted against the stimulus concentration.

used to analyze adaptation behavior of a chemotaxis system for now and both models have the following features (i) represented by 12 differential equation, (ii) chemoreceptors with four methylation sites and shift among five methylation states and active/inactive conformation, (iii) CheB doesn't interact with no-methylated receptor species and CheR doesn't interact with 4-methylated receptors.

The methylation state of each receptor affects its probability to be in active state. A more methylated receptor can be found in the active state with high probability and interact more frequently with CheBp than CheR.

We have implemented the biologically realistic model referred to in the reference[6] on E-Cell. We deducted the reference model to 375 elementary reactions. The model was simulated using ODE45Stepper. The Tar receptor complex has different binding states in regards to the methyl group and phosphate group (Fig. 4). Each state is implemented as a distinct simulation object on E-Cell 3.

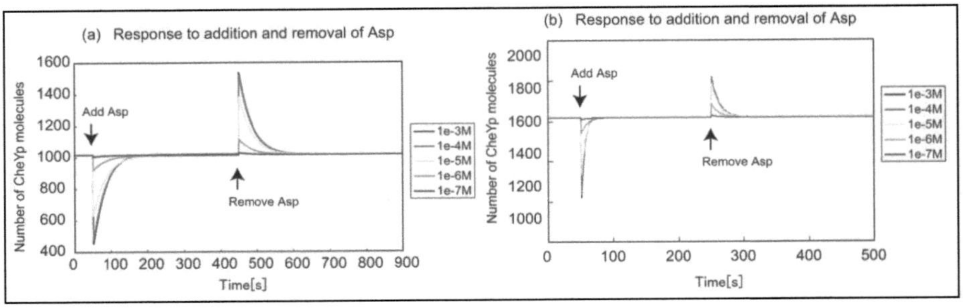


Figure 7. a) Response of CheYp molecule to the addition and removal of Asp. Stimulants were added at 50 simulation seconds and then removed after 400 seconds. b) Results of the model implemented on Mathematica, that perfectly adapts to the stimulation.

### Results

Figure 7 shows the simulation results of the model (ii). Phosphorylated CheY protein shows perfect adaptation for the stimulation by five orders of magnitude. Concentrations of each molecular species at a steady state was the same as the data shown in reference 6, Table IV.

For a reference, outputs from a mathematically strict model, which was implemented in Mathematica Version 4.2, is shown in Figure 7b. It shows exact adaptation at any concentration of 0.1 μM to 1.0 mM stimulant.

## *Stochastically Represented Perfect Adaptation Model (Based on Morton-Firth and Bray, 1999)*

### Methods

The model that reference[6] referred to as a biologically consistent model is originally a model on a stochastic simulator, StochSim, developed by Morton-Firth et al.[9,10] This stochastic model was also implemented on E-Cell as model (iii). This model can be used to analyze effects of random fluctuation of the system, which can't be discussed by deterministic models.

StochSim is a stochastic simulator for biological systems. It treats each molecule as distinct simulation objects. Simulation objects in StochSim models interact according to reaction rate constants and stochastic constants calculated by free energy and kinetic rate constants. In one simulation step, two objects are randomly selected. A generated random number will be compared with stochastic constants of the reaction. The system will calculate the reaction and update itself if the random number was larger than the stochastic constant.

Simulation with stochastic algorithm is suitable for analysis of biological systems in which the quantity of constitutive molecules are small, for example CheR.

The main feature of this reference model is the same as that described in model (ii). The imported model has an alteration from the original model: Tsr effects are not considered. This is for simplicity and to make comparison with model (ii) easier. Bindings of ligands are implicit in the rate of reactions. This is because the binding/dissociation reaction between ligand and receptors is very fast compared to other reactions in this system and can be assumed to be rapid equilibrium.

We imported this model using GillespieStepper, an implementation of Gillespie and Gibson's algorithm. Simulation outputs were compared with the results of StochSim calculation.[17]

### Results

The simulation outputs of E-Cell 3 and StochSim were consistent as shown in Figure 8.

This model also achieved perfect adaptation (Fig. 8). Also, the magnitude of the stimulation and adaptation time shows correlativity as in Model (i). In the stochastic model, response to 0.1 μM induction of the stimulus was concealed by the fluctuation (Fig. 9).

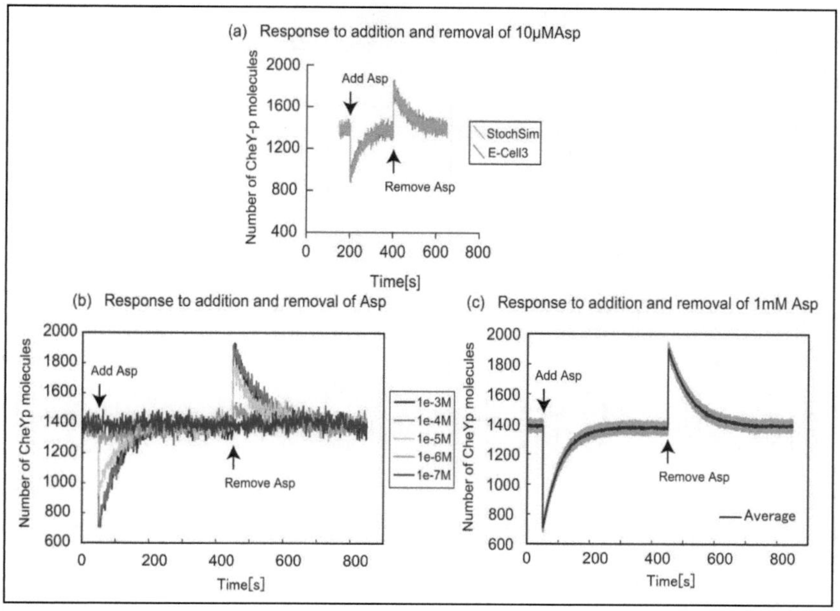


Figure 8. a) Comparison of simulation results by StochSim and E-Cell, in which 1mM Asp was added at 50 simulation seconds and then removed after 200 seconds. b,c) Results by E-Cell model, in which five orders of stimulant were added at 50 simulation seconds and removed after 400 seconds. c) Average and standard deviation of simulated number of CheYp molecules by 100 simulations, in response to 1mM Asp. Stimulants are added at 50 simulation seconds and removed after 400 seconds. The average number CheYp molecules is shown in the dark colored line and standard deviation is shown in the light colored line.

## Conclusion and Discussion

Model (i) demonstrates that a single methylation site is insufficient for perfect adaptation when activity-dependent kinetics is assumed. This result is consistent with the recent analysis by Shimizu et al.[12] The logarithmic dependence of adaptation time on stimulus size, however, can be reproduced even in this simplified model.

Model (ii), derived in an analytical study of the constraints required for exact adaptation, is presently the most detailed deterministic model for analyzing the adaptive behavior of the bacterial chemotaxis pathway. Because the model is a faithful reduction of the stochastic model of Morton-Firth et al,[10] it can be used to answer questions about perfect adaptation (except those pertaining to stochastic aspects) and can be solved much more efficiently than stochastic models.

Model (iii) ported to E-Cell 3 faithfully reproduced the behavior of the StochSim implementation. Interestingly, the time spent to run a 1500 second simulation was nearly the same between the two simulation systems. One of the reasons that StochSim was developed was to circumvent the difficulty that the time required for simulations using the Gillespie algorithm is proportional to the number of possible reactions in the system. The improved Gillespie-Gibson algorithm implemented in E-Cell 3, however, was expected to be faster than StochSim because it uses efficient data structures that make the execution time proportional to the logarithm of the number of reactions. It will be interesting to consider in more detail the conditions under which each algorithm outperforms the other.

Both deterministic and stochastic models of chemotaxis have been successfully implemented on E-Cell 3. In future work, it can be interesting to further exploit the flexibility of this system

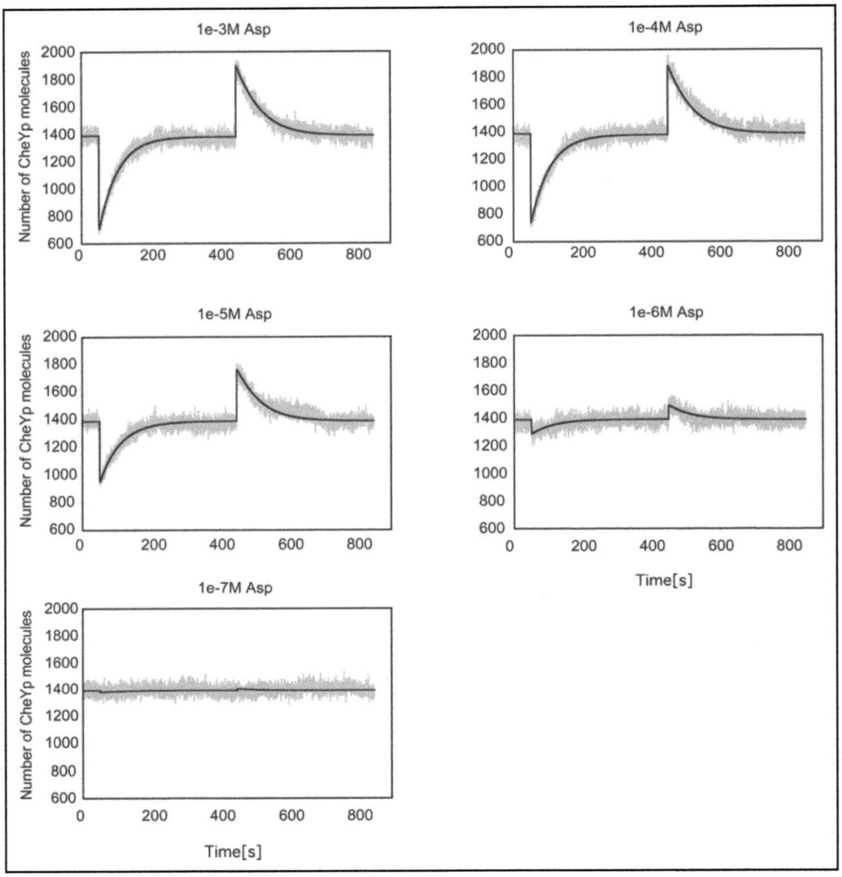


Figure 9. Simulation results of the stochastic and the deterministic model. Different amounts of Asp were added at 50 seconds and removed at 450 seconds. The simulation results by GillespieStepper are shown in gray lines. Those calculated by ODEStepper are shown in black (blue) lines.

to combine deterministic and stochastic computations within the same model. For example, we believe such a framework would be useful for studying the following problems: (i) the response of a stochastic model to various input signals that take the form of continuous functions, (ii) to combine dynamic models of the flagellar motor with the pathway models.

## References

1. Asakura S, Honda H. Two-state model for bacterial chemoreceptor proteins: the role of multiple methylation. J Mol Biol 1984; 176:349-367.
2. Barkai N, Leibler S. Robustness in simple biochemical networks. Nature 1997; 387:913-917.
3. Berg HC, Tedesco PM. Transient response to chemotactic stimuli in Escherichia coli. Proc Natl Acad Sci USA 1975; 72:3235-3239.
4. Borkovich KA, Kaplan N, Hess JF et al. Transmembrane signal transduction in bacterial chemotaxis involves ligand-dependent activation of phosphate group transfer. Proc Natl Acad Sci USA 1989; 86:1208-1212.
5. Bray D, Bourret RB, Simon MI. Computer simulation of the phosphorylation cascade controlling bacterial chemotaxis. Mol Biol Cell 1993; 4:469-482.

6. Le Novere N, Shimizu TS. Stochsim: modelling of stochastic biomolecular processes. Bioinformatics 2001; 17:575-576.
7. McNally DF, Matsumura P. Bacterial chemotaxis signaling complexes: formation of a CheA/CheW complex enhances autophosphorylation and affinity for CheY. Proc Natl Acad Sci USA 1991; 88:6269-6273.
8. Mello BA, Tu Y. Perfect and near-perfect adaptation in a model of bacterial chemotaxis. Biophys J 2003; 84:2943-2956.
9. Morton-Firth CJ, Bray D. Predicting temporal fluctuations in an intracellular signalling pathway. J Theor Biol 1998; 192:117-218.
10. Morton-Firth CJ, Shimizu TS, Bray D. A free-energy-based stochastic simulation of the tar receptor complex. J Mol Biol 1999; 286:1059-1074.
11. Ninfa EG, Stock A, Mowbray S et al. Reconstitution of the bacterial chemotaxis signal transduction system from purified components. J Biol Chem 1991; 266:9764-9770.
12. Shimizu TS, Aksenov SV, Bray D. A spatially extended stochastic model of the bacterial chemotaxis signaling pathway. J Mol Biol 2003; 329:291-309.
13. Takahashi K, Kaizu K, Bin H et al. A multi-algorithm, multi-timescale method for cell simulation. Bioinformatics 2004; 20:538-546.
14. Welch M, Oosawa K, Aizawa S et al. Phosphorylation-dependent binding of a signal molecule to the flagellar switch of bacteria. Proc Natl Acad Sci USA 1993; 90:8787-8791.
15. Wadhams GH, Armitage JP. Making sense of it all: bacterial chemotaxis. Nat Rev Mol Cell Biol 2004; 5:1024-1037.
16. E-Cell project website. http://www.e-cell.org/
17. Gibson MA, Bruck j. Effiecient exact stochastic simulation of chemical systems with many species and many channels. J. Phys. Chem. 2000; 104:1876-1889.

# Chapter 6

# Electrophysiological Simulation of Developmental Changes in Action Potentials of Cardiomyocytes

**Hitomi Itoh***

## Abstract

During cardiomyocyte development, early embryonic ventricular cells show spontaneous activity that disappears at a later stage. Dramatic changes in action potential are mediated by developmental changes in individual ionic currents. Hence, reconstruction of the individual ionic currents into an integrated mathematical model would lead to a better understanding of cardiomyocyte development. To simulate the action potential of the rodent ventricular cell, anecdotally reported developmental changes in individual ionic systems were integrated into two different cardiac electrophysiological models: the Kyoto model and the Luo-Rudy model. Quantitative changes in the ionic currents, pumps, exchangers and sarcoplasmic reticulum $Ca^{2+}$ kinetics were represented as relative activities, which were multiplied by conductance or conversion factors for individual ionic systems. The integrated models can simulate three representative stages in rodent development: early embryonic, late embryonic and neonatal stages. The simulated action potential of the early embryonic ventricular cell model exhibited spontaneous activity that ceased in the simulated action potential of the late embryonic and neonatal ventricular cell models. The simulations with our models reproduced action potentials consistent with the reported characteristics of the cells in vitro.

## Background

### *Cardiac Electrophysiological Model for Simulation of Action Potential*

The cardiac cell membrane contains various ionic channels, exchangers and pumps that allow specific ions to travel or be exchanged through the membrane (Fig. 1). Those ionic components in the cell membrane are utilized to maintain homeostasis of an intracellular and the extracellular environment; such gradient in ionic concentration causes an electrical voltage between the inside and outside of the cell, which is called a "membrane potential."

The membrane potential and the gradient in ionic concentration both mediate a passive transport of ions through the cell membrane. In addition to the passive force driven by the membrane potential and the gradient in ionic concentration, each ionic channel in the cardiomyocyte opens or closes in response to the shift in the membrane potential, represented as a gating property of the ionic current. All of the current components on the membrane are formulated on the basis of a basic mathematical expression of an ionic current that include three parameters: conductance

*Hitomi Itoh— Institute for Advanced Biosciences, Keio University, 5322 Endo, Fujisawa, Kanagawa, 252-8520, Japan. Email: ducky@sfc.keio.ac.jp

*E-Cell System: Basic Concepts and Applications*, edited by Satya Nanda Vel Arjunan, Pawan K. Dhar and Masaru Tomita. 

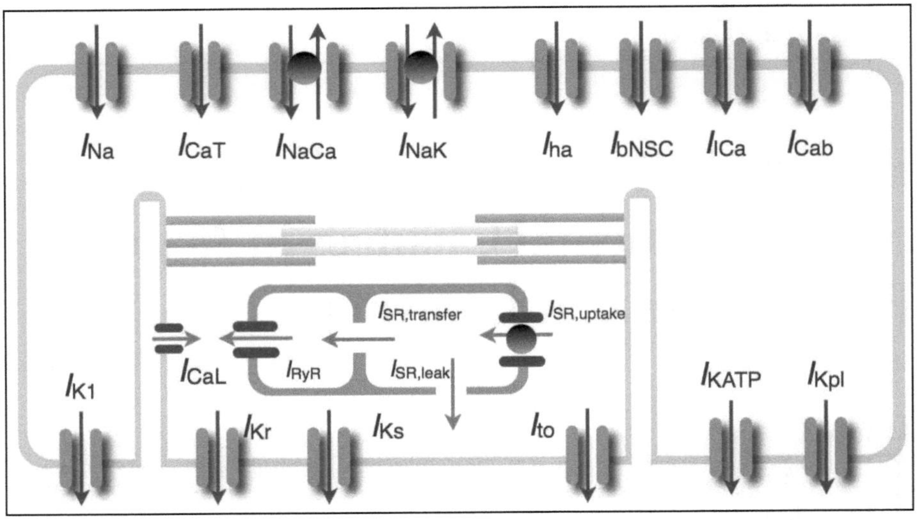


Figure 1. A schematic diagram describing the components of a cardiac electrophysiological model. The model contains more than ten ionic currents, pumps and exchangers; this model is called the Kyoto model.[8] Specific ions travel through ionic channels or are exchanged via exchangers or pumps between the intracellular and extracellular environments as well as between the cytosol and the sarcoplasmic reticulum (SR).

or a conversion factor, passive transport driven by membrane potential and gradient in ionic concentrations and gating properties.

The traveling of ions through the cell membrane causes either depolarization or hyperpolarization of the cell depending on the transport direction. In adult ventricular cells (Fig. 2), for example, opening of channels for $I_{Na}$ ($Na^+$ current) causes the membrane potential to rise to 40 mV; depolarization of the membrane then allows opening of channels for $I_{CaL}$ (L-type $Ca^{2+}$ current), which maintains the potential around 10 mV even after closing of the $Na^+$ channels; the membrane repolarizes to the resting potential level by opening various channels for outward potassium currents. The entire tracing of the transient change in membrane potential is called "action potential."

## *Developmental Changes in Electrophysiological Properties of Ventricular Cells*

The action potential properties of the ventricular cell have been broadly studied in various species at various stages of development. The early embryonic ventricular cells generally have spontaneous action potential in mouse,[1] rat[2,3] and chick[4]; representative in vitro recording of spontaneous action potential in early embryonic rat ventricular cells is shown as an example in Figure 3A.

The late embryonic and postnatal ventricular cells require external stimulation to fire the action potential.[5,6] Although several action potential parameters change among different stages, developmental changes in action potential duration (APD) are the most prominent; APD of guinea pig ventricular cells initially decreased in the neonatal stage and then increased until the adult period (Fig. 3B). Interestingly, the time courses of the changes are different among species; APD continues to decrease in postnatal development of mouse ventricular cells. The developmental changes and the species-specific differences in action potential are mediated by the ion channels of the cells.

Large amounts of data have been recorded via standard microelectrode techniques to describe electrophysiological properties of the ionic channels; several selected examples are reproduced

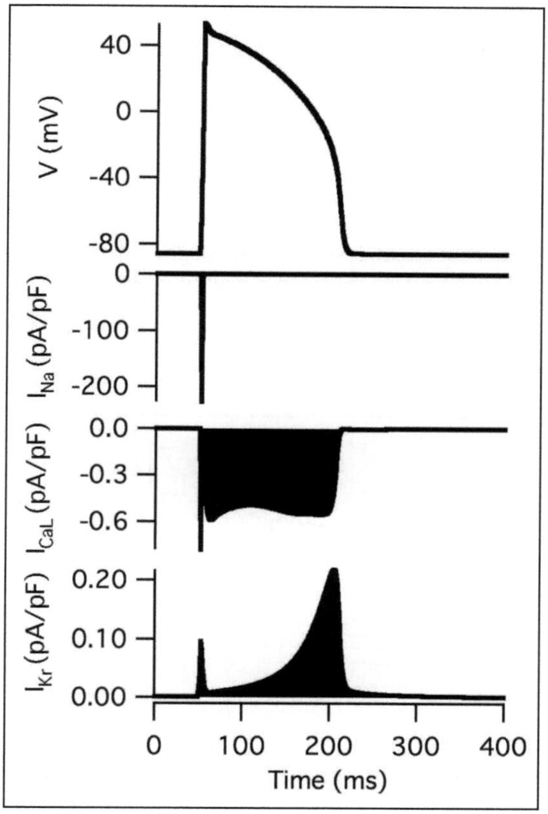


Figure 2. Simulated action potential of an adult ventricular cell with the Kyoto model and changes in $I_{Na}$, $I_{CaL}$ and $I_{Kr}$ accompanying the simulated action potential.

from literature and shown in Figure 4. The basic property of an ionic current can be obtained by shifting the membrane potential from a given holding potential to an arbitrary potential; tracings of $I_{CaL}$ and $I_{K1}$ (inward rectifier $K^+$ current) are recorded from ventricular cells at different developmental stages, wherein membrane is depolarized from a holding potential of −50 to 0 mV for recording of $I_{CaL}$ (Fig. 4A) and from a holding potential of −40 to −100, −90, −80 and −60 mV for recording of $I_{K1}$ (Fig. 4B). Current-voltage (*I-V*) curves of the currents can be drawn up by plotting selected points in the tracing that is obtained by shifting the membrane potential to different potentials (Fig. 4C, D).

## *Modeling Developmental Changes in Cardiomyocyte*

As shown above, developmental changes in cardiomyocyte have been anecdotally reported at various levels. This chapter summarizes the basic concept presented in a recently published paper[7] which aimed to integrate those anecdotally reported data from experiments in vivo or in vitro on the basis of comprehensive cardiac electrophysiological models. *I-V* curves of $I_{CaL}$ and $I_{K1}$ (Fig. 4C, D) indicate that the activity level of the ionic current changes among different stages while voltage dependencies of the current do not change. On the basis of these data, we have assumed that developmental changes in the ionic currents can be represented quantitatively as the activities of the channels in the developing rodent relative to those in the adult. Application of the integrated model for simulation of action potential showed that action potential at different developmental stages can be reproduced

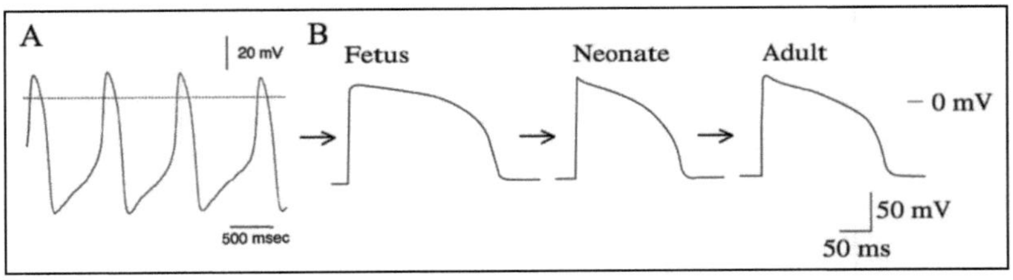


Figure 3. Action potential at different developmental stages in vitro. A) In vitro action potential recorded in ventricular myocytes of a 12-day fetal rat. [Reproduced from: Nagashima et al. J Mol Cell Cardiol 33(3):533-543; ©2001 with permission of Elsevier.[2]] B) In vitro action potential recorded in ventricular myocytes of fetal (1-5 days before birth), neonatal (1-5 days after birth) and adult (45-60 days after birth) guinea pigs. [Reproduced from: Kato et al. J Mol Cell Cardiol 28(7):1515-1522; ©1996 with permission of Elsevier.[12]]

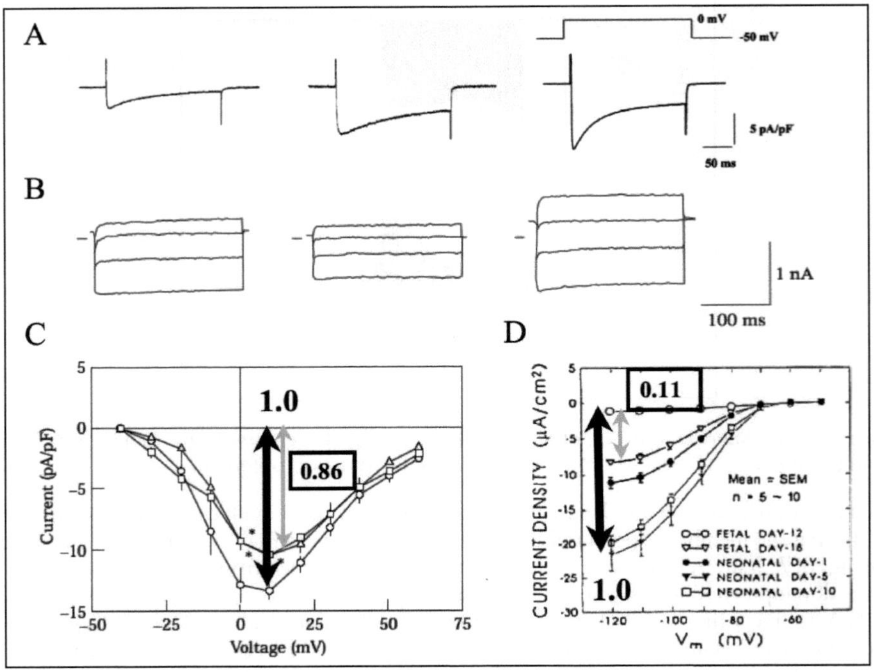


Figure 4. Various ionic currents recorded in different developmental stages. A) Representative tracing of $I_{CaL}$ recorded from ventricular myocytes of the mouse at 9.5-days postcoitum (dpc), 18-dpc and as an adult, wherein the membrane potential was depolarized from a holding potential of −50 mV to 0 mV. [Reproduced from: Liu et al. Life Sci 71(11):1279-1292;[18] ©2002 with permission of Elsevier.] B) Representative tracings of $I_{K1}$ recorded from ventricular myocytes of fetal (1-5 days before birth), neonatal (1-5 days after birth) and adult (45-60 days after birth) guinea-pigs, the membrane potential was polarized from a holding potential of −40 mV to −100, −90, −80 and −60 mV. [Reproduced from: Kato et al. J Mol Cell Cardiol 28(7):1515-1522; ©1996 with permission of Elsevier.[12]] C) Current-voltage (*I-V*) curves of $I_{CaL}$ for late embryonic (squares), neonatal (triangles) and adult (circles) ventricular cells. [Reproduced from: Kato et al. J Mol Cell Cardiol 1996; 28(7):8; with permission of Elsevier.] D) Current-voltage (*I-V*) curves of $I_{K1}$ for early embryonic (open circles), late embryonic (open triangles) and neonatal (close triangles) ventricular cells. [Reproduced from Masuda H, Sperelakis N. Am J Physiol Heart Circ Physiol 265(4):1108; [14] ©1993 with permission from the American Physiological Society.]

with common sets of mathematical models, wherein quantitative changes in the ionic currents, pumps, exchangers and sarcoplasmic reticulum (SR) $Ca^{2+}$ kinetics are expressed as relative activities.

## Methods

### *Implementation of Cardiac Electrophysiological Models to E-Cell Simulation Environment*

Models for simulating the action potential at different developmental stages were constructed on the basis of the Kyoto and Luo-Rudy models, electrophysiological models of the guinea pig cardiomyocyte.[8] The structures of the Kyoto and Luo-Rudy models are very similar and both models have been developed for simulation of guinea pig ventricular cells. The latest version of the Luo-Rudy model[9] was implemented in the E-Cell simulation environment version 3.1. All of the models are constructed on the basis of ElectrophysiologicalBaseProcess.hpp, which had been developed to facilitate further analysis via replacing mathematical equations of ionic currents from one electrophysiological model to the other and the models are available online at http://www.e-cell.org.*

### *General Approach to Modeling of Different Developmental Stages*

All ionic currents, pumps, exchangers and SR $Ca^{2+}$ kinetics are expressed in mathematical equations; as mentioned above, all of the equations include either a conversion factor (pA/mM) or conductance (pA/mV) as one of the parameters. For instance, $I_{CaL}$ and $I_{K1}$ in the Kyoto model are expressed as follow:

$$I_{CaL} = P_{CaL}\cdot(CF_{Ca} + 0.000365\cdot CF_K + 0.0000185\cdot CF_{Na})\cdot p(\text{open}_{CaL}) \quad (1)$$

$$I_{K1} = G_{K1}\cdot(V_m - E_K)\cdot(f_o^4 + 8/3\cdot f_o^3\cdot f_B + 2\cdot f_o^2\cdot f_B^2)\cdot y \quad (2)$$

In Equation (1), $CF_{Ca}$, $CF_K$ and $CF_{Na}$ represent constant field equations (mM) for $Ca^{2+}$, $K^+$ and $Na^+$, respectively; the open probability of three gates in the L-type $Ca^{2+}$ channel is expressed as $p(\text{open}_{CaL})$. Similarly in Equation (2), $V_m$ represents the membrane potential (mV); $E_K$ represents the equilibrium potential of $K^+$ (mV); $f_B$ and $f_O$ represent the fractions of blocked state and those of open state, respectively; $y$ represents the gating variable for a two-state gate. In order to simulate both ventricular cells and sinoatrial (SA) node cells by common mathematical equations, either the conversion factor ($P_{CaL}$ in Eq. 1) or conductance ($G_{K1}$ in Eq. 2) was adjusted based on electrophysiological experiments of each cell.[8]

Various in vitro experimental data, including *I-V* curves and Western blot analyses, were utilized to estimate the relative activities of ionic currents, pumps, exchangers and SR $Ca^{2+}$ kinetics. Those in vitro experimental studies that used guinea pigs were preferentially adopted, because both models were constructed using the adult guinea pig.[8,9] Although the guinea pig was the preferred experimental animal, data from the rat and mouse were also utilized, on the basis of the reported observation that the *I-V* relationships of the ionic channels are well conserved among different rodents.[10,11] In addition, the target stages for simulation of action potentials were set to early embryonic, late embryonic and neonatal, because plenty of literature was available for these stages. The early embryonic stage approximately represents the mouse at 9.5 days postcoitum (dpc) and the rat at 11.5 dpc; the late embryonic and neonatal stages correspond to 1-5 days before and after birth, respectively.

### *Ionic Currents*

It was assumed that developmental changes in ionic currents are determined mainly by their quantitative changes (Fig. 5), which can be represented as the activities of the current in developing stages relative to that of those in the adult stage.

The relative activities of ionic currents were either computed from *I-V* curves (Table 1) or estimated on the basis of qualitative observations (Table 2). It was confirmed that the *I-V* relationship did not change among different developmental stages for $I_{CaL}$,[12] $I_{CaT}$ (T-type $Ca^{2+}$ current),[13] $I_{K1}$,[12,14] $I_{Kr}$ (rapid component of delayed rectifier $K^+$ current),[15] $I_{Ks}$ (slow component of delayed rectifier $K^+$ current)[15] and $I_{Na}$.[15]

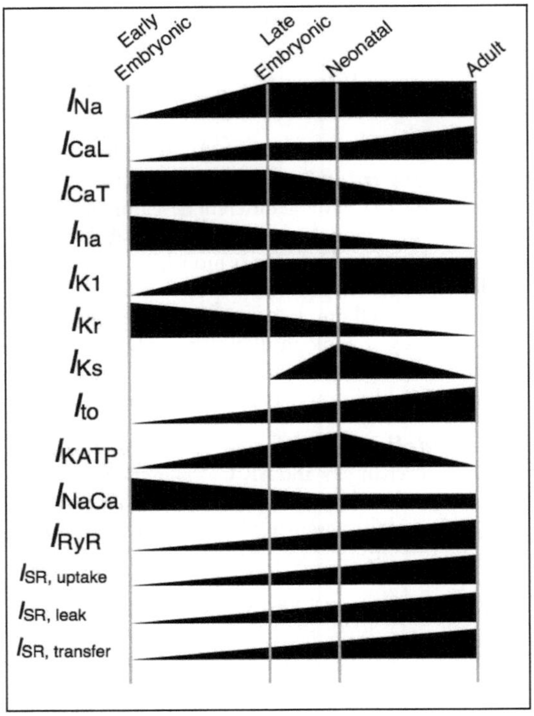


Figure 5. Schematic diagram for modeling rodent ventricular cells at different stages of development. The early embryonic stage approximately corresponds to 9.5-dpc mouse and 11.5-dpc rat. The late embryonic stage corresponds to 1-5 days before birth. The neonatal stage corresponds to 1-5 days after birth. The developmental changes are represented as relative activities, which are obtained or estimated from various in vitro experimental data. All of the relative activities are listed in Tables 1 to 3.

The relative activities were multiplied by the conversion factor or the conductance of the corresponding ionic current. In addition, all currents listed in Table 1 had to be normalized by the ratio of the cell capacitance ($C_m$) of individual myocytes at the corresponding developmental stages (Table 4) to that of adult ventricular cells (132 pF), because *I-V* relationships are usually reported as current density (pA/pF) and the Kyoto model presents current in pA. The ratios were 28/132 for the early embryonic ventricular cell model, 35/132 for the late embryonic ventricular cell model and 40/132 for the neonatal ventricular cell model.

***Table 1. Relative activities for ionic currents, as obtained from the literature***

| Current | Early Embryonic Ventricular Cell | Late Embryonic Ventricular Cell | Neonatal Ventricular Cell |
|---|---|---|---|
| $I_{Na}$ | 0.08 (Davies et al)[15] | 1.00 (Davies et al)[15] | 1.00 (Davies et al)[15] |
| $I_{CaL}$ | 0.46 (Liu et al)[18] | 0.78 (Kato et al;[12] Liu et al[18]) | 0.78 (Kato et al)[12] |
| $I_{CaT}$ | 4.50 (Ferron et al)[13] | 4.50 (Ferron et al)[13] | 2.90 (Ferron et al)[13] |
| $I_{K1}$ | 0.11 (Masuda & Sperelakis)[14] | 1.00 (Kato et al)[12] | 1.00 (Kato et al)[12] |
| $I_{KATP}$ | 0.32 (Xie et al)[17] | 0.88 (Xie et al)[17] | 1.60 (Xie et al)[17] |

***Table 2. Estimated relative activities of ionic currents***

| Current | Early Embryonic Ventricular Cell | Late Embryonic Ventricular Cell | Neonatal Ventricular Cell |
|---|---|---|---|
| $I_{ha}$ | 100.00 (Yasui et al)[1] | 18.00 (Yasui et al)[1] | 0.00 (n/a) |
| $I_{Kr}$ | 10.00 (Chun et al;[25] Spence et al[26]) | 2.00 (Kato et al;[12] Wang et al[5]) | 1.50 (Kato et al;[12] Wang et al[5]) |
| $I_{Ks}$ | 0.01 (Davies et al)[15] | 0.01 (Davies et al;[15] Kato et al.[12]) | 2.00 (Kato et al)[12] |
| $I_{to}$ | 0.01 (Davies et al)[15] | 0.27 (Kilborn & Fedida)[27] | 0.27 (Kilborn & Fedida)[27] |
| $I_{bNSC}$ | 0.35 (n/a) | 0.43 (n/a) | 0.49 (n/a) |

The Luo-Rudy model includes all ionic currents listed in Figure 5 except $I_{to}$ (transient outward current), $I_{KATP}$ (ATP-sensitive $K^+$ current) and $I_{ha}$ (hyperpolarization-activated cation current), all relative activities except those of $I_{to}$, $I_{KATP}$ and $I_{ha}$ were thus implemented in the Luo-Rudy model by the same procedure used in the Kyoto model. Unlike the Kyoto model, all of the currents in the Luo-Rudy model are presented as current density (pA/pF), so it was not necessary to normalize the activity of the currents by the ratio of the $C_m$ of individual myocytes at the corresponding developmental stages.

## *Background Ionic Currents*

$I_{bNSC}$ (background nonselective cation current) is known to have a higher current density in SA node cells than in ventricular cells.[16] Because we found that $I_{bNSC}$ plays an important role in the spontaneous action potential of both SA node cells and early embryonic ventricular myocytes, we scaled the current amplitudes at different stages according to the cell capacitances of the fetal and neonatal cells (Table 2).

$I_{KACh}$ (ACh-activated $K^+$ current) is known to have negligible effects on the action potential of ventricular cells during the course of development[15,17] and is not included in adult ventricular cell models.[8] Hence, we excluded $I_{KACh}$ from the models. Other background currents, including $I_{Kpl}$ (nonspecific, voltage-dependent outward current), $I_{l(Ca)}$ ($Ca^{2+}$-activated background cation current) and $I_{Cab}$ (background $Ca^{2+}$ current) were assumed to have steady current densities; as such, these currents were normalized to the corresponding cell capacitance by the method described above.

## *Exchangers, Pumps and SR $Ca^{2+}$ Kinetics*

The relative activities of exchangers, pumps and SR $Ca^{2+}$ kinetics were computed from a Western blot of SR-related proteins,[18,19] as listed in Table 3. Here, we assumed that the relative

***Table 3. Relative activities of exchangers, pumps and SR $Ca^{2+}$ kinetics***

| Current | Early Embryonic Ventricular Cell | Late Embryonic Ventricular Cell | Neonatal Ventricular Cell |
|---|---|---|---|
| $Na^+/Ca^{2+}$ exchange | 4.95 (Liu et al)[18] | 4.95 (Liu et al;[18] Artman[28]) | 1.00 (Liu et al;[18] Artman et al;[29]Artman[28]) |
| SR $Ca^{2+}$ pump | 0.03 (Liu et al)[18] | 0.21 (Chen et al.;[19] Liu et al[18]) | 0.21 (Chen et al;[19] Liu et al[18]) |
| RyR channel | 0.05 (Liu et al)[18] | 0.40 (Liu et al)[18] | 0.40 (Liu et al)[18] |
| SR transfer | 0.04 (Liu et al)[18] | 0.30 (Liu et al)[18] | 0.30 (Liu et al)[18] |
| SR leak | 0.04 (Liu et al)[18] | 0.30 (Liu et al)[18] | 0.30 (Liu et al)[18] |

***Table 4. Cell capacitances and volumes of cell compartments***

| Current | Early Embryonic Ventricular Cell | Late Embryonic Ventricular Cell | Neonatal Ventricular Cell |
|---|---|---|---|
| $C_m$ (pF) | 28 (Yasui et al)[1] | 35 (Kato et al;[12] Yasui et al[1]) | 40 (Kato et al)[12] |
| $V_i$ (μL) | $1.697 \times 10^{-3}$ (Huynh et al)[20] | $2.121 \times 10^{-3}$ (Huynh et al)[20] | $2.424 \times 10^{-3}$ (Huynh et al)[20] |
| $V_{rel}$ (μL) | $1.357 \times 10^{-6}$ (Liu et al)[18] | $1.273 \times 10^{-5}$ (Liu et al)[18] | $1.454 \times 10^{-5}$ (Liu et al)[18] |
| $V_{up}$ (μL) | $3.394 \times 10^{-6}$ (Liu et al)[18] | $3.182 \times 10^{-5}$ (Liu et al)[18] | $3.636 \times 10^{-5}$ (Liu et al)[18] |

expression level of the proteins directly reflected the relative activities of $Na^+/Ca^{2+}$ exchange, SR $Ca^{2+}$ pump, ryanodine receptor (RyR) channel and other SR $Ca^{2+}$ kinetics. The average relative expression values of SR-related proteins in the early embryonic stage (0.04), late embryonic stage (0.30) and neonatal stage (0.30) were adopted for estimating those values for $I_{SR,\,transfer}$ and $I_{SR,\,leak}$.

## *Cell Capacitance and Volume of Cell Compartments*

$C_m$ (cell capacitance) and volumes ($V_i$, $V_{rel}$, $V_{up}$) were computed on the basis of quantitative data obtained from the literature (Table 4). No significant differences were observed between the $C_m$ of mouse ventricular cells (31 ± 3.3 pF) and that of guinea pig ventricular cells (34.5 ± 2.72 pF) in the late embryonic stage;[1,12] as such, the $C_m$ values for mouse early embryonic ventricular cells (28 pF), guinea pig late embryonic ventricular cells (35 pF) and guinea pig neonatal ventricular cells (40 pF) were adopted.

The developmental change in $V_i$ (cell volume accessible for ion diffusion) in rabbit ventricular cells is roughly proportional to that of cell capacitance.[20] In addition, a positive linear correlation has been found between membrane capacitance and cell volume in several species.[21] Hence, cell volume was estimated by multiplying the adult $V_i$ ($8.0 \times 10^{-3}$ μL) by the corresponding $C_m$ (28, 35 or 40 pF) over the adult $C_m$ (132 pF).

In the Kyoto model, the volume fractions of $V_{rel}$ (volume of SR release site) and $V_{up}$ (volume of SR uptake site) were set to 2% and 5% of $V_i$, respectively.[8] The SR-mediated $Ca^{2+}$ transient is modeled by multiplying an estimated value called the "SA factor" by $V_{rel}$, $V_{up}$ and SR-related currents in the Kyoto model.[8] The same approach has been adopted for estimating $V_{rel}$ and $V_{up}$ in different developmental stages of ventricular cells; on the basis of quantitative changes in SR-related proteins,[18] the average relative expression values of those proteins in the early embryonic stage (0.04), late embryonic stage (0.30) and neonatal stage (0.30) were utilized for the estimation.

## *Simulation of Action Potential at Three Different Developmental Stages*

On the basis of the assumption that developmental changes in ionic currents are determined mainly by their quantitative changes (Fig. 5), the developmental changes in ionic components were represented as the activities of the components in the developing rodent relative to those in the adult; the relative activities were multiplied by either the conversion factor or conductance in corresponding mathematical equations. All of the models were simulated for 200 s to confirm that the spontaneous action potentials were stable or that the membrane potential had reached a quasi-steady state. Hence, the simulation results presented in this chapter were recorded after simulating the corresponding models for 200 s. In addition, an external current ($I_{ext}$) was applied in the late embryonic and neonatal ventricular cell models in order to fire the action potential of the cells. Because the Luo-Rudy model requires "pacing" of the action potential, the model was simulated for 600 s as instructed in the report.[9]

## Results

### *Simulated Action Potential at Three Representative Developmental Stages*

The implementation of relative activities of ionic components at early embryonic stage to both the Kyoto and Luo-Rudy models exhibited a spontaneous action potential (Fig. 6A,C). In the simulated action potential with the Kyoto model, the membrane slowly depolarized from the maximum diastolic potential (MDP) at −62.86 mV until it reached approximately −40 mV when spontaneous action potential was triggered. The membrane then started to repolarize after overshoot potential at 3.13 mV and completed the repolarization in less than 100 ms. The whole action potential was completed in a basic cycle length (BCL) of 492 ms. On the other hand, the membrane overshot to 13.74 mV from MDP at −71.16 mV in the simulation with the Luo-Rudy model; the whole action potential was completed in a BCL of 414 ms, which resulted from faster depolarization and repolarization of the membrane.

The spontaneous action potential ceased in the later stages of development in simulation of the corresponding stages with both the Kyoto model (Fig. 6B) and the Luo-Rudy model (Fig. 6D). In simulation with the Kyoto model, both late embryonic and neonatal ventricular cells showed resting membrane potentials that were more negative (−83.60 mV) than the MDP of the early embryonic ventricular cell. Repolarization of the membrane occurred more slowly in the late embryonic ventricular cell than in the neonatal ventricular cell; the APD was 140 ms in the late embryonic ventricular cell and 117 ms in the neonatal ventricular cell. The qualitative characteristics of the

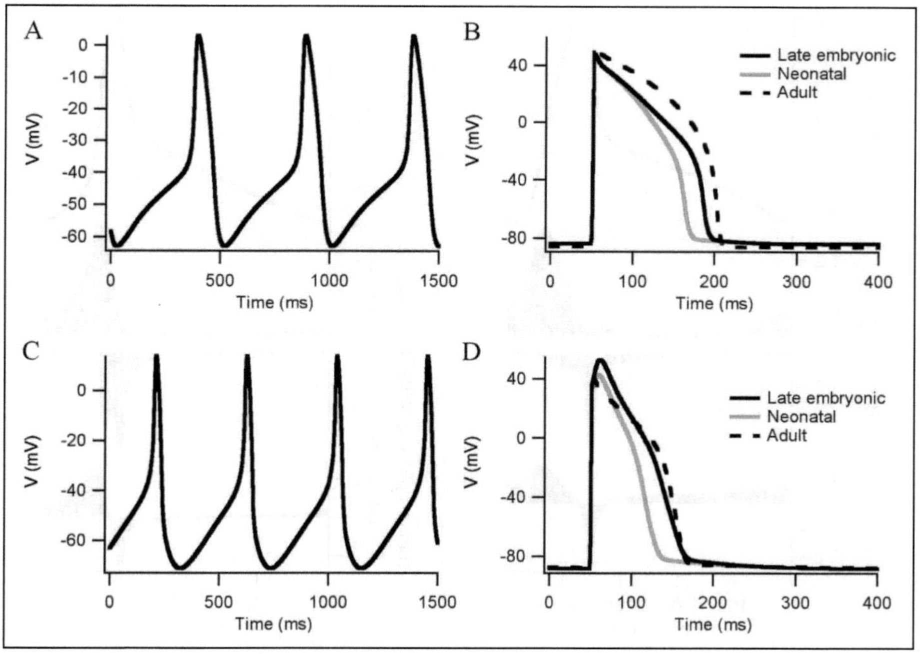


Figure 6. Simulated action potentials at different developmental stages with the Luo-Rudy model (B) in comparison with simulated action potential with the Kyoto model (A). A) Simulated action potential with the Kyoto model. B) Simulated action potential with the Luo-Rudy model at early embryonic stage (left), late embryonic stage (dark line in right) and neonatal stage (light line). Action potentials at adult stage (control) are shown as dashed line.

cells at those stages were well reproduced in the simulation with the Luo-Rudy model as well; the late embryonic and neonatal ventricular cells showed more negative resting membrane potentials than the MDP of the early embryonic ventricular cell and shorter APD in neonatal ventricular cells than in late embryonic ventricular cells.

### *Evaluation of Individual Ionic Currents in Two Different Models*

Comparison of the action potential tracings of early embryonic ventricular cell simulated with the Kyoto (Fig. 6A) and the Luo-Rudy model (Fig. 6C) clearly indicate that the Kyoto model reproduced the action potential recording in vitro (Fig. 3A) more consistently than did the Luo-Rudy model; the most prominent differences are the faster repolarization phase (RP) and diastolic slow depolarization (DSD) phase, both of which cause overall shortening of BCL. The differences in simulated action potential were determined by differences in mathematical equations of ionic currents, particularly $I_{Kr}$ that plays a predominant role in repolarization of the membrane during action potential. The dynamic behaviors of $I_{Kr}$ underlying the action potential were compared between the Kyoto and the Luo-Rudy models along with $I_{CaL}$ and sums of $I_{CaL}$ and $I_{Kr}$ (Fig. 7). Apparently, activation of $I_{Kr}$ in RP was faster in the Luo–Rudy model (Fig. 7B) than in the Kyoto model (Fig. 7A); the difference in $I_{CaL}$ in the inactivation phase is canceled out by the fast activation of $I_{Kr}$, illustrated as sum of $I_{CaL}$ and $I_{Kr}$. Hence, we made a working hypothesis that

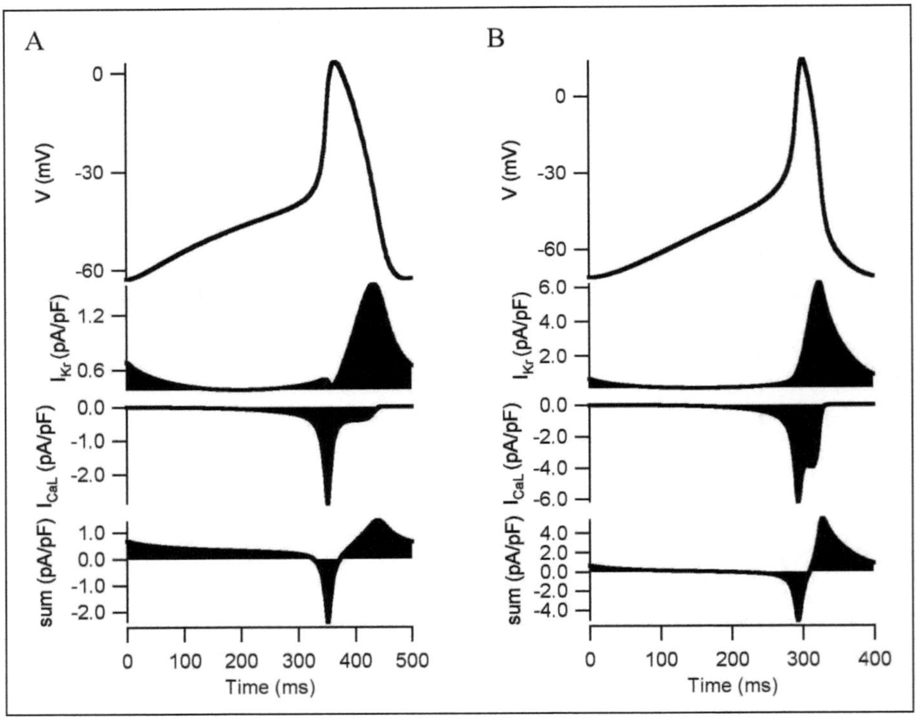


Figure 7. Simulated action potential, $I_{Kr}$ and $I_{CaL}$, at early embryonic stage with the Kyoto model (A) the Luo–Rudy model (B). The simulated action potential can be divided into three phases: diastolic slow depolarization (DSD), depolarization phase (DP) and repolarization phase (RP). Sum of $I_{Kr}$ and $I_{CaL}$ shows that the increase in outward (positive) current is slower in the Kyoto model than in the Luo–Rudy model.

the difference in the mathematical equations of $I_{Kr}$ in the two models undertakes more consistent simulated action potentials in the Kyoto model.

In order to assess the working hypothesis, mathematical equations of $I_{Kr}$ in the Luo-Rudy model was replaced with those of $I_{Kr}$ in the Kyoto model. Figure 8 illustrates simulated results of adult ventricular cell with original Luo-Rudy model (A) and the Luo-Rudy model whose $I_{Kr}$ is replaced with those of the Kyoto model (B); the conductance amplitude of $I_{Kr}$ ($G_{Kr}$) was adjusted to achieve approximately the same APD. The replaced model was then utilized for simulation of spontaneous action potential in early embryonic ventricular cell (Fig. 9A). Apparently, the replacement of the mathematical equations made all quantitative characteristics of the action potential less consistent with those of the cells in vitro; such characteristics are more negative MDP (−75.94 mV), more positive overshoot (21.03 mV) and longer BCL (697 ms).

Another difference between the Kyoto and Luo-Rudy models is that the Kyoto model successfully incorporated five known types of background current components. One of the defined background current is called $I_{bNSC}$ (background nonselective cation current), which shows ion selectivity of both $K^+$ and $Na^+$ and is determined by constant field equations of each ions. Because the balance of $I_{Kr}$ and $I_{bNSC}$ determines the MDP of the simulated spontaneous action potential of SA node cell with the Kyoto model[24] and the Luo-Rudy model lacks such nonselective current, model equations of $I_{bNSC}$ were augmented in addition to replacing $I_K$ equations (Fig. 9B). Varying the amplitude of $I_{bNSC}$ ($P_{bNSC}$) arbitrarily showed that $I_{bNSC}$ indeed plays an important role in both determining MDP and rate of DSD phase and all three quantitative characteristics, MDP (−71.15 mV), overshoot (18.20 mV) and BCL (510 ms), were thus improved compared to the $I_{Kr}$-replaced model without augmentation of $I_{bNSC}$.

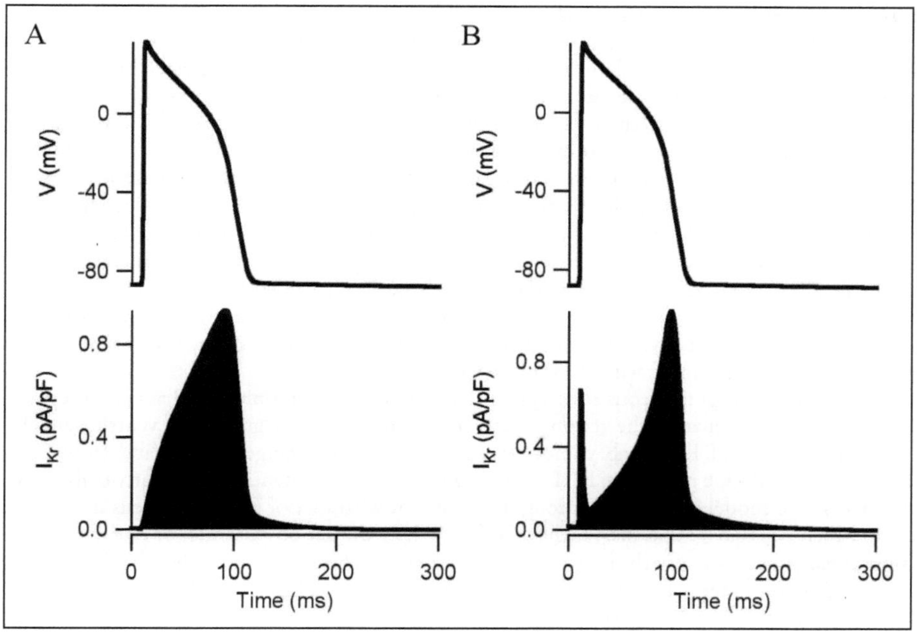


Figure 8. Simulated action potentials and tracings of $I_{Kr}$ of adult ventricular cell with the original Luo-Rudy model (A) and the Luo-Rudy model whose $I_{Kr}$ is replaced with those of the Kyoto model (B). Model equations of $I_{Kr}$ in the Luo-Rudy model were replaced with those of $I_{Kr}$ in the Kyoto model.

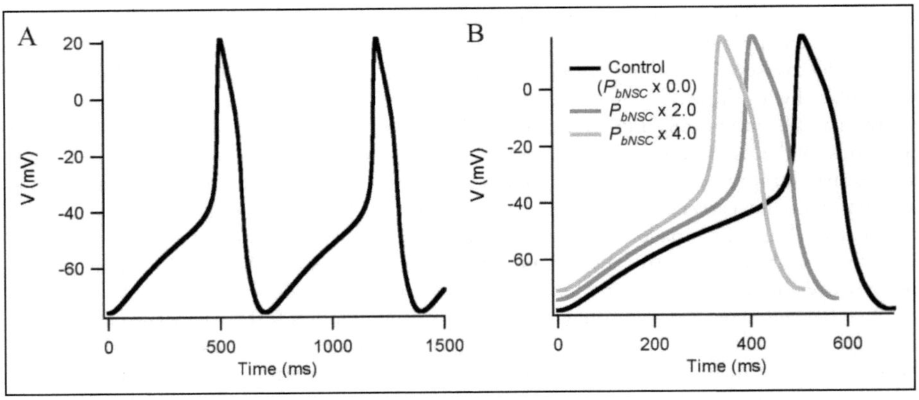


Figure 9. Simulated action potentials of early embryonic stage with various replacements. A) Simulated action potential with the Luo-Rudy model wherein the model equations of $I_{Kr}$ were replaced with those of $I_{Kr}$ in the Kyoto model. B) Simulated action potential with the Luo-Rudy model wherein the model equations of $I_{bNSC}$ were augmented in addition to replacement of $I_{Kr}$.

## Discussion

### *Spontaneous Action Potential In Vitro Was Well Simulated with the Early Embryonic Models*

The early embryonic ventricular cell model, which was constructed on the basis of the Kyoto model (Fig. 6A), reproduced well the spontaneous action potential that is generated by ventricular cells in 12-dpc rats.[2] Species-specific differences in spontaneous action potential waveforms have been observed between ventricular cells in 9.5-dpc mice[1] and those in 12-dpc rats.[2] The ventricular cells in 9.5-dpc mice generate a more hyperpolarized MDP (−71.2 ± 0.4 mV) than those in 12-dpc rats (−66.7 ± 3.6 mV). A spontaneous action potential is triggered when the membrane potential reaches approximately −60 mV in 9.5-dpc mice and approximately −40 mV in 12-dpc rats.[1,2] The simulated action potential in our early embryonic ventricular cell model constructed on the basis of the Kyoto model (Fig. 6A) was very similar to the action potential waveforms generated by the automatically beating cells in 12-dpc rats (Fig. 3A).[2] In addition, the MDP of the simulated action potential (−62.86 mV) was approximately consistent with that of the ventricular cells in 12-dpc rats. Hence, our early embryonic ventricular cell model could reproduce an action potential that was in reasonable agreement with those of previous studies.

The speed of the spontaneous action potential in the early embryonic stage has been a controversial issue. Unfortunately, the action potential of early embryonic guinea pig ventricular cells has not been reported. Early embryonic hearts have shown a large range of heart rates, from 61 to 219 min$^{-1}$ in 11.5-dpc rats.[22] The BCL of the simulated action potential of our early embryonic ventricular cell model (492 ms) was roughly consistent with that of ventricular cells in 9.5-dpc mice, which is 510.8 ± 32.8 ms.[1] Although the BCL of the action potential of our model was approximately consistent with those of previous studies, it should be noted that the BCL of the simulated action potential might not be quantitatively accurate, because early embryonic hearts have a large range of rates in vivo.

### *Developmental Changes in APD Were Reproduced Qualitatively with the Model*

APD changes over the course of rodent development. Although the duration and shape of the action potential in the adult rat are totally different from those in the adult guinea pig because of differences in the $I_{to}$, shortening of the APD between the late embryonic stage and the neonatal stage has been observed in both guinea pigs[2] and rats.[3] The rapid component ($I_{Kr}$) and slow component ($I_{Ks}$) of the delayed rectifier $K^+$ current play important roles in repolarization and thus control the length of the APD; both $I_{Kr}$ and $I_{Ks}$ undergo very complex changes in their activities between the late embryonic and neonatal stages (Fig. 5). As described in the Methods sections, I estimated the relative activities of both $I_{Kr}$ and $I_{Ks}$ on the basis of the qualitative characteristics of these currents, including the changes in APD in response to a selective $I_{Kr}$ blocker. Although qualitatively consistent, APD may not be quantitatively accurate because several relative activities were estimated on the basis of qualitative characteristics.

### *Evaluating the Role of Individual Ionic Currents for Better Simulation*

All of the simulated results with the Luo-Rudy model indicate that the Kyoto model reproduced the action potential in the early embryonic stage more consistently than the Luo–Rudy model. The role of individual ionic currents in the better simulation with the Kyoto model was evaluated by replacing mathematical models of specific ionic currents between the Kyoto model and the Luo-Rudy model.

Dynamic behavior was improved by replacement of the mathematical models for $I_{Kr}$. This result indicated that the fast repolarization in the Luo–Rudy model is determined by fast activation of $I_{Kr}$. The formulations of $I_{Kr}$ in the Luo-Rudy and Kyoto models are as follow:

$$I_{Kr} = G_{Kr} \cdot (V_m - E_K) \cdot X_r \cdot R \quad (3)$$

$$I_{Kr} = G_{Kr} \cdot C_m \cdot (V_m - E_K) \cdot (0.6 \cdot y_1 + 0.4 \cdot y_2) \cdot y_3 \quad (4)$$

Whereas $I_{Kr}$ in the Luo–Rudy model (Eq. 3) is described by a time-dependent activation gate ($X_r$) and a time-independent inactivation gate ($R$),[9] $I_{Kr}$ in the Kyoto model (Eq. 4) is described by two activation gates ($y_1, y_2$) and by one inactivation gate ($y_3$)[8]. In the Kyoto model, the equations were intentionally developed for two cell types, ventricular cells as well as SA node cells,[23] because no obvious difference has been observed in the electrophysiological properties of the currents in terms of their kinetics. In addition, the original paper[24] specifically mentioned that the balance of $I_{Kr}$ and $I_{bNSC}$ determines the MDP of the simulated spontaneous action potential of SA node cell with the Kyoto model; as such, the difference in background currents between the Kyoto and the Luo-Rudy models is one of the important differences contributing to the increased speed of the DSD phase. The Kyoto model may thus have been suitable for this study, because most currents in ventricular cells change quantitatively with similar kinetics throughout the stages of development.

## Conclusion

In the present chapter, developmental changes of the ion channels were represented quantitatively as the activities of the channels in the developing rodent relative to those in the adult. Multiplication of the relative activities by the corresponding mathematical equations reproduced the developmental changes in the action potential of the rodent ventricular cell. Although both the Kyoto and Luo–Rudy models represented various characteristics, the Kyoto model reproduced action potentials in the early embryonic stage more consistently than did the Luo–Rudy model, because of differences in mathematical model of $I_{Kr}$ and background currents.

## References


1. Yasui K, Liu W, Opthof T et al. I(f) current and spontaneous activity in mouse embryonic ventricular myocytes. Circ Res 2001; 88(5):536-542.
2. Nagashima M, Tohse N, Kimura K et al. Alternation of inwardly rectifying background K+ channel during development of rat fetal cardiomyocytes. J Mol Cell Cardiol 2001; 33(3):533-543.
3. Kojima M, Sada H, Sperelakis N. Developmental changes in beta-adrenergic and cholinergic interactions on calcium-dependent slow action potentials in rat ventricular muscles. Br J Pharmacol 1990; 99(2):327-333.
4. Satoh H, Sada H, Tohse N et al. Developmental aspects of electrophysiology in cardiac muscle. Nippon Yakurigaku Zasshi 1996; 107(5):213-223.

5. Wang L, Feng ZP, Kondo CS et al. Developmental changes in the delayed rectifier K+ channels in mouse heart. Circ Res 1996; 79(1):79-85.
6. Agata N, Tanaka H, Shigenobu K. Developmental changes in action potential properties of the guinea-pig myocardium. Acta Physiol Scand 1993; 149(3):331-337.
7. Itoh H, Naito Y, Tomita M. Simulation of developmental changes in action potentials with ventricular cell models. Systems and Synthetic Biology 2007; 1(1):11-23.
8. Matsuoka S, Sarai N, Kuratomi S et al. Role of individual ionic current systems in ventricular cells hypothesized by a model study. Jpn J Physiol 2003; 53(2):105-123.
9. Faber GM, Rudy Y. Action potential and contractility changes in [Na(+)](i) overloaded cardiac myocytes: a simulation study. Biophys J 2000; 78(5):2392-2404.
10. Linz KW, Meyer R. Profile and kinetics of L-type calcium current during the cardiac ventricular action potential compared in guinea-pigs, rats and rabbits. Pflugers Arch 2000; 439(5):588-599.
11. Zhang ZJ, Jurkiewicz NK, Folander K et al. K+ currents expressed from the guinea pig cardiac IsK protein are enhanced by activators of protein kinase C. Proc Natl Acad Sci USA 1994; 91(5):1766-1770.
12. Kato Y, Masumiya H, Agata N et al. Developmental changes in action potential and membrane currents in fetal, neonatal and adult guinea-pig ventricular myocytes. J Mol Cell Cardiol 1996; 28(7):1515-1522.
13. Ferron L, Capuano V, Deroubaix E et al. Functional and molecular characterization of a T-type Ca(2+) channel during fetal and postnatal rat heart development. J Mol Cell Cardiol 2002; 34(5):533-546.
14. Masuda H, Sperelakis N. Inwardly rectifying potassium current in rat fetal and neonatal ventricular cardiomyocytes. Am J Physiol 1993; 265(4 Pt 2):H1107-1111.
15. Davies MP, An RH, Doevendans P et al. Developmental changes in ionic channel activity in the embryonic murine heart. Circ Res 1996; 78(1):15-25.
16. Kiyosue T, Spindler AJ, Noble SJ et al. Background inward current in ventricular and atrial cells of the guinea-pig. Proc Biol Sci 1993; 252(1333):65-74.
17. Xie LH, Takano M, Noma A. Development of inwardly rectifying K+ channel family in rat ventricular myocytes. Am J Physiol 1997; 272(4 Pt 2):H1741-1750.
18. Liu W, Yasui K, Opthof T et al. Developmental changes of Ca(2+) handling in mouse ventricular cells from early embryo to adulthood. Life Sci 2002; 71(11):1279-1292.
19. Chen F, Ding S, Lee BS et al. Sarcoplasmic reticulum Ca(2+)ATPase and cell contraction in developing rabbit heart. J Mol Cell Cardiol 2000; 32(5):745-755.
20. Huynh TV, Chen F, Wetzel GT et al. Developmental changes in membrane Ca2+ and K+ currents in fetal, neonatal, and adult rabbit ventricular myocytes. Circ Res 1992; 70(3):508-515.
21. Satoh H, Delbridge LM, Blatter LA et al. Surface:volume relationship in cardiac myocytes studied with confocal microscopy and membrane capacitance measurements: species-dependence and developmental effects. Biophys J 1996; 70(3):1494-1504.
22. Couch JR, West TC, Hoff HE. Development of the action potential of the prenatal rat heart. Circ Res 1969; 24(1):19-31.
23. Ono K, Ito H. Role of rapidly activating delayed rectifier K+ current in sinoatrial node pacemaker activity. Am J Physiol 1995; 269(2 Pt 2):H453-462.
24. Sarai N, Matsuoka S, Kuratomi S et al. Role of individual ionic current systems in the SA node hypothesized by a model study. Jpn J Physiol 2003; 53(2):125-134.
25. Chun KR, Koenen M, Katus HA et al. Expression of the IKr components KCNH2 (rERG) and KCNE2 (rMiRP1) during late rat heart development. Exp Mol Med 2004; 36(4):367-371.
26. Spence SG, Vetter C, Hoe CM. Effects of the class III antiarrhythmic, dofetilide (UK-68,798) on the heart rate of midgestation rat embryos, in vitro. Teratology 1994; 49(4):282-292.
27. Kilborn MJ, Fedida D. A study of the developmental changes in outward currents of rat ventricular myocytes. J Physiol 1990; 430:37-60.
28. Artman M. Sarcolemmal Na(+)-Ca2+ exchange activity and exchanger immunoreactivity in developing rabbit hearts. Am J Physiol 1992; 263(5 Pt 2):H1506-1513.
29. Artman M, Ichikawa H, Avkiran M et al. Na+/Ca2+ exchange current density in cardiac myocytes from rabbits and guinea pigs during postnatal development. Am J Physiol 1995; 268(4 Pt 2):H1714-1722.

# Chapter 7

# Simulation of Human Erythrocyte Metabolism

**Ayako Kinoshita***

## Introduction

Since a mature mammalian erythrocyte is enucleated and it is void of mitochondria, gene expression does not take place, while glycolysis is the only mechanism to produce ATP. This simplicity makes its metabolism unique from other cells. Due to its simple structure and the traceability of the cell, erythrocyte metabolism and enzymology have been well studied over the last three to four decades. Although vast amounts of erythrocyte component information is available, the quantitative and physiological role of the metabolism is still an open question because the nature of the cellular function is the complex dynamics of components. Mathematical models for biochemical pathways comprising complex networks are of particular interest in order to identify the features of biological systems that cannot be investigated by the analysis of their individual components alone. Because of its simplicity, the robustness of the erythrocyte that enables the cell to circulate in the body for about 120 days and the abundance of knowledge, erythrocytes have been a good subject for numerous modeling and simulation studies. There is a long history of detailed metabolic models of erythrocyte metabolism with differential equations. The first mathematical models of erythrocyte metabolism were developed by Rapoport et al and the model by Heinrich et al, which only included the glycolytic pathway.[1-3] Ataullakhanov et al expanded the glycolytic model to represent the pentose phosphate pathway.[4] Subsequently, adenine nucleotide metabolism was first considered by Schauer et al.[5] The comprehensive biochemical network, which has been widely accepted as the complete network of the metabolic system in erythrocytes, was reconstructed by Joshi and Palsson in 1989-1990, involving membrane transports, the $Na^+/K^+$ pump and osmotic pressure.[6-9] Mulquiney and Kuchel developed a precise model that describes magnesium equilibrium, binding metabolites to oxyhemoglobin (oxyHb) considering the most detailed kinetics of glycolytic enzymes.[10,11] Based on these studies, several models focusing on human erythrocyte metabolism have been developed using E-Cell System, which is one of the leading simulation platforms for applying various modeling methods, mathematical analyses and multi-time/multi-size behaviors. The simulation analysis of these models predicted various aspects of the metabolism under physiological and pathological conditions: the importance of the de novo synthesis and transport of glutathione in glucose-6-phosphate dehydrogenase (G6PDH)-deficient cells,[12] the physiological significance of NADPH-dependent methemoglobin-reducing pathway[13] and the effectiveness of intracellular protein bindings in hypoxia-induced alterations of the metabolism through hemoglobin allostery.[14]

This chapter presents these applications of the metabolic model of human erythrocytes developed on E-Cell System in some detail.

*Ayako Kinoshita—Department of Biochemistry and Integrative Medical Biology School of Medicine, Keio University, 160-8582 Tokyo, Japan; Institute for Advanced Biosciences, Keio University, 252-8520 Fujisawa, Japan. Email: ayakosan@sfc.keio.ac.jp

*E-Cell System: Basic Concepts and Applications*, edited by Satya Nanda Vel Arjunan, Pawan K. Dhar and Masaru Tomita. 

## Simulation Analysis of Glucose-6-Phosphate Dehydrogenase (G6PDH) Deficiency

Using the metabolic model of human erythrocyte on E-Cell System, which consists of glycolysis, pentose phosphate pathways, nucleotide metabolism, simple membrane transport systems and the ATP dependent-$Na^+/K^+$ pump, we carried out a simulation analysis of G6PDH. The basic model was based on that developed by Joshi and Palsson.[6-9] G6PDH deficiency is the most common enzymopathy in human erythrocytes with more than two hundred million people affected by the disease. In serious cases, this disease causes chronic hemolytic anemia due to attenuated reducing potential. G6PDH, the initial step of the pentose-phosphate pathway (PPP), catalyzes the oxidation of glucose-6-phosphate (G6P) to 6-phosphoglucolactone (6PGL) concomitantly reducing NADP to NADPH (Fig. 1A) and is regulated by ATP and 2,3-BPG. NADPH is needed for conversion of GSH from GSSG, and GSH protects the cell membrane and any other proteins in a human erythrocyte from oxidative stress both directly and indirectly. We employed the initial metabolic model of human erythrocytes to reproduce the pathological condition of G6PDH deficiency. Figure 1B shows the kinetic equation of G6PDH and the corresponding parameter values of normal and deficient cells used in this study. In our first simulation of G6PDH deficiency, we substituted normal kinetic parameters with those obtained from the patients with the deficiency.

As a result, several sequential changes were observed in the simulation of G6PDH deficiency:reaction rate of G6PDH was very low, a decrease in NADPH occurred and GSH rapidly decreased (Fig. 2A, panel a-c). ATP kept its initial concentration for several simulation hours, because consumption and production of ATP in glycolysis was balanced. However, after approximately 55 hours, ATP began to decrease and glycolytic enzyme activities started to depress and finally depleted completely (Fig. 2A, panel d-f). It is experimentally known that in G6PDH-deficient cells, ATP and glycolytic enzyme activities keep their normal levels while the metabolites or metabolic fluxes in PPP are lowered;[15] however, the simulation results didn't agree with this metabolic feature of G6PDH deficiency.

After a precise survey of the metabolic pathways in erythrocytes, we hypothesized that the difference between the simulation model and the actual cell was caused by the lack of significant pathways in the model: de novo synthesizing GSH and excretion of GSSG. The first step of synthesis of GSH in human erythrocytes produces gamma-glutamyl cysteine (L_GC) from cysteine and glutamate using ATP. The reaction is catalyzed by gamma-glutamyl cysteine synthetase (L_GCS), the rate-limiting enzyme of glutathione synthesis. In the second step, GSH is produced from L_GC and glycine using ATP, which is catalyzed by glutathione synthetase (GSHsyn). Therefore, the GSH synthetic process involves the three kinds of amino acids which are transported through cell membrane and two molecules of ATP.[16] Due to the strong feedback inhibition of L_GCS by GSH, the synthesis of GSH is suppressed in the normal state in which GSH exists in high concentration. On the other hand, under abnormal conditions, e.g., suffering from oxidative stress or genetically deficient of steps in generating GSH, the pathway is speculated to be efficiently activated. In addition, erythrocytes have an ATP-dependent transport system of GSSG, which was first demonstrated by Srivastava and Beutler[17] and kinetically examined by Kondo and Beutler.[18] We added these pathways, which are neglected in former models, to the initial model. The rate equations and kinetic parameters of the expanded pathways were not shown here but presented in other models.[12]

Using the expanded model that contains the above pathways around GSH-GSSG, the following behaviors were predicted in the simulation of G6PDH deficiency: a lesser decrease in GSH, lower levels of GSSG and a higher NADP/NADPH ratio than that of the previous model (Fig. 2B, a-c). Note that the activities of glycolytic enzymes stayed at almost the initial rate, which was one of the most remarkable difference from the previous model, culminating in the retention of the ATP level (Fig. 2B, d-f). The lifetime predicted from the ATP level of the pathway-expanded model was much longer than that of the previous model. These results

A

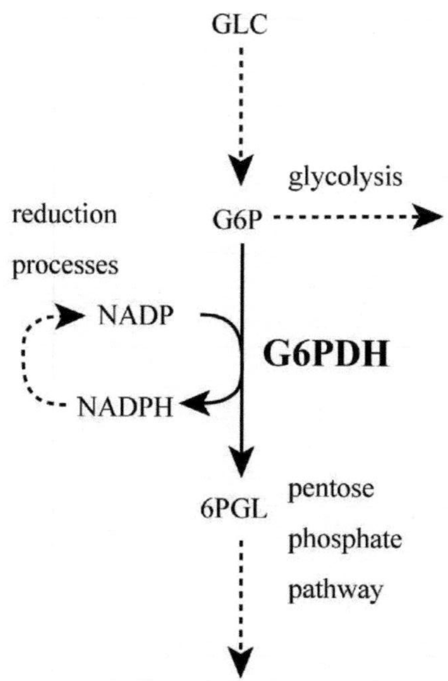


B

$$v_{G6PD} = \frac{V\max \dfrac{[NADP][G6P]}{Km_{NADP}\, Km_{G6P}}}{1 + \dfrac{[NADP]}{Km_{NADP}}\left(1 + \dfrac{[G6P]}{Km_{G6P}}\right) + \dfrac{[NADPH]}{Ki_{NADPH}} + \dfrac{[ATP]}{Ki_{ATP}} + \dfrac{[2,3\text{-}BPG]}{Ki_{2,3\text{-}BPG}}}$$

| | Half life (day) | Vmax (μkat/l cells) | $Km_{G6P}$ (μM) | $Km_{NADP}$ (μM) | $Ki_{NADPH}$ (μM) | $Ki_{ATP}$ (μM) | $Ki_{2,3\text{-}BPG}$ (μM) |
|---|---|---|---|---|---|---|---|
| Normal | 27 | 575 | 67 | 3.7 | 3.1 | 749 | 2289 |
| Deficiency | 2.5 | 10 | 152 | 3.8 | 0.62 | 180 | 520 |

Figure 1. G6PDH-catalyzing reaction and the corresponding parameters. A) A schematic representation of the reaction catalyzed by G6PDH. B) A kinetic equation of G6PDH in human erythrocytes (upper) and the corresponding parameters of the reaction from normal and G6PDH-deficient erythrocytes (lower).

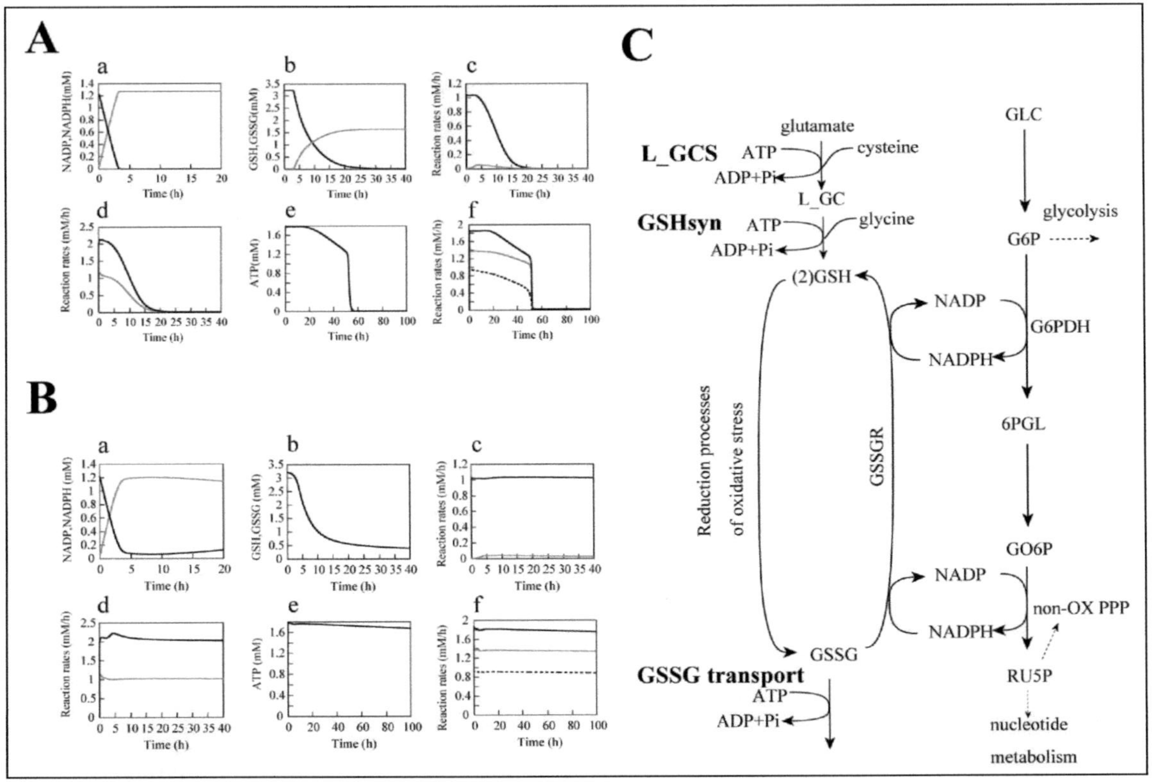


Figure 2. Simulation results of G6PDH deficiency. Simulation results of before (A) and after (B) expansion of the pathway of glutathione metabolism. Each panel shows the time-course in concentration of a) NADPH (black line), NADP (gray line), b) GSH (black line), GSH (gray line), and e) ATP and in reaction rate of c) HK (black line), G6PDH (gray line), d) PK (black line), PFK (gray line), f) GAPDH (black line), PGK (gray line), ALD (black-broken line), respectively. C) Schematic representation of the glutathione metabolism pathway including the de novo synthesis of glutathione catalyzed by L_GCS and GSHsyn and the transport of GSSG.

corresponded to the results by Ferretti et al that G6PDH-deficient cells have normal glycolytic activity and abnormally low activity of the pentose phosphate pathways.[15]

These results suggest that the expanded pathways, which have not so far been considered in modeling, play a significant role not only in keeping the GSH/GSSG ratio but also in retention of glycolytic activity, the ATP level in the G6PDH-deficient erythrocyte. Most patients of G6PDH deficiency are not anemic until the RBCs are exposed to strong oxidant stress. The compensatory effect of the expanded pathways, de novo GSH synthesis and GSSG transport, helps explain why many varieties of G6PDH deficiency have no significant phenotype in normal states. It is also well known that patients of G6PDH deficiency have significant resistance to severe malaria and due to its ability to protect against malaria, high frequency of G6PDH deficiency is shown. Under these circumstances, this study could also suggest that the compensatory mechanism may help the spread of G6PDH deficiency, thus decreasing its severity and promoting the propagation of the disease during evolution.

## Simulation Study for Methemoglobin Reduction Pathways

In circulating erythrocytes, hemoglobin oxidation to metHb continuously occurrs via intracellular and extracellular reactive oxygen species and via exogenous and endogenous nitrites/nitric oxide. The accumulation of intracellular metHb reduces the supply of oxygen to tissues. As the cycling of hemoglobin and metHb causes an associated persistent production of superoxide anions, metHb accumulation potentially results in additional oxidative stress.[19,20] In normal erythrocytes, metHb is maintained at a level of less than 1% of total hemoglobin through two metHb-reducing pathways.[21,22] One of these systems is the redox cycle consisting of cytochrome b5 (cytb5) and cytochrome b5-metHb reductase (b5R), which uses NADH as an electron transfer to cytb5 ("cytb5-NADH system"). The other pathway uses flavin as an electron carrier for the reduction of metHb coupled with NADPH oxidation, catalyzed by NADPH-dependent flavin reductase (FR) ("flavin-NADPH system"). The pathway schemes are shown in Figure 3A.

Cytb5-NADH system is estimated to be responsible for more than 95% of metHb-reducing capacity under experimental conditions.[23-25] In addition, hereditary methemoglobinemia, the condition where the level of metHb is greater than 1% of the total hemoglobin content of the cell,[26] is a congenital deficiency of b5R and/or cytb5.[27] Contrary to this, the contribution of flavin-NADPH system to the reduction of metHb has generally been considered to be negligible, as the deficiency of the flavin-NADPH system is not associated with a metHb-reduction-deficient phenotype.[28] On the other hand, FR is reported to be widely distributed in human tissues, but is most abundant in erythrocytes.[29,30] This appears to be an inefficient distribution pattern, given the potentially minor role of FR in metHb reduction.

NADH is produced by the reaction through GAPDH in glycolysis and is converted to NAD in the last step of glycolysis catalyzed by lactate dehydrogenase (LDH). These reactions are in a state of equilibrium, fully coupled to each other in human erythrocytes and the NADH/NAD ratio is kept very low for driving glycolysis. On the contrary, the ratio of NADPH/NADP is kept high by the metabolic property in the production of NADPH. The excess activity of G6PDH enables a high NADPH concentration and in an accute NADPH supply in response to naturally occurring oxidative challenges.[31,32] It has thus been accepted that NADPH is a main source of intracellular reductive power while NADH is not critical for redox status in the cell.

Under these circumstances, a question arises: what is the physiological role of the flavin-NADPH system and why do erythrocytes primarily use an NADH-dependent reduction process for the reduction of metHb?

To make predictions about the two pathways, in terms of their metHb-reducing behavior, a mathematical model was developed including both the above-mentioned two metHb-reducing systems and the major metabolic pathways (glycolysis, PPP) in human erythrocytes as a supplier of NADH or NADPH. The cytb5-NADH system consists of an enzymatic reduction of

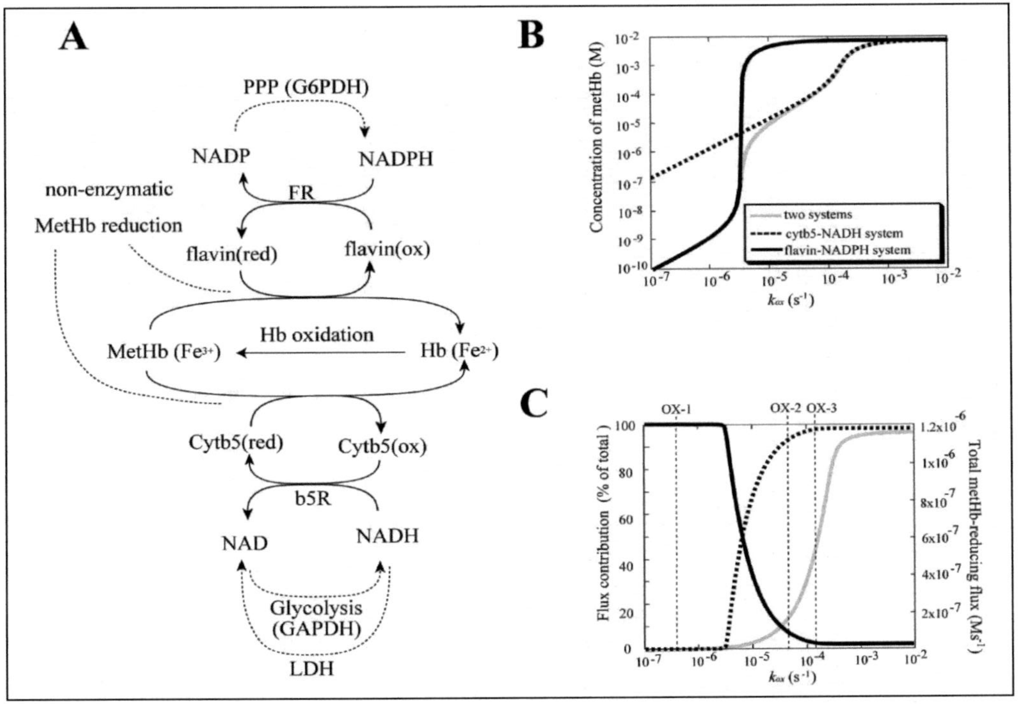


Figure 3. MetHb-reducing pathways included in the model and the simulation results. A) A schematic representation of the metHb-reducing pathways connected with the main metabolic pathways (PPP, glycolysis etc.). B) Steady-state concentrations of metHb with various *kox* predicted by the model with the two metHb-reducing systems (gray solid line), cytb5-NADH only system (black broken line) and flavin-NADPH only system (black solid line), respectively. C) Steady-state flux of metHb reduction and the percentage contribution of each pathway. Percentage contributions to total flux of metHb reduction for the cytb5-NADH pathway and the flavin-NADPH pathway are represented as the black broken and the black solid lines, respectively. The gray solid line represents the total metHb reduction rate with respect to oxidative load. Line OX-1 indicates the hemoglobin oxidation rate where the total metHb-reducing flux equals the reported rate of spontaneous hemoglobin oxidation ($2.78 \times 10^{-9}$ $Ms^{-1}$). Line OX-2 indicates the hemoglobin oxidation rates where the concentration of metHb reaches 1% of total hemoglobin, which is a diagnostic indicator of methemoglobinemia. OX-3 is that of 10%, the point where clinical symptoms are observed.

oxidized cytb5 by b5R using NADH as an electron carrier and the subsequent non-enzymatic reduction of metHb by the reduced cytb5. The kinetic equations used in the model were:

$$v_{b5R} = kcat[b5R]\left(\frac{[NADH^+]}{Km_{NADH^+} + [NADH^+]}\right)\left(\frac{[b5_{OX}]}{Km_{b5} + [b5_{ox}]}\right)$$

$$v_{b5-metHb} = k_1[b5_{red}][metHb] - k_{-1}[b5_{ox}][oxyHb]$$

where the corresponding parameters are: kcat, 418 $s^{-1}$; $Km_{NADH}$, 0.31 μM; $Km_{b5}$, 14.92 μM;[33] [b5R], 0.07 μM;[34] $k_1$, 6.2 × $10^3$ $M^{-1}s^{-1}$; and $k_{-1}$, 0.583 $M^{-1}s^{-1}$.[35] For the flavin-NADPH system, the electron transport from NADPH to oxidized flavin catalyzed by FR obeys an ordered BiBi mechanism.[36] MetHb is then reduced non-enzymatically by the reduced flavin:

$$v_{FR} = \frac{kcat[FR][NADPH][FMN_{ox}]}{\left(\begin{array}{l} Ki_{NADPH}Km_{FMN} + Km_{NADPH}\left(1 + \dfrac{[NADP^+]}{Ki_{NADP^+}}\right)[FMN_{ox}] \\ \qquad + Km_{FMN}[NADPH] + [FMN_{ox}][NADPH] \end{array}\right)}$$

$$v_{flavin-metHb} = k[FMN_{red}][metHb]$$

in which the parameter values used are: kcat, 0.099 $s^{-1}$; KmNADPH, 0.97 μM; $Km_{FMN}$, 52.76 μM; $Ki_{NADPH}$ 0.55 μM; $Ki_{NADP}$, 4.89 μM;[36] [FR], 9.09 μM;[25] and k, 5.5 × $10^6$ $M^{-1}s^{-1}$.[25] Total concentration of cytb5 and flavin was set to 0.812 μM[37] and 1.4 μM,[38] respectively. The hemoglobin oxidation was represented as a first-order reaction with respect to the concentration of oxyhemoglobin:

$$v_{Hbox} = k_{ox}[oxyHb]$$

where *kox* is a rate constant. In this model, the direct metHb-reducing effects by small molecules, such as ascorbic acid and GSH, were not included because the relative contribution of these molecules to the metHb-reducing rate is very small in comparison to those of the two above-mentioned metHb-reducing pathways.[39]

In addition, it was thought that the model should involve central energy metabolism which would account for NADH and NADPH production. The part of the model for glycolysis and PPP was taken from the model developed by Mulquiney and Kuchel.[10,11] The final model includes 87 reaction processes involving all of the binding processes and 63 metabolites involving all of the complex forms. It consists of the metHb-reduction pathways, glycolysis, 2,3-BPG metabolism, PPP and some transport processes of metabolites (e.g., pyruvate, lactate).

The results of the steady-state accumulation of metHb in response to increased hemoglobin oxidation (*kox*), are shown in Figure 3B. Each line represents the results from the model involving the two metHb-reducing systems (black solid line), the cytb5-NADH system alone (broken line) and the flavin-NADPH system alone (gray solid line), respectively. The accumulation of metHb in the flavin-NADPH-only model was significantly lower than that in the cytb5-NADH-only model when the *kox* was below 3.5 × $10^{-6}$ $s^{-1}$; however, when this rate was exceeded, an abrupt increase in metHb occurred in the flavin-NADPH-only model. The accumulation of metHb in the two-system model was similar to the flavin-NADPH-only model under the condition of slow hemoglobin oxidation; however, under conditions of fast hemoglobin oxidation it was similar to the cytb5-NADH-only model. From this result it was suggested that a switch from the flavin-NADPH system to the cytb5-NADH system occurs upon an increase in the oxidation rate of hemoglobin. The switching of the pathways' significance was also shown in the analysis of flux contribution. In Figure 3C, the overall flux of metHb reduction (gray solid line) and the flux contributions of the flavin-NADPH system (black solid line) and the cytb5-NADH system (black broken line) in proportion to total metHb-reducing flux are displayed. When *kox* was below $3.5 \times 10^{-6}\ s^{-1}$, most of the metHb-reducing flux was responsible for the flavin-NADPH system and the concentration of metHb was much lower than 1 μM. When *kox* was over $3.5 \times 10^{-6}\ s^{-1}$, an abrupt switch in flux contribution from the flavin-NADPH system to the cytb5-NADH system occurred.

In the model, under conditions where the cytb5-NADH system was responsible for greater than 95% of metHb reduction, the flux through the cytb5-NADH system (NADH consuming process) could potentially reach almost $1.2 \times 10^{-6}\ Ms^{-1}$, which is much higher than the rate reported for nonglycolytic NADH consumption in human erythrocytes which is reported to be approximately $2.78 \times 10^{-9}\ Ms^{-1}$.[40] Furthermore, the rate of constitutive methemoglobin formation in normal erythrocytes is reported to be 3% of the total amount of hemoglobin in the cell per day,[41] equal to $2.78 \times 10^{-9}\ Ms^{-1}$ of a spontaneous rate of hemoglobin oxidation. This rate is significantly lower than $3.5 \times 10^{-6}\ s^{-1}$, where the flavin-NADPH system exceeds its flux capacity. Under such low levels of oxidative stress, the flavin-NADPH system would be responsible for most of the metHb reduction, because the rate constant of the non-enzymatic system which directly reduces metHb is 1000-fold higher than in the cytb5-NADH system. From these results, it is suggested that either the two systems are active under distinct conditions of hemoglobin oxidation and make different contributions to the tolerance of oxidative stress: The flavin-NADPH system works mainly to provide reduction potential under normal conditions, while the cytb5-NADH system functions to reduce metHb under conditions of excess oxidation, such as during the intake of oxidant drugs. In addition, it is speculated that the oxidative rate under physiological conditions is estimated to be much lower than that of experimental and abnormal conditions. One reason why the contribution of flavin-NADPH system has not been uncovered may be because of difficulties in measuring the trace levels of oxidation occurring normally in vivo, whereas it is much easier to observe conditions of excess oxidative stress in which the cytb5-NADH system may play a major role.

NADPH is supplied from the pentose-phosphate pathway and the primary use of NADPH in erythrocytes is reducing GSSG into GSH catalyzed by GSSGR. It is known that the high enzyme activities of G6PDH and GSSGR in human erythrocyte are evolutionarily maintained because they are necessary to avoid strong NADPH depletion and GSSG accumulation under oxidative stress.[31,32] One possible explanation for the use of NADH as a major source of reducing equivalents for metHb in abnormal oxidative stress may be to avoid competition for NADPH among glutathione and hemoglobin. Interestingly, the expression levels of soluble cytb5 and soluble b5R are significantly increased just prior to loss of the nucleus at the late stage of erythroid maturation.[42] Moreover, in nucleated erythrocytes containing TCA cycles (e.g., avian erythrocytes), the NADPH-dependent pathway has a dominant role in reducing metHb, even under conditions of excess oxidation of hemoglobin.[43] It can be speculated that the preference of nucleated erythrocytes for the flavin-NADPH system is related to the lower availability of NADH-coupled reducing equivalents in the cytoplasm, which would result from their preferential transfer to mitochondria for the respiratory chain and/or for high malate dehydrogenase activity, resulting in a large flux of NADPH regeneration.

In the simulation model, the increased demand for NADH was met by the reverse reaction of lactate dehydrogenase (LDH), rather than by the increased glycolytic flux (Fig. 4). In other words, the vast amount of NADH is supplied by the lactate/pyruvate shuttle: a combination of the reverse reaction of LDH and the lactate/pyruvate transport process. It can thus be supposed that NADH production via reverse flux of LDH results in an increase in intracellular pyruvate concentration, which could then be released into the plasma. In fact, it has been reported that excess oxidative stress causes an accumulation of pyruvate in plasma, due to its release from erythrocytes coupling with the increase in metHb.[44,45] It has been reported that, in some tissues including neurons, plasma pyruvate is rapidly transported from plasma into the tissue under excess oxidative stress caused by $H_2O_2$.[46,47] Furthermore, it has been recently suggested that the lactate/pyruvate shuttle in astrocytes plays an important role in preventing oxidative injury in neurons by supplying pyruvate from plasma.[48] These circumstances allow us to hypothesize that plasma pyruvate is partially supplied by erythrocytes via the reduction of metHb under high oxidative stress and these synergistic effects

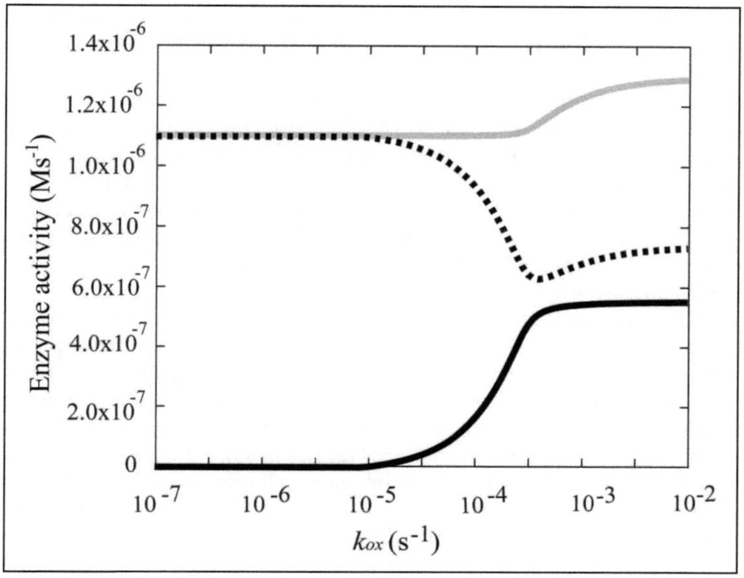


Figure 4. Steady state enzyme activities that utilize NAD/NADH Steady state activities of b5R (solid line in black), LDH (dotted line) and GAPDH (solid line in gray) are plotted as a function of $k_{ox}$.

may be another story of the benefit to the existence and the oxidation level-dependent switching of this "hybrid system:flavin-NADPH and cytb5-NADH systems".

## Prediction by Mathematical Modeling and Its Verification by Metabolome Analysis for Oxygen Sensing Mechanism in Human Erythrocytes

In human erythrocytes, an extremely high concentration of Hb exists in the cell that enables oxygen ($O_2$) delivery from the lungs to every tissue through the blood stream. The ability of Hb to carry $O_2$ is modulated through allosteric regulation of Hb affected by a variety of metabolites, such as protons ($H^+$), 2,3-BPG, nitric oxide (NO) and ATP. The behavior of the metabolism in erythrocytes is thus directly and highly related to the ability to deliver oxygen. Erythrocytes are known to accelerate glucose consumption in response to hypoxic exposure, which results from acceleration of glycolysis.[49] As the increase in 2,3-BPG stabilizes the T-state of Hb and thereby facilitates $O_2$ dissociation from the cells, the increment of 2,3-BPG should lead to a further T-state Hb stabilization. Furthermore, as T-state Hb has a higher affinity to 2,3-BPG and ATP than the R-state Hb, stabilization of hemoglobin into T-state would reduce amounts of free 2,3-BPG and ATP. A decrease in free ATP reduces the availability of maintenance of cellular homeostasis and deformability of the cells. From the fact that the initial steps of glycolysis (e.g., used by hexokinase (HK) and phosphofructokinase (PFK)) require ATP in triggering ATP synthesis itself, researchers have hypothesized that erythrocytes might have suitable mechanisms for responding quickly to hypoxia to up-regulate de novo ATP synthesis and glycolytic flux, leading to the increase in 2,3-BPG.

Meanwhile, evidence of compensatory mechanisms to maintain intracellular ATP levels through the interaction of Hb with Band III (BIII), a major transmembrane protein in erythrocytes,[50] has been reported. The cytoplasmic domain of BIII binds to Hb with a greater affinity for T-state-Hb rather than R-state-Hb[51] and also binds to some glycolytic enzymes such as PFK, aldolase (ALD) and GAPDH.[52] The activity of these enzymes disappears while making complex with BIII, but is recovered upon dissociation from BIII.[52] This evidence led us to hypothesize that Hb stabilized in the T-state upon hypoxia serves as a trigger to increase the activity of these glycolytic enzymes and to accelerate glucose consumption to increase the synthesis of ATP and 2,3-BPG. However, the dynamics of sequential glycolytic reactions based on the mechanistic features of the coordination and the alterations in intracellular metabolites resulting from such dynamics are not comprehensively understood. Moreover, the link between the metabolism and the Hb regulation is not fully understood, nor does mathematical model taking them into consideration simultaneously exist. Here, we further expanded the mathematical model of metabolism in erythrocytes, involving the $O_2$-sensing mechanisms of Hb, to predict temporal alterations in intracellular metabolites and cellular energetics in response to hypoxia and to verify the predictions derived from the model through metabolome analyses.

The reversible binding of the glycolytic enzymes (PFK, ALD and GAPDH) and two allosteric forms of Hb (R- and T-states) to BIII on the membrane, also known as anion exchanger Type I, were modeled on the basis of the individual association constants[14] by adding the basal metabolic model.

The metabolic model covers comprehensive metabolic pathways including not only glycolysis, but also pentose phosphate pathways, adenine nucleotide metabolism, membrane transport of metabolites, the ion pump, the above-mentioned GSH metabolism since the pathways determine levels of such as GSH, AMP and Pi, which are known allosteric regulators of HK, PFK and GAPDH, respectively. In the model we also considered effects of Hbs (T-state Hb and R-state Hb) binding to intracellular metabolites (2,3-BPG, MgATP, ATP, ADP and 1,3-BPG) and magnesium ion ($Mg^{2+}$) binding to ATP, ADP, AMP, 1,3-BPG, 2,3-BPG, F-1,6BP and GDP. BIII accounts for about 25% of the total erythrocyte membrane protein and its cytoplasmic domain displays a greater affinity for Hb in the T-state rather than the R-state:[51] T-state Hb has 100-fold greater affinity to BIII and is much more likely to associate with this anion transporter than R-state Hb. Based on the recent observations,[52] these three enzymes were modeled to be inactivated upon formation of the complex and activated reversibly upon dissociation in the model. Consequently, the competitive association of Hb and the glycolytic enzymes with BIII and the subsequent changes in glycolysis could be calculated in response to alterations in partial $O_2$ tension ($pO_2$). In this mathematical model, we can then manipulate $pO_2$ as a parameter to predict glycolytic metabolism as an outcome. The oxygenation status alters the T-R transition of Hb according to a reversible Hill-type equation[53] that is also dictated by $pCO_2$, intracellular pH, concentrations of 2,3-BPG and ATP and temperature. To adapt the model to hypoxic conditions, $pO_2$, which was initially set to 100 mm Hg, was reduced to 30 mm Hg, for desired lengths of time. As seen in previous studies, circulating erythrocytes may be exposed to such a $pO_2$ value when they travel through capillaries under physiological conditions or when they traverse low-flow or static microvessels belonging to post-ischemic damaged regions in the liver.[54,55]

The simulation results of hypoxia-induced metabolic alterations in human erythrocytes and the measurement result of metabolomics under a similar condition to the simulation are shown in **Fig**ure 5A (see 14 for the details of experimental procedure). The differences in time-courses between the BIII(+) model, involving interactions between BIII and the intracellular proteins (Hb and the glycolytic enzymes) and the BIII(−) model, without these interactions, were predicted (Fig. 5A, left two lines). As expected, in the BIII(+) model, the activities of PFK, ALD and GAPDH were evaluated immediately by their release from BIII upon alteration of Hb allostery, while they did not change significantly in the BIII(−) model. Such effects of protein-interactions with BIII made distinct profiles in metabolite concentrations and the subsequent enzyme activities. In the BIII(−)model, G6P and F6P increased slightly while F1,6BP, DHAP, 3PG and PEP decreased modestly versus the steady-state baseline levels. In contrast, an opposite pattern to the BIII(−) model was displayed in the BIII(+) model: decreases in G6P and F6P by 50% and increases in F1,6BP, DHAP, 3PG and PEP by 40% versus the corresponding baseline levels (Fig. 2B) were shown. The decrease in G6P in the BIII(+) model resulted in further activation compared to the BIII(−) model through a product inhibition for HK by G6P. This would lead to help accelerate the first step of glycolysis. Moreover, hypoxia-triggered activation of GAPDH

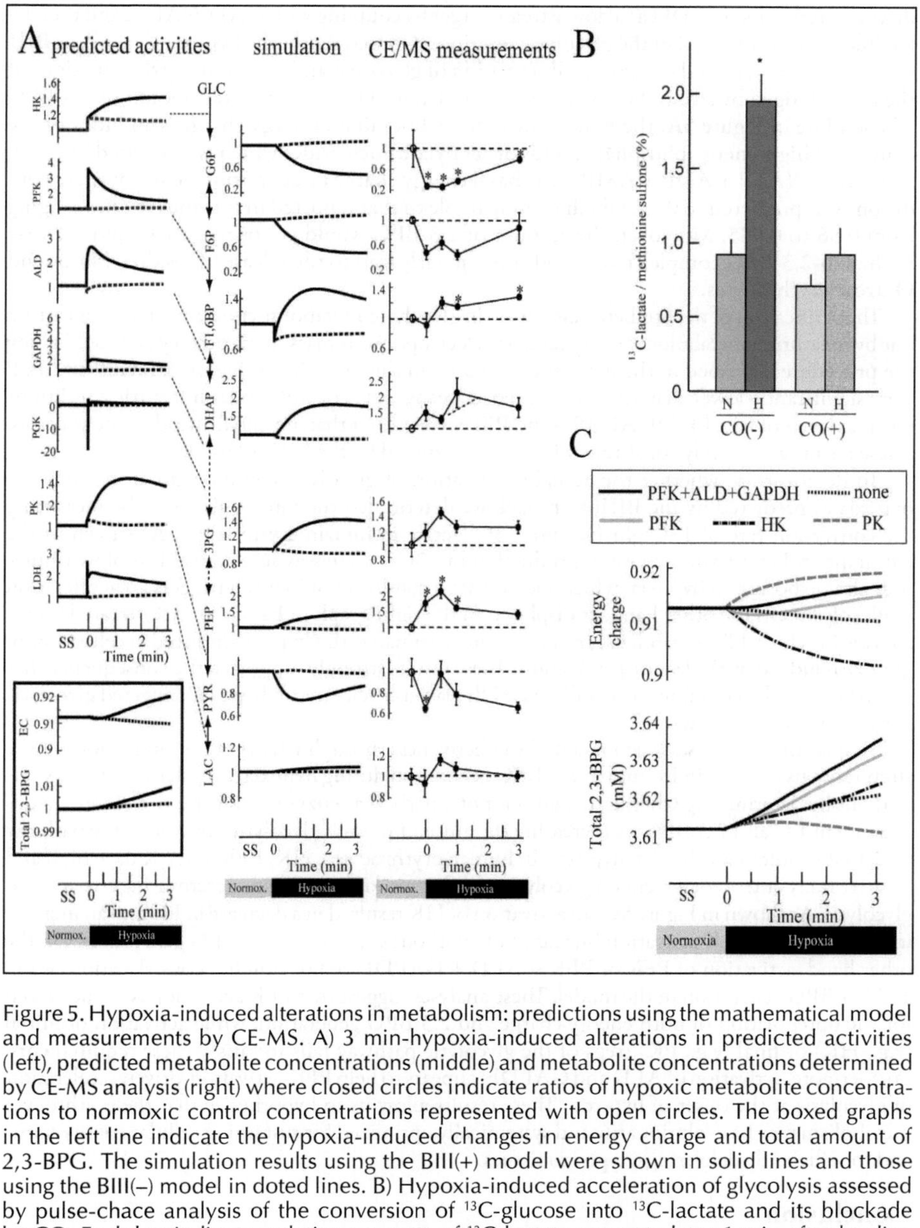


Figure 5. Hypoxia-induced alterations in metabolism: predictions using the mathematical model and measurements by CE-MS. A) 3 min-hypoxia-induced alterations in predicted activities (left), predicted metabolite concentrations (middle) and metabolite concentrations determined by CE-MS analysis (right) where closed circles indicate ratios of hypoxic metabolite concentrations to normoxic control concentrations represented with open circles. The boxed graphs in the left line indicate the hypoxia-induced changes in energy charge and total amount of 2,3-BPG. The simulation results using the BIII(+) model were shown in solid lines and those using the BIII(–) model in doted lines. B) Hypoxia-induced acceleration of glycolysis assessed by pulse-chace analysis of the conversion of $^{13}$C-glucose into $^{13}$C-lactate and its blockade by CO. Each bar indicates relative amounts of $^{13}$C-lactate converted per 1 min after loading with $^{13}$C-glucose at 5mM under normoxic (N) and hypoxic (H) conditions. CO(–) and CO(+) indicate erythrocytes pretreated without and with CO, respectively. C) Prediction of beneficial effects of enzyme-BIII interaction in changes in energy charge (upper graph) and total amount of 2,3-BPG (lower graph). Each line indicates the results under different hypoxic conditions when the amounts of the following enzymes were increased by 2-fold, PFK, HK, PK and their combinations, in corresponding line types shown in the upper box. Experimental values are the mean ± S.E. (n = 4). Asterisks, $p < 0.05$ versus the base-line values.

drives an activation of LDH as a downstream target by coupling with NAD-NADH and thereby facilitates the second half of the glycolytic reactions. Consequently, the hypoxia-dependent BIII interactions contributed to the overall activation of glycolysis and to sustaining the functions of the cell as judged by two indicators: the energy charge (EC) and the total amount of 2,3-BPG (the left line in Figure 5A, the figures enclosed by bold line). Energy charge is an index of the content of high-energy phosphate bonds of adenylate nucleotides which is calculated by (ATP + 0.5ADP)/(ATP + ADP + AMP). The basal energy charge under normoxic steady-state conditions was predicted to 0.91, which is comparable to that reported in previous studies ranging from 0.86 to 0.935. Moreover, the amount of 2,3-BPG would contribute to a rapid increase in the Hb-2,3-BPG complex that could consequently lead to the release of residual Hb-bound $O_2$ from erythrocytes.

The verification of the predicted alteration in glycolytic-metabolite concentrations was carried out by measuring metabolome using capillary electrophoresis mass spectrometry (CE-MS) along the procedure described in the literature.[14] As seen in the right line in Figure 5A, G6P and F6P were significantly lower than those measured as steady-state controls under normoxic conditions whereas levels of F1,6BP, DHAP, 3PG and PEP were greater than normoxic steady-state controls. These results are entirely consistent with those predicted by the BIII(+) model.

To demonstrate whether the actual acceleration of glycolysis could occurr in response to hypoxia as predicted by the BIII(+) model, we determined the rate of glycolysis by measuring the conversion rate of 13C-glucose into 13C-lactate in human erythrocytes. As shown in the left graph in Figure 5B, the rate of production of 13C-lactate was accelerated 1.8-fold within 1 min after exposure to hypoxia, which means that a condition of hypoxia triggers an acceleration of glycolysis. On the other hand, as displayed in the right graph in Figure 5B, CO-treated erythrocytes in which Hb is stabilized in the R-state attenuated the hypoxia-induced acceleration of glycolysis judged by the lactate production. These results strongly supported the consequence that the hypoxia-induced stabilization of T-state Hb plays a crucial role in hypoxia-triggered glycolytic activation in erythrocytes.

To quantitatively assess such metabolic effectiveness through BIII-protein interactions of the simultaneous increase in EC and in 2,3-BPG generation during hypoxia, a model analysis was carried out by determining whether the amount of a particular enzyme can achieve a simultaneous increase in EC and 2,3-BPG by increasing the amount of each glycolytic enzyme in the pathway by 2-fold simultaneously with hypoxia. In human erythrocytes, HK, PFK and PK have high and positive flux control coefficient on glycolysis and they are known as "rate-determining enzymes" in glycolysis. As shown in Figure 5C, an activation of HK resulted in a decrease in EC and an increase in 2,3-BPG, while PK activation increased EC without stimulating 2,3-BPG generation. On the other hand, activation of PFK or PFK + ALD + GAPDH led to simultaneous elevation of EC and 2,3-BPG generation in the model. These analyses suggest that PFK activation is a crucial step for the upregulation of both energy charge and 2,3-BPG generation, while activation of initial (e.g., HK) or final (e.g., PK) steps of the glycolytic pathway fails to satisfy these requirements. Furthermore, activation of ALD and GAPDH appears to help PFK-activation-driven acceleration of glycolysis at the onset of hypoxia. These results allow us to hypothesize that the erythrocyte metabolism may be evolutionarily and systemically optimized for sustaining cellular energy status and for efficiently delivering oxygen to tissues.

## Conclusion

In the previous sections, practical examples of using mathematical models focusing on human erythrocyte metabolism on E-Cell System were presented.

In *Simulation Analysis of Glucose-6-Phosphate Dehydrogenase (G6PDH) Deficiency*, an expansion was added to the model by introducing a GSH synthesis pathway and a GSSG export system. With this expansion, the model maintained high ATP concentrations even in the simulated condition of G6PDH deficiency. This suggests that these pathways may play an important role in alleviating the consequences of G6PDH deficiency and that these sub-pathways that are normally not particularly highly activated may play important roles in abnormal conditions. Models sufficient for representing the normal state can become inadequate for simulating irregular conditions such as deficiencies, because they lack alternative pathways that may normally not be particularly active but can compensate for the deficiency to some extent. This study also suggested that resolving the discrepancies between experimentally validated knowledge and the simulation results allows us to improve our understanding of the underlying mechanisms making fragility of the cells under particular conditions.

The next section discussed the rational design of metHb-reducing pathways in human erythrocytes with kinetic modeling. Erythrocytes are continuously subjected to oxidative stress and exposure to nitrite, which results in spontaneous formation of metHb, which is an oxidized form of hemoglobin preventing binding and carrying oxygen. To avoid accumulation of metHb, reductive pathways mediated by two substrates coupled with NADH- and NADPH-dependent metHb reductases keep the level of metHb in erythrocytes at less than 1% of the total hemoglobin under normal conditions. The results of simulation experiments suggest that NADH- and NADPH-dependent methemoglobin-reducing pathways have different but important roles: one has a high-elasticity, small-capacity reducing flux while the other has a low elasticity, high-capacity flux. This section also showed the necessity and effectiveness of using mathematical models to predict when and how the particular pathways work as a system in the various physiological conditions where experimental verification is difficult.

In *Prediction by Mathematical Modeling and its Verification by Metabolome Analysis for Oxygen Sensing Mechanism in Human Erythrocytes*, the example for the intercommunication between the simulation and the experiment was shown. Temporal alterations in metabolites predicted in the mathematical model, including the effects of BIII interactions with Hb and the glycolytic enzymes, are in good agreement with results obtained from the metabolome analyses using CE-MS, which has recently emerged as a powerful tool for the global analysis of charged metabolites.[56] In contrast, the virtual model lacking the effects of the Hb-BIII interaction was unable to reproduce actual alterations in the metabolites, suggesting a pivotal role for this molecular interaction in the maintenance of erythrocyte energetics. Furthermore, a coordinated increase in the energy charge and 2,3-BPG was predicted when the mid-way glycolytic enzymes, but not up- or down-stream rate-limiting enzymes, are activated in response to the hypoxia-induced Hb binding to BIII. Furthermore, the hypoxia-induced activation of glycolysis was not observed when Hb was stabilized in R-state by treating the cells with CO. Under these circumstances, it can be suggested that Hb allostery in erythrocytes serves as an oxygen-sensing trigger that drives glycolytic acceleration to sustain intracellular energetics and to promote the ability to release oxygen from the cells through the rational design of metabolism.

The above simulation studies enabled us to see the rational design of metabolic pathways in human erythrocytes as an evolutionarily optimized system. Mathematical models can be applied not only for straightforward simulations, but also for explanations of the nature of network properties complying nonlinear dynamics in the cell.

On the other hand, the models do not include certain aspects of red blood cell metabolism, such as the oxidation of membrane proteins which are rapidly oxidized during elimination of $H_2O_2$, the direct inhibition of G6PDH by reactive oxygen species. Furthermore, many physical viewpoints have not yet been considered: the maintenance of cellular status through regulating intracellular pH, membrane potential, cell volume in connection with ion balances and cell shapes. They may be significant for considering the in vivo state of the cell.[57] Another limitation of the current models is the lack of spatial information and diffusion processes. Because erythrocytes do not contain any cell organelle in cytoplasm, the intracellular system has been assumed as homogeneous in space. However, recent observations showed that glycolytic enzymes form a macromolecular complex and the complex changes its localization in response to oxygen availability,[52] suggesting the importance of considering the spatial effect even when the model focuses on the metabolic reactions. E-Cell System will be a suitable platform for considering these features in more precise modeling.

## *Acknowledgments*

I sincerely acknowledge my gratitude to Prof. Makoto Suematsu at the school of medicine of Keio University and to Prof. Tomoyoshi Soga for critical discussions and providing new perspectives, especially for the interrelation between experimental and simulation studies. The works in this chapter were carried out in association with Yoichi Nakayama (section 2 and 3), Tomoya Kitayama (section 3), Dr. Kosuke Tsukada (section 4) and Dr. Takako Hishiki (section 4). These works were supported by grants from the Japan Society for the Promotion of Science (JSPS), supported in part by the Ministry of Education, Culture, Sports, Science and Technology, with a Grant-in-Aid for the 21st Century Center of Excellence (COE) Program entitled "Understanding and Control of Life's Function via Systems Biology (Keio University)" and by Core Research for Evolutional Science and Technology (CREST) of Japan Science and Technology Agency (JST).


## References


1. Rapoport TA, Otto M, Heinrich R. An extended model of the glycolysis in erythrocytes. Acta Biol Med Ger 1997; 36:461-8.
2. Heinrich R, Rapoport SM, Rapoport TA. Metabolic regulation and mathematical models. Prog Biophys Mol Biol 1977; 32:1-82.
3. Rapoport TA, Heinrich R, Rapoport SM. The regulatory principles of glycolysis in erythrocytes in vivo and in vitro. A minimal comprehensive model describing steady states, quasi-steady states and time-dependent processes. Biochem J 1976; 154:449-69.
4. Ataullakhanov FI, Vitvitsky VM, Zhabotinsky AM et al. The regulation of glycolysis in human erythrocytes. The dependence of the glycolytic flux on the ATP concentration. Eur J Biochem 1981; 115:359-65.
5. Schauer M, Heinrich R, Rapoport SM. [Mathematical modelling of glycolysis and adenine nucleotide metabolism of human erythrocytes. I. Reaction-kinetic statements, analysis of in vivo state and determination of starting conditions for in vitro experiments]. Acta Biol Med Ger 1981; 40:1659-82.
6. Joshi A, Palsson BO. Metabolic dynamics in the human red cell. Part I--A comprehensive kinetic model. J Theor Biol 1989; 141:515-28.
7. Joshi A, Palsson BO. Metabolic dynamics in the human red cell. Part II--Interactions with the environment. J Theor Biol 1989; 141:529-45.
8. Joshi A, Palsson BO. Metabolic dynamics in the human red cell. Part III--Metabolic reaction rates. J Theor Biol 1990; 142:41-68.
9. Joshi A, Palsson BO. Metabolic dynamics in the human red cell. Part IV--Data prediction and some model computations. J Theor Biol 1990; 142:69-85.
10. Mulquiney PJ, Bubb WA, Kuchel PW. Model of 2,3-bisphosphoglycerate metabolism in the human erythrocyte based on detailed enzyme kinetic equations: in vivo kinetic characterization of 2,3-bisphosphoglycerate synthase/phosphatase using 13C and 31P NMR. Biochem J 1999; 342 Pt 3: 567-80.
11. Mulquiney PJ, Kuchel PW. Model of 2,3-bisphosphoglycerate metabolism in the human erythrocyte based on detailed enzyme kinetic equations: equations and parameter refinement. Biochem J 1999; 342 Pt 3:581-96.
12. Nakayama Y, Kinoshita A, Tomita M. Dynamic simulation of red blood cell metabolism and its application to the analysis of a pathological condition. Theor Biol Med Model 2005; 2:18.
13. Kinoshita A, Nakayama Y, Kitayama T et al. Simulation study of methemoglobin reduction in erythrocytes. Differential contributions of two pathways to tolerance to oxidative stress. Febs J 2007; 274:1449-58.
14. Kinoshita A, Tsukada K, Soga T et al. Roles of hemoglobin Allostery in hypoxia-induced metabolic alterations in erythrocytes: simulation and its verification by metabolome analysis. J Biol Chem 2007; 282:10731-41.
15. Ferretti A, Bozzi A, Di Vito M et al. 13C and 31P NMR studies of glucose and 2-deoxyglucose metabolism in normal and enzyme-deficient human erythrocytes. Clin Chim Acta 1992; 208:39-61.
16. Meister A. Glutathione, metabolism and function via the gamma-glutamyl cycle. Life Sci 1974; 15:177-90.
17. Srivastava SK, Beutler E. The transport of oxidized glutathione from human erythrocytes. J Biol Chem 1969; 244:9-16.
18. Kondo T, Beutler E. Developmental changes in glucose transport of guinea pig erythrocytes. J Clin Invest 1980; 65:1-4.
19. Hebbel RP. Erythrocyte antioxidants and membrane vulnerability. J Lab Clin Med 1986; 107:401-4.
20. Rice-Evans C, Omorphos SC, Baysal E. Sickle cell membranes and oxidative damage. Biochem J 1986; 237:265-9.
21. Jaffe ER. Methaemoglobinaemia. Clin Haematol 1981; 10:99-122.
22. Mansouri A, Lurie AA. Concise review: methemoglobinemia. Am J Hematol 1993; 42:7-12.

23. Yubisui T, Takeshita M. Purification and properties of soluble NADH-cytochrome b5 reductase of rabbit erythrocytes. J Biochem (Tokyo) 1982; 91:1467-77.
24. Yubisui T, Murakami K, Shirabe K et al. Structural analysis of NADH-cytochrome b5 reductase in relation to hereditary methemoglobinemia. Prog Clin Biol Res 1989; 319:107-19; discussion 120-1.
25. Yubisui T, Takeshita M, Yoneyama Y. Reduction of methemoglobin through flavin at the physiological concentration by NADPH-flavin reductase of human erythrocytes. J Biochem (Tokyo) 1980; 87:1715-20.
26. Hultquist DE, Passon PG. Catalysis of methaemoglobin reduction by erythrocyte cytochrome B5 and cytochrome B5 reductase. Nat New Biol 1971; 229:252-4.
27. Wang Y, Wu YS, Zheng PZ et al. A novel mutation in the NADH-cytochrome b5 reductase gene of a Chinese patient with recessive congenital methemoglobinemia. Blood 2000; 95:3250-5.
28. Yubisui T, Matsuki T, Takeshita M et al. Characterization of the purified NADPH-flavin reductase of human erythrocytes. J Biochem (Tokyo) 1979; 85:719-28.
29. Quandt KS, Hultquist DE. Flavin reductase: sequence of cDNA from bovine liver and tissue distribution. Proc Natl Acad Sci U S A 1994; 91:9322-6.
30. Zhu H, Qiu H, Yoon HW et al. Identification of a cytochrome b-type NAD(P)H oxidoreductase ubiquitously expressed in human cells. Proc Natl Acad Sci U S A 1999; 96:14742-7.
31. Salvador A, Savageau MA. Quantitative evolutionary design of glucose 6-phosphate dehydrogenase expression in human erythrocytes. Proc Natl Acad Sci U S A 2003; 100:14463-8.
32. Salvador A, Savageau MA. Evolution of enzymes in a series is driven by dissimilar functional demands. Proc Natl Acad Sci U S A 2006; 103:2226-31.
33. Higasa K, Manabe JI, Yubisui T et al. Molecular basis of hereditary methaemoglobinaemia, types I and II: two novel mutations in the NADH-cytochrome b5 reductase gene. Br J Haematol 1998; 103:922-30.
34. Kuma F. Properties of methemoglobin reductase and kinetic study of methemoglobin reduction. J Biol Chem 1981; 256:5518-23.
35. Abe K, Sugita Y. Properties of cytochrome b5 and methemoglobin reduction in human erythrocytes. Eur J Biochem 1979; 101:423-8.
36. Cunningham O, Gore MG, Mantle TJ. Initial-rate kinetics of the flavin reductase reaction catalysed by human biliverdin-IXbeta reductase (BVR-B). Biochem J 2000; 345 Pt 2:393-9.
37. Kuma F, Inomata H. Studies on methemoglobin reductase. II. The purification and molecular properties of reduced nicotinamide adenine dinucleotide-dependent methemoglobin reductase. J Biol Chem 1972; 247:556-60.
38. Yubisui T, Matsukawa S, Yoneyama Y. Stopped flow studies on the nonenzymatic reduction of methemoglobin by reduced flavin mononucleotide. J Biol Chem 1980; 255:11694-7.
39. Curry S. Methemoglobinemia. Ann Emerg Med 1982; 11:214-21.
40. Grimes A. Human Red Cell Metabolism. In: Blackwell Scientific Publications, Oxford: 1980.
41. Nagababu E, Rifkind JM. Reaction of hydrogen peroxide with ferrylhemoglobin: superoxide production and heme degradation. Biochemistry 2000; 39:12503-11.
42. Bulbarelli A, Valentini A, DeSilvestris M et al. An erythroid-specific transcript generates the soluble form of NADH-cytochrome b5 reductase in humans. Blood 1998; 92:310-9.
43. Board PG, Agar NS, Gruca M et al. Methaemoglobin and its reduction in nucleated erythrocytes from reptiles and birds. Comp Biochem Physiol B 1977; 57:265-7.
44. Sullivan SG, Stern A. Glucose metabolism of oxidatively stressed human red blood cells incubated in plasma or medium containing physiologic concentrations of lactate, pyruvate and ascorbate. Biochem Pharmacol 1984; 33:1417-21.
45. Zerez CR, Lachant NA, Tanaka KR. Impaired erythrocyte methemoglobin reduction in sickle cell disease: dependence of methemoglobin reduction on reduced nicotinamide adenine dinucleotide content. Blood 1990; 76:1008-14.
46. Desagher S, Glowinski J, Premont J. Pyruvate protects neurons against hydrogen peroxide-induced toxicity. J Neurosci 1997; 17:9060-7.
47. Lee YJ, Kang IJ, Bunger R et al. Enhanced survival effect of pyruvate correlates MAPK and NF-kappaB activation in hydrogen peroxide-treated human endothelial cells. J Appl Physiol 2004; 96:793-801; discussion 792.
48. Cerdan S, Rodrigues TB, Sierra A, Benito M et al. The redox switch/redox coupling hypothesis. Neurochem Int 2006; 48:523-30.
49. Murphy JR. Erythrocyte metabolism. II. Glucose metabolism and pathways. J Lab Clin Med 1960; 55:286-302.
50. Ellsworth ML, Forrester T, Ellis CG et al. The erythrocyte as a regulator of vascular tone. Am J Physiol 1995; 269:H2155-61.
51. Tsuneshige A, Imai K, Tyuma I. The binding of hemoglobin to red cell membrane lowers its oxygen affinity. J Biochem (Tokyo) 1987; 101:695-704.

52. Campanella ME, Chu H, Low PS. Assembly and regulation of a glycolytic enzyme complex on the human erythrocyte membrane. Proc Natl Acad Sci U S A 2005; 102:2402-7.
53. Dash RK, Bassingthwaighte JB. Blood HbO2 and HbCO2 dissociation curves at varied O2, CO2, pH, 2,3-DPG and temperature levels. Ann Biomed Eng 2004; 32:1676-93.
54. Suganuma K, Tsukada K, Kashiba M et al. Erythrocytes with T-state-stabilized hemoglobin as a therapeutic tool for postischemic liver dysfunction. Antioxid Redox Signal 2006; 8:1847-55.
55. Tsai AG, Johnson PC, Intaglietta M. Oxygen gradients in the microcirculation. Physiol Rev 2003; 83:933-63.
56. Soga T, Baran R, Suematsu M et al. Differential metabolomics reveals ophthalmic acid as an oxidative stress biomarker indicating hepatic glutathione consumption. J Biol Chem 2006; 281:16768-76.
57. Kuchel PW. Current status and challenges in connecting models of erythrocyte metabolism to experimental reality. Prog Biophys Mol Biol 2004; 85:325-42.

# Chapter 8

# Dynamic Kinetic Modeling of Mitochondrial Energy Metabolism

**Katsuyuki Yugi***

## Abstract

Computer simulations can be used to predict the dynamic behaviour of metabolic pathways and to provide evidence in support of clinical treatments for metabolic disorders. Here, we performed dynamic kinetic simulations of mitochondrial energy metabolism using the E-Cell Simulation Environment. The simulation model was developed as a reconstruction of publicly available kinetic studies on the enzymes of the respiratory chain, the TCA cycle, fatty acid β-oxidation and the inner-membrane metabolite transporters.[1] Rate equations for the 58 enzymatic reactions and 286 of the 471 kinetic parameters were taken from 36 and 45 articles, respectively. Approximately 80% of the articles that contributed to the kinetic properties of the mitochondrial model have "kinetics" and the enzyme name as their MeSH terms. The published data were mainly obtained from various tissues in five mammals (human, bovine, pig, rabbit and rat). The other kinetic parameters were estimated numerically using a genetic algorithm module of E-Cell to satisfy the Lineweaver-Burk plot of each enzyme. The simulations indicated that increasing coenzyme Q and succinate promotes the total activity of the respiratory chain without affecting other pathways. This result agrees qualitatively with a clinical case report of treatment with coenzyme Q and succinate.[2] In another case, oxoglutarate supplementation also activated the respiratory chain, but mainly through activation by Complex I. This contrasts with the electron donation through the succinate dehydrogenase complex in the case of coenzyme Q + succinate. These results support the utility of the mitochondrial metabolism model in elucidating action mechanism of clinical treatments.

## Background

Computer simulations of metabolic pathways have been employed as a method to predict the dynamic behaviour of metabolic pathways since the 1960s and have recently been revisited in the context of systems biology. In their pioneering work, Chance et al calculated the time evolution of carbon metabolism in ascites tumour cells from numerical integration of 22 rate equations.[3] While Chance et al employed the law of mass action to approximate the reactions, later metabolic pathway simulations have often been based on kinetic studies on each enzyme. These attempts resulted in simulations on the whole-cell scale, such as the human red blood cell model by Joshi and Palsson.[4]

Mitochondrial energy metabolism has also been simulated, with a focus on its central role in eukaryotic energy metabolism and the pathology of mitochondrial dysfunction. For example, the respiratory chain was modelled by Korzeniewski and Froncisz[5] to analyze the

*Katsuyuki Yugi—Department of Biophysics and Biochemistry, University of Tokyo, Tokyo, Japan. Email: yugi@bio.keio.ac.jp

*E-Cell System: Basic Concepts and Applications*, edited by Satya Nanda Vel Arjunan, Pawan K. Dhar and Masaru Tomita. 

control of ATP production. Another example, the TCA cycle of *Dictyostelium discoideum*, was simulated and analyzed in terms of metabolic control analysis.[6] However, these previous mitochondrial models simulated groups of pathways one by one, rather than several pathways cooperating in the organelle. We constructed a mitochondrial model that includes the respiratory chain, the TCA cycle, fatty acid β-oxidation and the metabolite transport system at the inner-membrane.[1] All the rate equations of the model were obtained from published enzyme kinetics. The model is capable of calculating the time evolution of mitochondrial energy metabolism on a whole-organelle scale. Here we have applied this model in two simulation experiments.

## Construction of the Model

Our mitochondrial model includes 58 enzymatic reactions and 117 metabolites to represent the respiratory chain, the TCA cycle, fatty acid β-oxidation and the inner-membrane metabolite transporters. The inner-membrane metabolite transporters were included to allow simulation of metabolite administration from outside the mitochondrion (Fig. 1). The TCA cycle and the fatty acid β-oxidation process the metabolites transported by the membrane carriers and provide NADH for the respiratory chain.

Kinetic properties of the enzymes, such as Km values and reaction mechanisms, were collected through comprehensive searches of literature databases and enzyme databases such as PubMed (in http://www.ncbi.nlm.nih.gov) and BRENDA (http://www.brenda-enzymes.info). Rate equations for all 58 of the reactions were obtained from 36 articles. Of the 471 total kinetic parameters, 286 were obtained from 45 articles. The other parameters were estimated numerically using the genetic algorithm module to satisfy the Lineweaver-Burk plot of each enzyme.

Ideally, all of the kinetic properties would be derived from experiments on a single cell line under similar conditions in order to faithfully reconstruct the reaction network. However, a homogeneous data set is not available at present. Thus, these data were collected in diverse tissues, mostly obtained from five species of mammal (human, bovine, pig, rabbit and rat).

The data set was implemented as a simulation model of E-Cell, a simulation platform developed to facilitate mixed-mode calculations.[7] In the standard way of modelling with E-Cell, the mathematical description of a chemical reaction, such as a rate equation, is described in the source file of a small program referred to as "Reactor" ("Process" in version 3), following the grammar and the semantics of the programming language C++. Kinetic parameters and initial metabolite concentrations are described in the "Rulefile", which determines the reaction network and initial condition of the model. To extend the model, the user has only to add Reactors and descriptions of initial metabolite concentrations for newly involved reactions and metabolites, respectively. This feature of E-Cell allows facile integration of independently constructed models. For example, the mitochondrial model is reusable as a module for the simulation of eukaryotic cell metabolism. In the mitochondrial model, the metabolites and enzymes were assigned to one of five compartments: matrix, inner-membrane, outer-membrane, inter-membrane space and cytosol.

PubMed provides a system of keywords called MeSH (Medical Subject Headings), which are embedded in all references included in the database. PubMed users are able to find articles by combining MeSH terms. The search efficiency of comprehensive literature searches is improved when the pattern of MeSH terms embedded in the "HIT" articles (the articles from which the kinetic properties of the mitochondrial model were obtained) is clear. Table 3 shows that "kinetics", the enzyme name and the substrate name are the MeSH terms involved in "HIT" articles in most cases. Combining these three keywords made the identification of published articles on kinetics more efficient. For example, "kinetics AND enzyme name" and "kinetics AND substrate name" cover 81% and 74% of the useful articles, respectively.

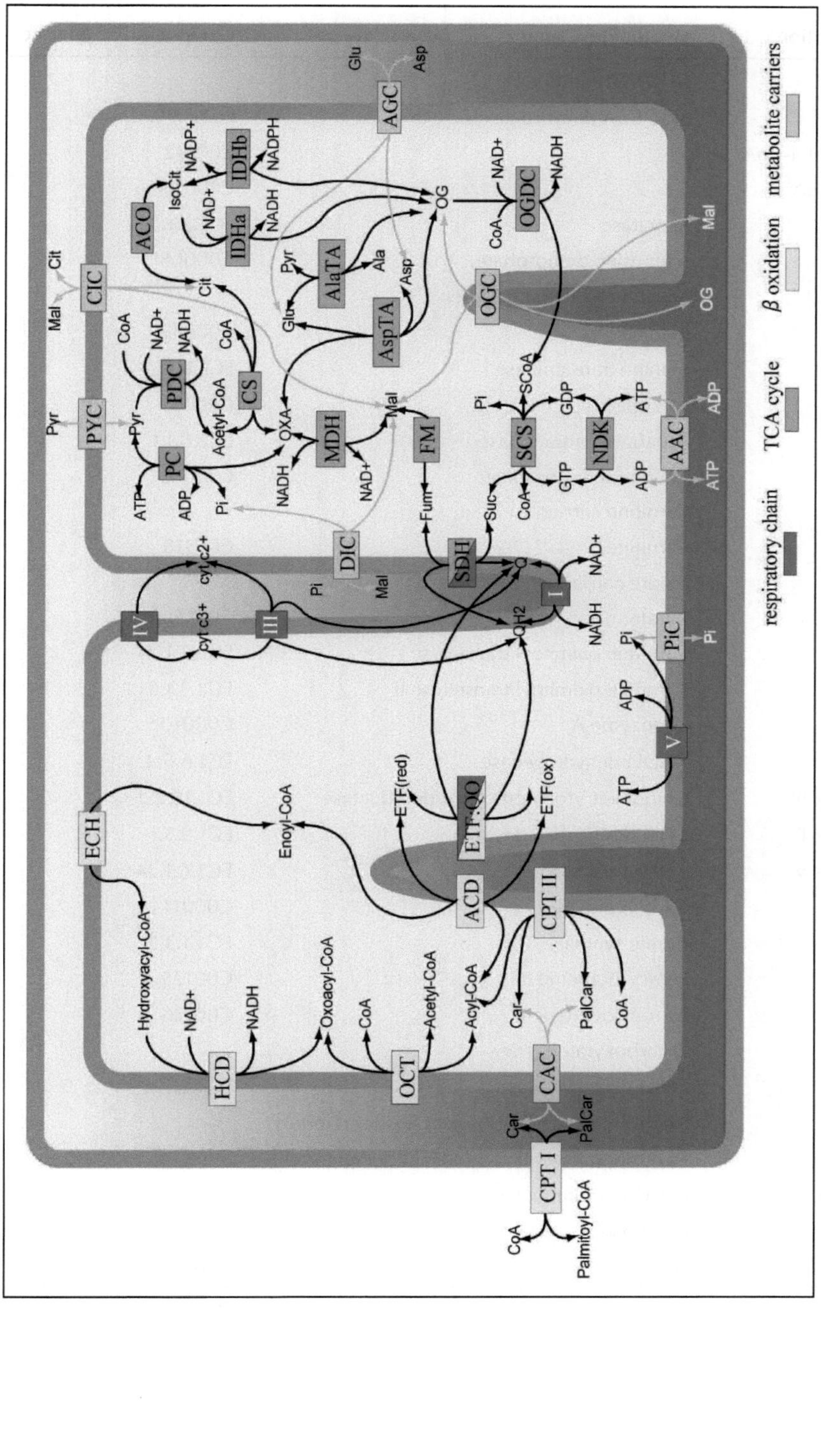


Figure 1. A map of the simulated mitochondrial metabolic pathway. A single mitochondrion is represented. Rectangles in the pathway map represent enzymes. The enzymes with bidirectional and unidirectional arrows catalyze reversible and irreversible reactions, respectively. See Tables 1 and 2 for the abbreviations.

***Table 1. Abbreviations of the compound names (A-N)***

| Abbreviation | Metabolite Name | Compound/EC Number |
|---|---|---|
| AAC | ATP/ADP carrier | |
| ACD | Acyl-CoA dehydrogenase | EC1.3.99.3 |
| Acetoacetyl-CoA | | C00332 |
| Acetyl-CoA | | C00024 |
| ACO | Aconitase | EC4.2.1.3 |
| ADP | Adenosine diphosphate | C00008 |
| AGC | Aspartate/glutamate carrier | |
| Ala | Alanine | C00041 |
| AlaTA | Alanine transaminase | EC2.6.1.2 |
| Asp | Aspartate | C00049 |
| AspTA | Aspartate transaminase | EC2.6.1.1 |
| ATP | Adenosine triphosphate | C00002 |
| CAC | Carnitine carrier | |
| Car | Carnitine | C00318 |
| CIC | Citrate carrier | |
| Cit | Citrate | C00158 |
| CPT-I | Carnitine palmitoyl transferase I | EC2.3.1.21 |
| CPT-II | Carnitine palmitoyl transferase II | EC2.3.1.21 |
| CoA | Coenzyme A | C00010 |
| Complex-I | NADH dehydrogenase | EC1.6.5.3 |
| Complex-III | Ubiquino:Cytochrome c oxidoreductase | EC1.10.2.2 |
| Complex-IV | Cytochrome c oxidase | EC1.9.3.1 |
| Complex-V | ATP synthetase | EC3.6.1.34 |
| $CO_2$ | Carbon dioxide | C00011 |
| CS | Citrate synthase | EC4.1.3.7 |
| cyt-$c^{2+}$ | Ferricytochrome c | C00125 |
| cyt-$c^{3+}$ | Ferrocytochrome c | C00126 |
| DIC | Dicarboxyrate carrier | |
| ECH | Enoyl-CoA hydratase | EC4.2.1.17 |
| ETFox | Electron transfer flavoprotein (oxidised form) | |
| ETFred | Electron transfer flavoprotein (reduced form) | |
| ETF-QO | ETF:Q oxidoreductase | |
| FM | Fumarase | EC4.2.1.2 |
| Fum | Fumarate | C00122 |

*continued on next page*

***Table 1. Continued***

| Abbreviation | Metabolite Name | Compound/EC Number |
|---|---|---|
| GDP | Guanosine diphosphate | C00035 |
| Glu | Glutamate | C00025 |
| GTP | Guanosine triphosphate | C00044 |
| HCD | Hydroxyacyl-CoA dehydrogenase | EC1.1.1.35 |
| $H^+$ | Hydrogen ion (proton) | C00080 |
| IDHa | Isocitrate dehydrogenase ($NAD^+$) | EC1.1.1.41 |
| IDHb | Isocitrate dehydrogenase ($NADP^+$) | EC1.1.1.42 |
| IsoCit | Isocitrate | C00311 |
| Mal | Malate | C00149 |
| MDH | Malate dehydrogenase | EC1.1.1.37 |
| $NAD^+$ | | C00003 |
| NADH | | C00004 |
| $NADP^+$ | | C00006 |
| NADPH | | C00005 |
| NDK | Nucleoside diphosphate kinase | EC2.7.4.6 |

## Simulation Results

The dynamic behaviour of the metabolic pathway was calculated by the numerical integration of the rate equations programmed into the Reactors, employing the fourth-order Runge-Kutta method implemented in E-Cell. Simulated time courses of enzyme activities and metabolite concentrations are observable by means of a graphical interface named "TracerWindow". Another interface, "SubstanceWindow", allows users to increase or decrease metabolite concentrations while running simulations.

### *Simulation Experiment 1*

Clinically, several metabolites are widely administered to patients with mitochondrial disorders.[8,9] The rationales for these metabolic treatments, however, are still unclear in many cases. In our previous study,[1] we showed the example that increasing coenzyme Q and succinate supplies sufficient electrons to the respiratory chain through the succinate dehydrogenase complex. The evidence supporting this conclusion is presented in Figure 2: increasing coenzyme Q and succinate results in higher reduction of cytochrome c (Fig. 2A) and activation of the succinate dehydrogenase complex and subsequent respiratory enzymes (SDH, Complex III, IV in Fig. 2B).

In this study, we also examined the effect of this metabolic treatment on the peripheral pathways. Figure 2C,D are time courses of the metabolite concentrations and the enzyme activities of the pathways around coenzyme Q and succinate. No significant concentration change was observed in metabolites such as fumarate, malate and citrate (Fum, Mal and Cit in Fig 2C, respectively), which are within a few enzyme steps of succinate. Similarly, the enzyme activities of the peripheral pathway were not influenced by coenzyme Q and succinate with the exception of fumarase (FM in Fig. 2D), which is adjacent to succinate dehydrogenase complex in the TCA cycle.

***Table 2. Abbreviations of the compound names (O–)***

| Abbreviation | Metabolite Name | Compound/EC Number |
|---|---|---|
| OCT | Oxoacyl-CoA thiolase | EC2.3.1.16 |
| OG | Oxoglutarate | C00026 |
| OGC | Oxoglutarate carrier | |
| OGDC | Oxoglutarate dehydrogenase complex | EC1.2.4.2 etc. |
| OXA | Oxaloacetate | C00036 |
| PalCar | Palmitoylcarnitine | C02990 |
| PC | Pyruvate carboxylase | EC6.4.1.1 |
| PDC | Pyruvate dehydrogenase complex | EC1.2.4.1 etc. |
| Pi | Phosphate | C00009 |
| PiC | Pi carrier | |
| Pyr | Pyruvate | C00022 |
| PYC | Pyruvate carrier | |
| Q | Ubiquinone | C00399 |
| $QH_2$ | Ubiquinol | C00390 |
| SCoA | Succinyl-CoA | C00091 |
| SCS | Succinyl-CoA synthetase | EC6.2.1.4 |
| SDH | Succinate dehydrogenase | EC1.3.5.1 |
| Suc | Succinate | C00042 |
| 10Acyl-CoA | Decanoyl-CoA | C05274 |
| 10Enoyl-CoA | Trans-Dec-2-enoyl-CoA | C05275 |
| 10Hydroxyacyl-CoA | (S)-3-Hydroxydedecanoyl-CoA | C05264 |
| 10Oxoacyl-CoA | 3-Oxodecanoyl-CoA | C05265 |
| 12Acyl-CoA | Lauroyl-CoA | C01832 |
| 12Enoyl-CoA | Trans-Dodec-2-enoyl-CoA | C03221 |
| 12Hydroxyacyl-CoA | (S)-3-Hydroxydodecanoyl-CoA | C05262 |
| 12Oxoacyl-CoA | 3-Oxodo decanoyl-CoA | C05263 |
| 14Acyl-CoA | Myristoyl-CoA | C02593 |
| 14Enoyl-CoA | Trans-Tetradec-2-enoyl-CoA | C05273 |
| 14Hydroxyacyl-CoA | (S)-3-Hydroxytetradecanoyl-CoA | C05260 |
| 14Oxoacyl-CoA | 3-Oxotetradecanoyl-CoA | C05261 |
| 16Acyl-CoA | Palmitoyl-CoA | C00154 |
| 16Enoyl-CoA | Trans-Hexadec-2-enoyl-CoA | C05272 |
| 16Hydroxyacyl-CoA | (S)-3-Hydroxyhexadecanoyl-CoA | C05258 |
| 16Oxoacyl-CoA | 3-Oxohexadecanoyl-CoA | C05259 |
| 4Acyl-CoA | Butanoyl-CoA | C00136 |
| 4Enoyl-CoA | Crotonyl-CoA | C00877 |

*continued on next page*

***Table 2. Continued***

| Abbreviation | Metabolite Name | Compound/EC Number |
|---|---|---|
| 4Hydroxyacyl-CoA | (S)-3-Hydroxybutanoyl-CoA | C01144 |
| 6Acyi-CoA | Hexanoyl-CoA | C05270 |
| 6Enoyl-CoA | Trans-Hex-2-enoyl-CoA | C05271 |
| 6Hydroxyacyl-CoA | (S)-3-Hydroxyhexanoyl-CoA | C05268 |
| 6Oxoacyl-CoA | 3-Oxohexanoyl-CoA | C05269 |
| 8Acyl-CoA | Octanoyl-CoA | C01944 |
| 8Enoyl-CoA | Trans-Oct-2-enoyl-CoA | C05276 |
| 8Hydroxyacyl-CoA | (S)-3-Hydroxyoctanoyl-CoA | C05266 |
| 8Oxoacyl-CoA | 3-Oxooctaanoyl-CoA | C05267 |

***Table 3. The pattern of MeSH terms embedded in the "HIT" articles. "Kinetics and enzyme name" and "kinetics and substrate name" accounted for 81% and 74% of the "HIT" articles, respectively.***

| | Kinetics | Models | Mathematics | Enzyme Name | Substrate Name |
|---|---|---|---|---|---|
| Ref. 13 | + | +, Chemical | + | – | + |
| Ref. 14 | + | – | – | + | – |
| Ref. 15 | + | – | + | + | + |
| Ref. 16 | + | +, Biological | – | + | + |
| Ref. 17 | – | – | – | + | – |
| Ref. 18 | + | – | – | + | – |
| Ref. 19 | + | – | – | + | + |
| Ref. 20 | – | – | – | + | – |
| Ref. 21 | + | – | – | + | + |
| Ref. 22 | + | – | – | + | + |
| Ref. 23 | + | – | – | + | + |
| Ref. 24 | + | – | – | + | + |
| Ref. 25 | + | – | – | + | + |
| Ref. 26 | + | + | – | + | + |
| Ref. 27 | + | – | – | + | + |
| Ref. 28 | + | – | – | + | + |
| Ref. 29 | + | – | – | + | + |
| Ref. 30 | + | – | – | + | + |
| Ref. 31 | + | – | + | + | + |
| Ref. 32 | + | – | – | – | + |
| Ref. 33 | + | – | – | + | – |
| Ref. 34 | – | – | – | – | + |
| Ref. 35 | + | +, Chemical | + | + | + |
| Ref. 36 | + | – | – | + | + |
| Ref. 37 | + | – | – | + | + |
| Ref. 38 | + | – | – | + | – |
| Ref. 39 | + | +, Theoretical | + | + | + |
| Hit frequency | 24/27 | 5/27 | 5/27 | 24/27 | 21/27 |

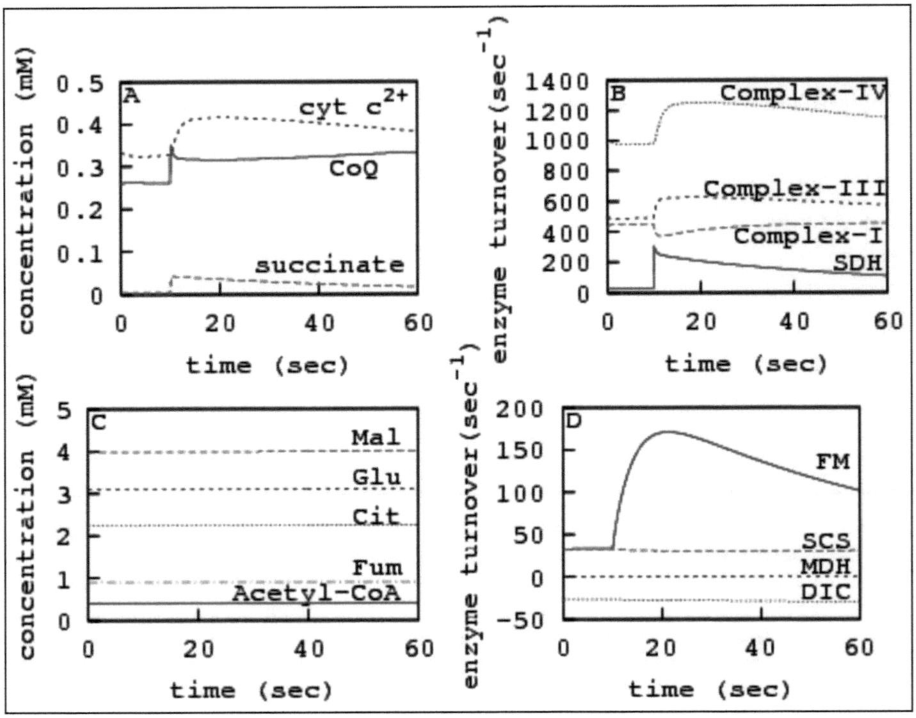


Figure 2. The time courses calculated by Simulation experiment 1. An increase in coenzyme Q and succinate promotes the total activity of the respiratory chain through activation of the succinate dehydrogenase complex (SDH in B). The influence of coenzyme Q and succinate is limited to the respiratory chain except for the activation of fumarase (FM in D). See Tables 1 and 2 for the other abbreviations. (Panels A and B are from ref. 1 by permission of Oxford University Press.)

### *Simulation Experiment 2*

In a second simulation, we administered 0.15 mM oxoglutarate to the matrix in a quasi-steady-state. Oxoglutarate increased the activity of one of the respiratory enzymes (Complex I in Fig. 3D) and the concentration of reduced electron transporters (Fig. 3B), ATP (Fig. 3C) and other metabolites such as succinate and 16Acyl-CoA (Figs. 3A and C, respectively). Of all the enzymes that catalyze reactions in which oxoglutarate is a substrate or a product, aspartate transaminase showed the highest activity, 40-fold greater than that of the oxoglutarate dehydrogenase complex, the second largest.

## Discussion

### *Modelling*

Our model was based on published kinetic equations. By extracting a pattern of MeSH terms we were able to construct a more efficient literature-based model and to comprehensively detect a suitable number of papers for kinetic modelling. However, the kinetic properties of enzymes are not being characterised as actively now as in the 1960-70s. Thus, literature-based modelling will be confronted with the practical obstacle that enzymes of interest that have not already been studied might never be examined. To overcome this bottleneck for the simulation of larger pathways, novel

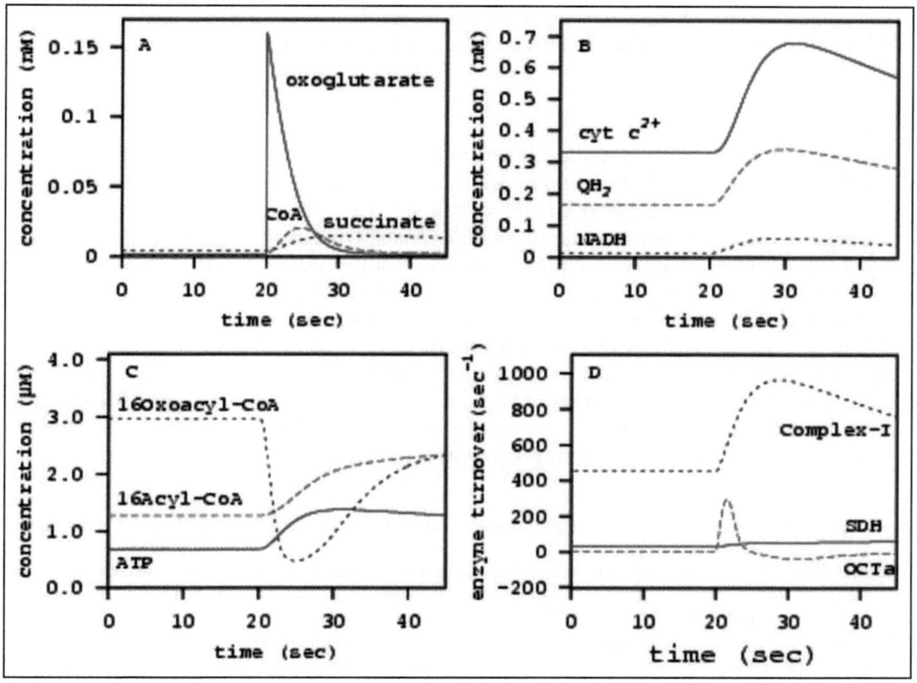


Figure 3. The time courses calculated by Simulation experiment 2. Administration of oxoglutarate promotes NADH production (B) which consequently causes activation of Complex I (D). Oxoglutarate affects a broader pathway (A,C,D) than coenzyme Q + succinate, whose influence was limited to the respiratory chain (Simulation experiment 1, Fig. 2). See Tables 1 and 2 for the abbreviations.

methods for comprehensive and high-throughput characterisation of kinetic properties of enzymes will be necessary. A solution to this problem is discussed in reference 10.

### *Simulation Experiment 1*

We found an increase in the total activity of the respiratory chain following an increase in coenzyme Q + succinate, which is qualitatively in agreement with the report of successful clinical treatment with coenzyme Q + succinate.[2] The simulated time courses suggest a hypothetical rationale for this metabolic treatment: the increase of succinate promotes the respiratory chain by electron donation through the succinate dehydrogenase complex. The activation of the succinate dehydrogenase complex compensated for a decrease in the Complex I activity. The influence of the coenzyme Q + succinate supplementation was observed specifically in the respiratory chain.

### *Simulation Experiment 2*

The activity of the total respiratory chain also increased in Simulation experiment 2; however, the mechanism of the activation was different from that of Simulation experiment 1. The activation of Complex I (Fig. 3D) indicates that NADH oxidation by Complex I is the primary electron donor to the respiratory chain in the condition of Simulation experiment 2, while electrons were mainly supplied through the succinate dehydrogenase complex in Simulation experiment 1.

Another difference between Simulation experiments 1 and 2 is that the oxoglutarate in Simulation experiment 2 affected broader pathways than the coenzyme Q + succinate in Simulation

1. The administration of oxoglutarate influenced metabolite concentrations in the TCA cycle and fatty acid β-oxidation, while the effect of coenzyme Q + succinate was observed specifically around the respiratory chain.

## Conclusion

As shown above, simulation studies of metabolic pathways are capable of deriving hypotheses about the dynamics of metabolite concentrations and enzyme activities. However, validation by wet experiments will be required for a more realistic simulation of mitochondria.

At present, there are experimentally observable variables that can be used to check the consistency of the model. Robinson et al reported a method for the quantitative measurement of ATP production of mitochondria using a luminometer.[11] With this method, it is possible to compare mitochondrial ATP production in vivo and in silico. Moreover, recent advancements in metabolome measurement will facilitate not only the quantification of ATP production but also the comprehensive profiling of intracellular/organellar metabolite concentration.[12] In cases where only qualitative results are necessary, staining of cytochrome c oxidase can be used to provide qualitative measurements of the enzyme activity. Revision of the mitochondrial model after these experimental validations will provide a more realistic prediction of mitochondrial energy metabolism.

## Reference

1. Yugi K, Tomita M. A general computational model of mitochondrial metabolism. Bioinformatics 2004; 20:1795-1796.
2. Shoffner JM et al. Spontaneous Kearns-Sayre/chronic external ophthalmoplegia plus syndrome associated with a mitochondrial DNA deletion: a slip-replication model and metabolic therapy. Proc Natl Acad Sci USA 1989; 86:7952-7956.
3. Chance B, Garfinkel D, Higgins J et al. Metabolic control mechanisms V: A solution for the equations representing interaction between glycolysis and respiration in ascites tumor cells. J Biol Chem 1960; 235:2426-2439.
4. Joshi A, Palsson BO. Metabolic dynamics in the human red cell: Part I. A comprehensive kinetic model. J Theor Biol 1989; 141:515-528.
5. Korzeniewski B, Froncisz W. A dynamic model of mitochondrial respiration. Stud Biophys 1989; 132:173-187.
6. Wright BE, Butler MH, Albe KR. Systems analysis of the tricarboxylic acid cycle in dictyostelium discoideum. I. The basis for model construction. J Biol Chem 1992; 267:3101-3105.
7. Takahashi K et al. Computational challenges in cell simulation. IEEE Intelligent Systems 2002; 17:64-71.
8. Przyrembel H. Therapy of mitochondrial disorders. J Inherit Metab Dis 1987; 10:129-146.
9. Luft R. The development of mitochondrial medicine. Proc Natl Acad Sci USA 1994; 91:8731-8738.
10. Yugi K, Nakayama Y, Kinoshita A et al. Hybrid dynamic/static method for large-scale simulation of metabolism. Theoretical Biology and Medical Modelling 2005; 2:42.
11. Robinson BH et al. The use of skin fibroblast cultures in the detection of respiratory chain defects in patients with lacticacidemia. Pediatr Res 1990; 28:549-555.
12. Soga T et al. Pressure-assisted capillary electrophoresis electrospray ionization mass spectrometry for analysis of multivalent anions. Anal Chem 2002; 74:6224-6229.
13. Barden RE, Fung CH, Utter MF et al. Pyruvate carboxylase from chicken liver. J Biol Chem 1972; 247:1323-1333.
14. Beckmann JD, Frerman FE. Reaction of electron transfer flavoprotein with electron-transfer flavoprotein-ubiquinone oxidoreductase. Biochemistry 1985; 24:3922-3925.
15. Crow KE, Braggins TJ, Hardman MJ. Human liver cytosolic malate dehydrogenase: purification, kinetic properties and role in ethanol metabolism. Arch Biochem Biophys 1983; 225:621-629.
16. Davisson VJ, Schulz AR. The purification and steady-state kinetic behaviour of rabbit heart mitochondrial NAD(P)+ malic enzyme. Biochem J 1985; 225:335-342.
17. De Rosa G, Burk TL, Swick RW. Isolation and characterization of mitochondrial alanine aminotransferase from porcine tissue. Biochim Biophys Acta 1979; 567:116-124.
18. Dierks T, Kramer R. Asymmetric orientation of the reconstituted aspartate/glutamete carrier from mitochondria. Biochim Biophys Acta 1988; 937:112-126.
19. Fato R et al. Steady-state kinetics of the reduction of coenzyme Q analogs by complex I (NADH:ubiquinone oxidoreductase) in bovine heart mitochondria and submitochondrial particles. Biochemistry 1996; 35:2705-2716.

20. Grivennikova VG, Gavrikova EV, Timoshin AA et al. Fumarate reductase activity of bovine heart succinate-ubiquinone reductase. New assay system and overall properties of the reaction. Biochim Biophys Acta 1993; 1140:282-292.
21. Guarriero-Bobyleva V, Masini A, Volpi-Becchi MA et al. Kinetic studies of cytoplasmic and mitochondrial aconitate hydratases from rat liver. Ital J Biochem 1978; 27:287-299.
22. Hamada M et al. A kinetic study of the alpha-keto acid dehydrogenase complexes from pig heart mitochondria. J Biochem (Tokyo) 1975; 77:1047-1056.
23. Indiveri C, Dierks T, Kramer R et al. Reaction mechanism of the reconstituted oxoglutarate carrier from bovine heart mitochondria. Eur J Biochem 1991; 198:339-347.
24. Indiveri C, Tonazzi A, Prezioso G et al. Kinetic characterization of the reconstituted carnitine carrier from rat liver mitochondria. Biochim Biophys Acta 1991; 1065:231-238.
25. Indiveri C, Tonazzi A, Palmieri F. The reconstituted carnitine carrier from rat liver mitochondria: evidence for a transport mechanism different from that of the other mitochondrial translocators. Biochim Biophys Acta 1994; 1189:65-73.
26. Kholodenko BN. Kinetic models of coupling between H+ and Na(+)-translocation and ATP synthesis/hydrolysis by FoF1-ATPases: can a cell utilize both delta mu H+ and delta mu Na+ for ATP synthesis under in vivo conditions using the same enzyme? J Bioenerg Biomembr 1993; 25:285-295.
27. Kramer R, Klingenberg M. Electrophoretic control of reconstituted adenine nucleotide translocation. Biochemistry 1982; 21:1082-1089.
28. Kubota T, Yoshikawa S, Matsubara H. Kinetic mechanism of beef heart ubiquinol: cytochrome c oxidoreducase. J Biochem (Tokyo) 1992; 111:91-98.
29. Malmstrom BG, Andreasson LE. The steady-state rate equation for cytochrome c oxidase based on a minimal kinetic scheme. J Inorg Biochem 1985; 23:233-242.
30. Mann WR, Yan B, Dragland CJ et al. Kinetic, circular dichroism and fluorescence studies on heterologously expressed carnitine palmitoyltransferase II. J Enzym Inhib 1995; 9:303-308.
31. Matsuoka Y, Srere PA. Kinetic studies of citrate synthase from rat kidney and rat brain. J Biol Chem 1973; 248:8022-8030.
32. McKean MC, Frerman FE, Mielke DM. General acyl-CoA dehydrogenase frome pig liver. J Biol Chem 1979; 254:2730-2735.
33. Miyazawa S, Furuta S, Osumi T et al. Properties of peroxisomal 3-ketoacyl-CoA thiolase from rat liver. J Biochem (Tokyo) 1981; 90:511-519.
34. Mukherjee A, Srere PA. Purification of and mechanism studies on citrate synthase. J Biol Chem 1976; 251:1476-1480.
35. Plaut GWE, Schramm VL, Aogaichi T. Action of magnesium ion on diphosphopyridine nucleotide-linked isocitrate dehydrogenase from bovine heart. J Biol Chem 1974; 249:848-1856.
36. Ramsay RR, Derrick JP, Friend AS et al. Purification and properties of the soluble carnitine palmitoyltransferase from bovine liver mitochondria. Biochem J 1987; 244:271-278.
37. Sluse FE et al. Kinetic study of the aspartate/glutamate carrier in intact rat heart mitochondria and comparison with a reconstituted system. Biochim Biophys Acta 1991; 1058:329-338.
38. Stappen R, Kramer R. Kinetic mechanism of phosphate/phosphate and phosphate/OH- antiports catalyzed by reconstituted phosphate carrier from beef heart mitochondria. J Biol Chem 1994; 269:11240-11246.
39. Yang SY, Schulz H. Kinetics of coupled enzyme reactions. Biochemistry 1987; 26:5579-5584.
40. Velick SF, Vavra J. A kinetic and equilibrium analysis of the glutamic oxaloacetate transaminase mechanism. J Biol Chem 1962; 237:2109-2122.
41. Henson CP, Cleland WW. Kinetic studies of glutamic oxaloacetic transaminase isozymes. Biochemistry 1964; 3:338-345.
42. Bisaccia F, De Palma A, Dierks T et al. Reaction mechanism of the reconstituted tricarboxylate carrier from rat liver mitochondria. Biochim Biophys Acta 1993; 1142:139-145.
43. Matsuno-Yagi A, Hatefi Y. Studies on the mechanism of oxidative phosphorylation: catalytic site cooperativity in ATP synthesis. J Biol Chem 1985; 260:14424-14427.
44. Woeltje KF, Kuwajima M, Foster DW et al. Characterization of the mitochondrial carnitine palmitoyltransferase enzyme system. J Biol Chem 1987; 262:9822-9827.
45. Shepherd D, Garland PB. The kinetic properties of citrate synthase from rat liver mitochondria. Biochem J 1969; 114:597-610.
46. Indiveri C, Prezioso G, Dierks T et al. Kinetic characterization of the reconstituted dicarboxylate carrier from mitochondria: a four-binding-site sequential transport system. Biochim Biophys Acta 1993; 1143:310-318.
47. Hill RL, Teipel JW. The Enzymes volume V. In: Boyer PD, ed. New York and London: Academic Press, 1970; 539-571.

48. Ehrlich RS, Hayman S, Ramachandran N et al. F. Re-evaluation of molecular weight of pig heart NAD-specific isocitrate dehydrogenase. J Biol Chem 1981; 256:10560-10564.
49. Londesborough JC, Dalziel K. Pyridine nucleotide dependent dehydrogenases. In: Sund H, ed. New York: Springer-Verlag 1970; 315-324.
50. Colomb MG, Cheruy A, Vignais PV. Nucleoside diphosphatekinase from beef heart mitochondria: purification and properties. Biochemistry 1969; 8:1926-1939.
51. Garces E, Cleland WW. Kinetic studies of yeast nucleoside diphosphate kinase. Biochemistry 1969; 8:633-640.
52. Cleland WW. Derivation of rate equations of multisite ping-pong mechanisms with ping-pong reactions at one or more sites. J Biol Chem 1973; 248:8353-8355.
53. Kiselevsky YV, Ostrovtsova SA, Strumilo SA. Kinetic characterization of the pyruvate and oxoglutarate dehydrogenase complexes from human heart. Acta Biochim Pol 1990; 37:135-139.
54. Heckert LL, Butler MH, Reimers JM et al. Purification and characterization of the 2-oxoglutarate dehydrogenase complex from Dictyostelium discoideum. J Gen Microbiol 1989; 135:155-161.
55. Nalecz KA. Molecular biology of mitochondrial transport systems. In: Forte M, Colombini M, eds. Springer-Verlag Berlin Heidelberg 1994; 67-79.
56. Capuano F, Di Paola M, Azzi A et al. The monocarboxylate carrier from rat liver mitochondria: purification and kinetic characterization in a reconstituted system. FEBS Lett 1990; 261:39-42.
57. Cha S, Parks Jr, RE. Succinic thiokinase II. kinetic studies: Initial velocity, product inhibition and effect of arsenate. J Biol Chem 1964; 239:1968-1977.

# Appendix A

***Supporting Table 1. Initial concentrations of metabolites and enzymes***

| Enzyme | Localisation | Number of Molecules |
|---|---|---|
| Complex-I | MT-IM | 1000 |
| Complex-III | MT-IM | 3000 |
| Complex-IV | MT-IM | 7000 |
| Complex-V | MT-IM | 900 |
| CS | MATRIX | 100 |
| ACO | MATRIX | 100 |
| IDHa | MATRIX | 100 |
| IDHb | MATRIX | 100 |
| OGDC | MATRIX | 100 |
| SCS | MATRIX | 100 |
| SDH | MT-IM | 100 |
| FM | MATRIX | 100 |
| MDH | MATRIX | 100 |
| AlaTA | MATRIX | 100 |
| AspTA | MATRIX | 100 |
| NDK | MATRIX | 100 |
| PDC | MATRIX | 100 |
| PC | MATRIX | 100 |
| CPT-I | MT-OM | 100 |
| CAC | MT-IM | 100 |
| ACD | MT-IM | 100 |
| ECH | MT-IM | 100 |
| HCD | MT-IM | 100 |
| OCT | MT-IM | 100 |
| ETF-QO | MT-IM | 100 |
| AAC | MT-IM | 1000 |
| AGC | MT-IM | 1000 |
| PiC | MT-IM | 1000 |
| PYC | MT-IM | 1000 |
| OGC | MT-IM | 1000 |
| DIC | MT-IM | 1000 |
| CIC | MT-IM | 1000 |

*continued on next page*

**Supporting Table 1. Continued**

| Compound | Localisation | Concentration |
|---|---|---|
| Q | MT-IMS | 0.26 mM |
| $QH_2$ | MT-IMS | 28 μM |
| cyt-$c^{3+}$ | MT-IMS | 3 μW |
| cyt-$c^{2+}$ | MT-IMS | 0.11 mM |
| $H^+$ | MT-IMS | 1 μM |
| $H^+$ | MATRIX | 10 nM |
| Cit | MT-IMS | 0.42 mM |
| Cit | MATRIX | 0.42 mM |
| IsoCit | MATRIX | 0.42 mM |
| OG | MT-IMS | 21 μM |
| OG | MATRIX | 21 μM |
| SCoA | MATRIX | 0.29 mM |
| Suc | MATRIX | 2.95 mM |
| Fum | MATRIX | 65.00 μM |
| Mal | MT-IMS | 0.50 mM |
| Mal | MATRIX | 0.50 mM |
| OXA | MATRIX | 4.00 μM |
| Asp | MATRIX | 1.14 mM |
| Asp | MT-IMS | 1.14 mM |
| Glu | MATRIX | 3.03 mM |
| Glu | MT-IMS | 3.03 mM |
| Ala | MATRIX | 3.44 mM |
| Pyr | MT-IMS | 0.10 mM |
| Pyr | MATRIX | 0.10 mM |
| CoA | MT-IMS | 0.27 mM |
| CoA | MATRIX | 0.27 mM |
| Acetyi-CoA | MATRIX | 30.00 μM |
| NADH | MATRIX | 72.00 μM |
| $NAD^+$ | MATRIX | 0.17 mM |
| NADPH | MATRIX | 72.00 μM |
| $NADP^+$ | MATRIX | 0.17 mM |
| $CO_2$ | MATRIX | 1.63 mM |
| ATP | MT-IMS | 4.50 mM |

*continued on next page*

***Supporting Table 1. Continued***

| Compound | Localisation | Concentration |
|---|---|---|
| ATP | MATRIX | 4.50 mM |
| ADP | MT-IMS | 0.45 mM |
| ADP | MATRIX | 0.45 mM |
| GTP | MATRIX | 4.50 mM |
| GDP | MATRIX | 0.45 mM |
| Pi | MT-IMS | 4.00 mM |
| Pi | MATRIX | 4.00 mM |
| Car | MT-IMS | 0.20 mM |
| Car | MATRIX | 0.95 mM |
| PalCar | MT-IMS | 0.60 mM |
| PalCar | MATRIX | 12.00 μM |
| ETFred | MATRIX | 0.31 μM |
| ETFox | MATRIX | 0.32 μM |
| 16Acyl-CoA | MATRIX | 39.00 μM |
| 16Enoyl-CoA | MATRIX | 17.00 μM |
| 16Hydroxyacyl-CoA | MATRIX | 12.00 μM |
| 160xoacyl-CoA | MATRIX | 1.10 μM |
| 14Acyl-CoA | MATRIX | 39.00 μM |
| 14Enoyl-CoA | MATRIX | 17.00 μM |
| 14 Hydroxyacyl-CoA | MATRIX | 12.00 μM |
| 140xoacyl-CoA | MATRIX | 1.10 μM |
| 12Acyl-CoA | MATRIX | 87.00 μM |
| 12Enoyl-CoA | MATRIX | 17.00 μM |
| 12Hydroxyacyl-CoA | MATRIX | 12.00 μM |
| 120xoacyl-CoA | MATRIX | 1.30 μM |
| 10Acyl-CoA | MATRIX | 87.00 μM |
| 10Enoyl-CoA | MATRIX | 17.00 μM |
| 10Hydroxyacyl-CoA | MATRIX | 12.00 μM |
| 10Oxoacyl-CoA | MATRIX | 2.10 μM |
| 3Acyl-CoA | MATRIX | 87.00 μM |
| 8Enoyl-CoA | MATRIX | 17.00 μM |
| 8Hydroxyacyl-CoA | MATRIX | 12.00 μM |
| 8Oxoacyl-CoA | MATRIX | 3.20 μM |

*continued on next page*

***Supporting Table 1. Continued***

| Compound | Localisation | Concentration |
|---|---|---|
| 6Acyl-CoA | MATRIX | 87.00 μM |
| 6Enoyl-CoA | MATRIX | 17.00 μM |
| 6Hydroxyacyl-CoA | MATRIX | 12.00 μM |
| 60xoacyl-CoA | MATRIX | 6.70 μM |
| 4Acyl-CoA | MATRIX | 87.00 μM |
| 4Enoyl-CoA | MATRIX | 17.00 μM |
| 4Hydroxyacyl-CoA | MATRIX | 12.00 μM |
| Aceloacetyl-CoA | MATRIX | 12.40 μM |

**Supporting Table 2. Steady-state amounts of metabolites and enzymes**

| Compound | Localisation | Number of Molecules |
|---|---|---|
| Q | MT-IMS | 77547 |
| $QH_2$ | MT-IMS | 500 |
| cyt-$c^{3+}$ | MT-IMS | 29624 |
| cyt-$c^{2+}$ | MT-IMS | 999 |
| $H^+$ | MT-IMS | 3 |
| $H^+$ | MATRIX | 3 |
| Cit | MT-IMS | 1265 |
| Cit | MATRIX | 583455 |
| IsoCit | MATRIX | 74758 |
| OG | MT-IMS | 63 |
| OG | MATRIX | 424 |
| SCoA | MATRIX | 32 |
| Suc | MATRIX | 1133 |
| Fum | MATRIX | 231567 |
| Mal | MT-IMS | 1506 |
| Mal | MATRIX | 1028383 |
| OXA | MATRIX | 302 |
| Asp | MATRIX | 244090 |
| Asp | MT-IMS | 3433 |
| Glu | MATRIX | 801482 |
| Glu | MT-IMS | 9124 |
| Ala | MATRIX | 1016709 |
| Pyr | MT-IMS | 27777 |
| Pyr | MATRIX | 309 |
| CoA | MT-IMS | 700 |
| CoA | MATRIX | 286 |
| Acetyl-CoA | MATRIX | 104498 |
| NADH | MATRIX | 3672 |
| $NAD^+$ | MATRIX | 61909 |
| NADPH | MATRIX | 7508 |
| $NADP^+$ | MATRIX | 58073 |
| $CO_2$ | MATRIX | 42631671 |
| ATP | MT-IMS | 13550 |
| ATP | MATRIX | 180 |
| ADP | MT-IMS | 1355 |
| ADP | MATRIX | 121948 |
| GTP | MATRIX | 2579 |

*continued on next page*

***Supporting Table 2. Continued***

| Compound | Localisation | Number of Molecules |
|---|---|---|
| GDP | MATRIX | 1338852 |
| Pi | MT-IMS | 12044 |
| Pi | MATRIX | 2507395 |
| Car | MT-IMS | 602 |
| Car | MATRIX | 47418 |
| PalCar | MT-MS | 1807 |
| PalCar | MATRIX | 213280 |
| 16Acyl-CoA | MT-MS | 117 |
| ETFred | MATRIX | 89 |
| ETFox | MATRIX | 82 |
| 16Acyl-CoA | MATRIX | 331 |
| 16Enoyl-CoA | MATRIX | 698 |
| 16Hydroxyacyl-CoA | MATRIX | 3 |
| 16Oxoacyl-CoA | MATRIX | 769 |
| 14Acyl-CoA | MATRIX | 331 |
| 14Enoyl-CoA | MATRIX | 699 |
| 14Hydroxyacyl-CoA | MATRIX | 3 |
| 14Oxoacyl-CoA | MATRIX | 771 |
| 12Acyl-CoA | MATRIX | 330 |
| 12Enoyl-CoA | MATRIX | 700 |
| 12Hydroxyacyl-CoA | MATRIX | 2 |
| 12Oxoacyl-CoA | MATRIX | 763 |
| 10Acyl-CoA | MATRIX | 331 |
| 10Enoyl-CoA | MATRIX | 700 |
| 10Hydroxyacyl-CoA | MATRIX | 2 |
| 10Oxoacyl-CoA | MATRIX | 762 |
| BAcyl-CoA | MATRIX | 332 |
| 8Enoyl-CoA | MATRIX | 701 |
| 8Hydroxyacyl-CoA | MATRIX | 2 |
| 80xoacyl-CoA | MATRIX | 763 |
| 6Acyl-CoA | MATRIX | 332 |
| 6Enoyl-CoA | MATRIX | 701 |
| 6Hydroxyacyl-CoA | MATRIX | 3 |
| 6Oxoacyl-CoA | MA | 764 |
| 4Acyl-CoA | MATRIX | 331 |
| 4Enoyl-CoA | MATRIX | 702 |
| 4Hydroxyacyl-CoA | MATRIX | 2 |
| Acetoacetyl-CoA | MATRIX | 239686 |

***Supporting Table 3. Parameter classification***

| Class | Definition | Example |
|---|---|---|
| Class 0 | Found in the literature | Km = 2.3 mM |
| Class 1 | Estimated around the values in the literature | Km = 2.3 mM → Km = 2.6 mM |
| Class 2 | Estimated around the values of analogous metabolites | KmATP = 2.3 mM → 0 < KmGTP <3.0 mM |
| Class 3 | Estimated arbitrarily | ? < k < ?→ k = $1.2 \times 10^9$ $sec^{-1}$ |

***Supporting Table 4. The kinetic properties of AAC***

| | | | |
|---|---|---|---|
| Reaction | | ATP(MAT) → ATP(IMS), ADP(MAT) → ADP(IMS) | |
| Mechanism | | See ref. 27 | |
| Rate equation | | Eqn. 1 | |
| Species, organ | | Rat heart mitochondria | |
| **Parameter** | | **Class** | **Notice** |
| kf0 | 0.9 | Class 0 | Velocity model (mp = 0, kf0 = kr0) |
| kr0 | 0.9 | Class 0 | Velocity model (mp = 0) |
| Normalize | 2.21 | Class 0 | Normalizing factor of kf0 and kr0 |
| Kd1 | $5.9 \times 10^{-4}$ | Class 3 | Kd1 → Kd velocity model, Kd1 = Kd2 |
| Kd2 | $5.9 \times 10^{-4}$ | Class 3 | Kd1 → Kd′<br>Kd is not effected by the membrane potential |
| Cf | 3.30 | Class 0 | Kf0 × exp(Cf × ΔΨ) = kf(ΔΨ) |
| Cf | –3.34 | Class 0 | Kr0 × exp(Cr × ΔΨ) = kr(ΔΨ) |
| T | 310.0 K | – | Absolute temperature |

Source of parameter estimation: Figure 2(B) $V^{D}_{\rightarrow}$(ΔΨ = 0mV, 180mV) in reference 27.

***Supporting Table 5. The kinetic properties of ACD***

| | | | |
|---|---|---|---|
| Reaction | | Acyl-CoA + ETFox ⇔ Enoyl-CoA + ETFred | |
| Mechanism | | Ordered Bi Bi[32] | |
| Rate equation | | | |
| Species, organ | | Pig liver mitochondria | |
| **Parameter** | | **Class** | **Notice** |
| KmS1 | $39 \times 10^{-6}$ | Class 0 | Ref. 32 Table 1 |
| KmS2 | $0.12 \times 10^{-6}$ | Class 0 | |
| KmP1 | $1.08 \times 10^{-6}$ | Class 2 | |
| KmP2 | $2.42 \times 10^{-5}$ | Class 2 | |
| KiS1 | $76 \times 10^{-6}$ | Class 0 | |
| KiS2 | $0.24 \times 10^{-6}$ | Class 0 | |
| KiP1 | $7.53 \times 10^{-5}$ | Class 2 | |
| KiP2 | $1.19 \times 10^{-5}$ | Class 2 | |
| Keq | 8.99 | Class 3 | |
| KcF | 2.18 | Class 0 | |
| KcR | 0.30 | Class 2 | |

Source for parameter estimation: reference 32.

***Supporting Table 6. The kinetic properties of ACO***

| | | | |
|---|---|---|---|
| Reaction | | Cit ⇔ IsoCit | |
| Mechanism | | Uni uni reversible[21] | |
| Rate equation | | | |
| Species, organ | | Rat liver mitochondria | |
| **Parameter** | **Class** | **Notice** | |
| Ks | $0.50 \times 10^{-3}$ | Class 0 | |
| Kp | $0.11 \times 10^{-3}$ | Class 0 | |
| KcF | 20.47 | Class 0 | Calculated from the graph |
| KcR | 31.44 | Class 0 | Calculated from the graph |

***Supporting Table 7. The kinetic properties of AGC***

| | | | |
|---|---|---|---|
| Reaction | | Asp(IMS) + Glu (MAT) ⇔ Asp(MAT) + Glu(IMS) | |
| Mechanism | | Rapid equilibrium Random Bi Bi[37] | |
| Rate equation | | | |
| Species | | Rat heart mitochondria | |
| **Parameter** | | **Class** | **Notice** |
| KiS1 | $80 \times 10^{-6}$ | Class 0 | Ref. 18 |
| KiS2 | $3.2 \times 10^{-3}$ | Class 0 | Ref. 18 |
| KiP1 | $180 \times 10^{-6}$ | Class 0 | Ref. 18 |
| KiP2 | $2.8 \times 10^{-3}$ | Class 0 | Ref. 18 |
| KcF | 10.0 | Class 3 | |
| KcR | 10.0 | Class 3 | |
| Alpha | 1.0 | Class 0 | |
| Beta | 1.0 | Class 0 | |
| Gamma | 1.0 | Class 0 | |
| Delta | 1.0 | Class 0 | |

***Supporting Table 8. The kinetic properties of AlaTA***

| | | | |
|---|---|---|---|
| Reaction | | Ala + OG ⇔ Glu + Pyr | |
| Mechanism | | Ping-pong Bi Bi[17] | |
| Rate equation | | | |
| Species, organ | | Pig liver | |
| **Parameter** | | **Class** | **Notice** |
| KmS1 | 0.002 | Class 0 | |
| KmS2 | 0.0004 | Class 0 | |
| KmP1 | 0.032 | Class 0 | |
| KmP2 | 0.0004 | Class 0 | |
| KiS1 | 0.0087 | Class 2 | KiP2 |
| KiP2 | 0.012 | Class 0 | |
| Keq | 0.69 | Class 2 | 0.16, AspTA |
| | | | At MW = 78000 |
| KcF | 337 | Class 0 | Activity = 210 micromol/min/mg |
| KcR | 0.15 | Class 3 | |

Source for parameter estimation: Figure 3 with 5 mM glutamate in reference 17.

***Supporting Table 9. The kinetic properties of AspTA***

| | | | |
|---|---|---|---|
| Reaction | | Asp + OG ⇔ O × A + Glu | |
| Mechanism | | Ping-pong Bi Bi[40,41] | |
| Rate equation | | | |
| Species, organ | | Pig heart | |
| **Parameter** | | **Class** | **Notice** |
| KmS1 | $0.9 \times 10^{-3}$ | Class 0 | Ref. 40, Table II |
| KmS2 | $0.1 \times 10^{-3}$ | Class 0 | Ref. 40, Table II |
| KmP1 | $0.04 \times 10^{-3}$ | Class 0 | Ref. 40, Table II |
| KmP2 | $4 \times 10^{-3}$ | Class 0 | Ref. 40, Table II |
| KiS1 | $2 \times 10^{-3}$ | Class 0 | Ref. 40, Table II |
| KiP2 | $8.3 \times 10^{-3}$ | Class 0 | Ref. 40, Table II |
| Keq | 6.2 | Class 0 | |
| KcF | 300 | Class 0 | |
| KcR | 1000 | Class 0 | From k4 and k 10 |

## Supporting Table 10. The kinetic properties of CAC

| | | | |
|---|---|---|---|
| Reaction | | PalCar(IMS) + Car(MAT) ↔ PalCar(MAT) + Car(IMS) | |
| Mechanism | | Ping-pong Bi Bi[25] | |
| Rate equation | | | |
| Species | | Rat liver mitochondria | |
| **Parameter** | | **Class** | **Notice** |
| KmS1 | $0.6 \times 10^{-3}$ | Class 0 | Ref. 25 |
| KmS2 | $9.4 \times 10^{-3}$ | Class 0 | Ref. 25 |
| KmP1 | $43.4 \times 10^{-6}$ | Class 1 | $11.6 \times 10^{-6}$, the value of Car/Car reaction |
| KmP2 | $0.4 \times 10^{-3}$ | Class 1 | $1.2 \times 10^{-3}$, the value of Car/Car reaction |
| KiS1 | $8.7 \times 10^{-6}$ | Class 1 | $5.1 \times 10^{-6}$, ref. 24 |
| KiP2 | $250 \times 10^{-6}$ | Class 1 | $510 \times 10^{-6}$, ref. 24 |
| Keq | 243.3 | Class 3 | |
| KcF | 1.22 | Class 2 | |
| KcR | 1.08 | Class 1 | 0.92, ref. 24 |

Source for parameter estimation: Figure 4 with 13 mM acetylcarnitine in reference 24.

## Supporting Table 11. The kinetic properties of CIC

| | | | |
|---|---|---|---|
| Reaction | | Cit(IMS) + Mal(MAT) ⇔ Cit(MAT) + Mal(IMS) | |
| Mechanism | | Rapid equilibrium random Bi Bi[42] | |
| Rate equation | | | |
| Species | | Rat liver mitochondria | |
| **Parameter** | | **Class** | **Notice** |
| KiS1 | $1.3 \times 10^{-4}$ | Class 2 | |
| KiS2 | $4.4 \times 10^{-4}$ | Class 2 | |
| KiP1 | $3.3 \times 10^{-4}$ | Class 0 | |
| KiP2 | $4.18 \times 10^{-5}$ | Class 0 | |
| KcF | 5.6 | Class 0 | 11.2 mmol/min/g prot. × 30 kDa |
| KcR | 3.5 | Class 1 | KcR = 2.1 (ref. 42, Table II) |
| Alpha | 1.0 | Class 0 | |
| Beta | 1.0 | Class 0 | |
| Gamma | 1.0 | Class 0 | |
| Delta | 1.0 | Class 0 | |

Source for parameter estimation: Figure 1(A) with 0.05 mM citrate, (C) with 0.05 mM malate in reference 42.

***Supporting Table 12. The kinetic properties of complex I***

| | | | |
|---|---|---|---|
| Reaction | | $NADH + Q + 5H^+ (MAT) \Leftrightarrow NAD^+ + QH_2 + 4H^+ (IMS)$ | |
| Mechanism | | Ping-pong Bi Bi[19] | |
| Rate equation | | Eqn. 11 | |
| Species, organ | | Bovine heart mitochondria | |
| **Parameter** | | **Class** | **Notice** |
| KmS1 | $9.2 \times 10^{-6}$ | Class 0 | |
| KmS2 | $2.6 \times 10^{-4}$ | Class 0 | |
| KmP1 | $9.9 \times 10^{-6}$ | Class 2 | |
| KmP2 | $5.9 \times 10^{-5}$ | Class 2 | |
| KiS1 | $2.1 \times 10^{-8}$ | Class 0 | KiS1 = 1/Kmin |
| KiP2 | $9.8 \times 10^{-8}$ | Class 2 | |
| Keq | 407.9 | Class 3 | |
| KcF | 498 | Class 0 | |
| KcR | 229 | Class 2 | |

Source of parameter estimation: Figure 1C with 2.4 μM reduced $CoQ_2$ in reference 19.

***Supporting Table 13. The kinetic properties of complex III***

| | | | |
|---|---|---|---|
| Reaction | | $QH_2 + 2cyt\ c^{3+} + 2H^+ (MAT) \rightarrow Q + 2cyt\ c^{2+} + 4H^+ (IMS)$ | |
| Mechanism | | See ref. 28 scheme 3 | |
| Rate equation | | Eqn. 3 | |
| Species, organ | | Bovine heart mitochondria | |
| **Parameter** | | **Class** | **Notice** |
| KmA | $2.8 \times 10^{-5}$ | Class 0 | K5 × KcF |
| KmB | $3.0 \times 10^{-6}$ | Class 0 | K6 × KcF |
| Kb1 | $5.4 \times 10^{-6}$ | Class 2 | k5/k4, K3 = K4 × Kb1 |
| Kb2 | $5.7 \times 10^{-6}$ | Class 2 | k10/k9, K1 = K2 × Kb2 |
| Kq1 | $2.8 \times 10^{-6}$ | Class 2 | k7/k6, K4 = Kq1/ks |
| Kq2 | $1.9 \times 10^{-6}$ | Class 2 | k12/k11, K2 = K5 × Kq2 |
| K8 | 622.1 | Class 2 | |
| KcF | 426.8 | Class 0 | 1/K7 |

Source for parameter estimation: Figure 6 with 15 μM $Q_2H_2$ in reference 28.

***Supporting Table 14. The kinetic properties of complex IV***

| | | | |
|---|---|---|---|
| Reaction | | $4cyt\ c^{2+} + O_2 + 8H^+(MAT) \rightarrow 4cyt\ c^{3+} + 2H_2O + 4H^+(IMS)$ | |
| Mechanism | | Michaelis-menten ref. 29 | |
| Rate equation | | Eqn. 6 | |
| Species, organ | | | |
| **Parameter** | | **Class** | **Notice** |
| Ks | $110 \times 10^{-6}$ | Class 0 | Value at pH = 7 |
| KcF | 93.5 | Class 0 | Value at pH = 7, $d[cyt\ c^{2+}]/dt \times 1/4$ |

***Supporting Table 15. The kinetic properties of complex V***

| | | | |
|---|---|---|---|
| Reaction | | ADP + Pi + $3H^+$(IMS) ⇔ ATP + $H_2O$ + $3H^+$ (MAT) | |
| Mechanism | | See ref. 26 | |
| Rate equation | | Eqn. 3 | |
| Species, organ | | | |
| **Parameter** | | **Class** | **Notice** |
| Kd | $2.67 \times 10^{-7}$ | Class 3 | |
| Kp | $9.02 \times 10^{-5}$ | Class 3 | |
| Kt | $4.33 \times 10^{-5}$ | Class 3 | |
| KcF | 14.5 | Class 0 | 2340 nmol/min/mg × 371 kDa |
| Khx | $1.3 \times 10^{-4}$ | Class 3 | |
| Khy | $1.6 \times 10^{-4}$ | Class 3 | |
| Klt f | $1.35 \times 10^{8}$ | Class 3 | |
| Klt r | 0.00018 | Class 3 | |
| Ax | 0.1 | Class 3 | |
| Ay | 0.6 | Class 3 | |
| Beta | 0.3 | Class 3 | |
| T | 310 | – | |

Source for parameter estimation: Figure 2 with NADH respiration in reference 43.

***Supporting Table 16. The kinetic properties of CPT I***

| | | | |
|---|---|---|---|
| Reaction | | 16Acyl-CoA + Car ⇔ CoA + PalCar | |
| Mechanism | | Rapid equilibrium random Bi Bi[36] | |
| Rate equation | | | |
| Species, organ | | Bovine liver mitochondria | |
| **Parameter** | | **Class** | **Notice** |
| KiS1 | $182 \times 10^{-6}$ | Class 0 | Ref. 36 |
| KiS2 | $0.82 \times 10^{-6}$ | Class 0 | |
| KiP1 | $6.7 \times 10^{-6}$ | Class 0 | |
| KiP2 | $21 \times 10^{-6}$ | Class 0 | |
| KcF | 61.4 | Class 0 | |
| KcR | 32.8 | Class 0 | |
| Alpha | 1.0 | Class 0 | |
| Beta | 1.0 | Class 0 | |
| Gamma | 1.0 | Class 0 | |
| Delta | 1.0 | Class 0 | |

### Supporting Table 17. The kinetic properties of CPT II

| | | | |
|---|---|---|---|
| Reaction | | CoA + PalCar ⇔ 16Acyl-CoA + Car | |
| Mechanism | | Ordered Bi Bi[30] | |
| Rate equation | | Eqn. 8 | |
| Species, organ | | Rat liver mitochondira | |
| **Parameter** | | **Class** | **Notice** |
| KmS1 | $6.3 \times 10^{-4}$ | Class 2 | |
| KmS2 | $3.3 \times 10^{-4}$ | Class 2 | |
| KmP1 | $950 \times 10^{-6}$ | Class 0 | |
| KmP2 | $34 \times 10^{-6}$ | Class 0 | |
| KiS1 | $2.4 \times 10^{-4}$ | Class 2 | |
| KiS2 | $2.7 \times 10^{-4}$ | Class 2 | |
| KiP1 | $41 \times 10^{-6}$ | Class 0 | |
| KiP2 | $7 \times 10^{-6}$ | Class 0 | |
| Keq | 23540 | Class 3 | |
| KcF | 8.0 | Class 2 | |
| KcR | 2.4 | Class 0 | 1.8 Unit/mg × 80kDa, refs. 30,44 |

Source for parameter estimation: Figure 1 with 0 μM SDZ in reference 30.

### Supporting Table 18. The kinetic properties of CS

| | | | |
|---|---|---|---|
| Reaction | | OXA + Acetyl-CoA ⇔ Cit + CoA | |
| Mechanism | | Random Bi Bi[31,34,45] | |
| Rate equation | | | |
| Species, organ | | Rat kidney, rat brain | |
| **Parameter** | | **Class** | **Notice** |
| k1 | $6.8 \times 10^{10}$ | Class 3 | |
| k_1 | $8.1 \times 10^{8}$ | Class 3 | |
| k2 | $3.0 \times 10^{10}$ | Class 3 | |
| k_2 | $7.2 \times 10^{8}$ | Class 3 | |
| k3 | $6.2 \times 10^{10}$ | Class 3 | |
| k_3 | $5.1 \times 10^{8}$ | Class 3 | |
| k4 | $1.2 \times 10^{10}$ | Class 3 | |
| k_4 | $4.0 \times 10^{8}$ | Class 3 | |
| k5 | $1.4 \times 10^{9}$ | Class 3 | |
| k_5 | $2.4 \times 10^{8}$ | Class 3 | |
| k6 | $4.1 \times 10^{10}$ | Class 3 | |
| k_6 | $1.1 \times 10^{8}$ | Class 3 | |
| k7 | $5 \times 10^{10}$ | Class 3 | |
| k_7 | $9.8 \times 10^{8}$ | Class 3 | |
| k8 | $5.3 \times 10^{10}$ | Class 3 | |
| k_8 | $7.7 \times 10^{8}$ | Class 3 | |

Source for parameter estimation: reference 31.

### *Supporting Table 19. The kinetic properties of DIC*

| | | | |
|---|---|---|---|
| Reaction | | Mal(IMS) + Pi(MAT) ⇔ Mal(MAT) + Pi(IMS) | |
| Mechanism | | Rapid equilibrium random Bi Bi[46] | |
| Rate equation | | Eqn. 12 | |
| Species, organ | | Rat liver mitochondria | |
| **Parameter** | | **Class** | **Notice** |
| KiS1 | $0.20 \times 10^{-3}$ | Class 0 | Ref. 46, Fig.5 |
| KiS2 | $0.72 \times 10^{-3}$ | Class 0 | Ref. 46, Fig.5 |
| KiP1 | $9.0 \times 10^{-4}$ | Class 2 | |
| KiP2 | $7.6 \times 10^{-4}$ | Class 2 | |
| KcF | 2.7 | Class 0 | $6.7 \times 10^{-6}$ mol/min/mg × 28 kDa |
| KcR | 4.1 | Class 1 | |
| Alpha | 1.0 | Class 0 | |
| Beta | 1.0 | Class 0 | |
| Gamma | 1.0 | Class 0 | |
| Delta | 1.0 | Class 0 | |

Source for parameter estimation: Figure 5A with 0.05 mM phosphate, (C) with 0.10 mM malate in reference 46.

### *Supporting Table 20. The kinetic properties of ECH*

| | | | |
|---|---|---|---|
| Reaction | | Enoyl-CoA + $H_2O$ ⇔ 3-hydroxyacyl-CoA | |
| Mechanism | | Uni uni reversible[39] | |
| Rate equation | | Eqn. 14 | |
| Species, organ | | Bovine liver | |
| **Parameter** | | **Class** | **Notice** |
| Ks | $16.9 \times 10^{-6}$ | Class 0 | |
| Kp | $12.1 \times 10^{-6}$ | Class 0 | |
| KcF | 8.9166667 | Class 0 | |
| KcR | 2154.1667 | Class 0 | |

***Supporting Table 21. The kinetic properties of ETF-QO***

| | | | |
|---|---|---|---|
| Reaction | | ETFred + Q ⇔ ETFox + $QH_2$ | |
| Mechanism | | Ping-pong Bi Bi[14] | |
| Rate equation | | Eqn. 11 | |
| Species, organ | | Pig liver mitochondria | |
| **Parameter** | | **Class** | **Notice** |
| KmS1 | $0.31 \times 10^{-6}$ | Class 0 | |
| KmS2 | $0.39 \times 10^{-6}$ | Class 2 | |
| KmP1 | $0.32 \times 10^{-6}$ | Class 0 | |
| KmP2 | $4.2 \times 10^{-9}$ | class 2 | |
| KiS1 | $0.31 \times 10^{-6}$ | Class 0 | |
| KiP2 | $0.3 \times 10^{-6-6}$ | Class 2 | |
| Keq | 0.66 | Class 0 | |
| KcF | 78 | Class 0 | |
| KcR | 101 | Class 2 | |

Source for parameter estimation: Figure 4 with 1.5 μM ETF hydroquinone in reference 14.

***Supporting Table 22. The kinetic properties of FM***

| | | | |
|---|---|---|---|
| Reaction | | Fum ⇔ Mal | |
| Mechanism | | Uni uni reversible | |
| Rate equation | | Eqn. 14 | |
| Species, organ | | | |
| **Parameter** | | **Class** | **Notice** |
| Ks | $0.5 \times 10^{-5}$ | Class 0 | Ref. 47, Table V |
| Kp | $2.5 \times 10^{-5}$ | Class 0 | |
| KcF | 800 | Class 0 | |
| KcR | 900 | Class 0 | |

***Supporting Table 23. The kinetic properties of HCD***

| | | | |
|---|---|---|---|
| Reaction | | 3-hydroxyacyl-CoA + $NAD^+$ ⇔ 3-oxoacyl-CoA + NADH | |
| Mechanism | | Michaelis-menten[39] | |
| Rate equation | | Eqn. 6 | |
| Species, organ | | Pig heart | |
| **Parameter** | | **Class** | **Notice** |
| Ks | $1.5 \times 10^{-6}$ | Class 0 | |
| KcF | 41.483333 | Class 0 | |

***Supporting Table 24. The kinetic properties of IDHa***

| | | | |
|---|---|---|---|
| Reaction | | $IsoCit + NAD^+ \rightarrow OG + NADH$ | |
| Mechanism | | Ref. 35 | |
| Rate equation | | Eqn. 5 | |
| Species, organ | | Bovine heart | |
| **Parameter** | | **Class** | **Notice** |
| KcF | 105 | Class 0 | 28 U/mg × 224000 Da (refs. 35,48) |
| b | 29.6 | Class 3 | |
| c | 0.00023 | Class 3 | |
| d | $7.8 \times 10^{-5}$ | Class 3 | |
| E | 0.00064 | Class 3 | |
| F | 0.00036 | Class 3 | |

Source for parameter estimation: Figure 4 with 1.0 mM ADP in reference 35.

***Supporting Table 25. The kinetic properties of IDHb***

| | | | |
|---|---|---|---|
| Reaction | | $IsoCit + NADP^+ \Leftrightarrow OG + NADPH$ | |
| Mechanism | | See ref. 49 | |
| Rate equation | | Eqn. 5 | |
| Species, organ | | Bovine heart mitochondria | |
| **Parameter** | | **Class** | **Notice** |
| Phi0 | $5.1 \times 10^{-2}$ | Class 0 | Ref. 49, Table 1 |
| Phi1 | $9.5 \times 10^{-8}$ | Class 0 | |
| Phi2 | $0.96 \times 10^{-6}$ | Class 0 | |
| Phi12 | $9 \times 10^{-8}$ | Class 0 | |
| Phir0 | $6.6 \times 10^{-2}$ | Class 0 | |
| Phir1 | $0.37 \times 10^{-6}$ | Class 0 | |
| Phir2 | $29 \times 10^{-6}$ | Class 0 | |
| Phir3 | $2.5 \times 10^{-4}$ | Class 0 | |
| Phir12 | $6 \times 10^{-12}$ | Class 0 | |
| Phir13 | $1.3 \times 10^{-10}$ | Class 0 | |
| Phir23 | $9.4 \times 10^{-8}$ | Class 0 | |
| Phir123 | $4.6 \times 10^{-14}$ | Class 0 | |

### *Supporting Table 26. The kinetic properties of MDH*

| | | | |
|---|---|---|---|
| Reaction | | Mal + $NAD^+$ ⇔ OXA + NADH | |
| Mechanism | | Ordered Bi Bi ref. 15 | |
| Rate equation | | Eqn. 9 | |
| Species, organ | | Human liver cytosol | |
| **Parameter** | | **Class** | **Notice** |
| KmS1 | $72 \times 10^{-6}$ | Class 0 | |
| KmS2 | $110 \times 10^{-6}$ | Class 0 | |
| KmP1 | $1600 \times 10^{-6}$ | Class 0 | |
| KmP2 | $170 \times 10^{-6}$ | Class 0 | |
| KiS1 | $11 \times 10^{-6}$ | Class 0 | |
| KiS2 | $100 \times 10^{-6}$ | Class 0 | |
| KiP1 | $7100 \times 10^{-6}$ | Class 0 | |
| KiP2 | $1900 \times 10^{-6}$ | Class 0 | |
| KcF | 0.390 | Class 0 | Specific activity = 0.33 U/mg, MW = 72000 (ref. 15, Table I) |
| KcR | 0.040 | Class 0 | Vf/Vr = 9.8 (ref. 15, Table III) |

### *Supporting Table 27. The kinetic properties of NDK*

| | | | |
|---|---|---|---|
| Reaction | | ATP + GDP ⇔ ADP + GTP | |
| Mechanism | | Ping-pong Bi Bi[50,51] | |
| Rate equation | | Eqn. 11 | |
| Species, organ | | Yeast | |
| **Parameter** | | **Class** | **Notice** |
| KmS1 | $0.31 \times 10^{-3}$ | Class 0 | Ref. 51 |
| KmS2 | $0.043 \times 10^{-3}$ | Class 0 | Ref. 51, UDP |
| KmP1 | $0.050 \times 10^{-3}$ | Class 0 | Ref. 51 |
| KmP2 | $0.25 \times 10^{-3}$ | Class 0 | Ref. 51, UTP |
| KiS1 | $0.21 \times 10^{-3}$ | Class 2 | Ref. 51 |
| KiP2 | $0.35 \times 10^{-3}$ | Class 2 | Ref. 51, UTP |
| Keq | 1.28 | Class 0 | Ref. 51 |
| KcF | 6883 | Class 0 | MW = 70000 Da, ref. 50 |
| KcR | 5950 | Class 0 | MW = 70000 Da, ref. 50 |

Source for parameter estimation: Figure 4 with 0.18 mM ATP in reference 50.

**Supporting Table 28. The kinetic properties of OCT**

| | | | |
|---|---|---|---|
| Reaction | | 3-oxoacyl-CoA + CoA ⇔ Acyl-CoA + Acetyl-CoA | |
| Mechanism | | Ping-pong Bi Bi[33] | |
| Rate equation | | Eqn. 11 | |
| Species, organ | | Rat liver mitochondria | |
| **Parameter** | | **Class** | **Notice** |
| KmS1 | $1.1 \times 10^{-6}$ | Class 0 | OCTa |
| | $1.10 \times 10^{-6}$ | Class 0 | OCTb, value for 16Oxoacyl-CoA |
| | $1.30 \times 10^{-6}$ | Class 0 | OCTc |
| | $2.10 \times 10^{-6}$ | Class 0 | OCTd |
| | $3.20 \times 10^{-6}$ | Class 0 | OCTe |
| | $6.70 \times 10^{-6}$ | Class 0 | OCTf |
| | $1.24 \times 10^{-6}$ | Class 0 | OCTg |
| KmS2 | $28.6 \times 10^{-6}$ | Class 0 | |
| | $2.86 \times 10^{-6}$ | Class 0 | OCTb, value for 16Oxoacyl-CoA |
| | $3.84 \times 10^{-6}$ | Class 0 | OCTc |
| | $3.57 \times 10^{-6}$ | Class 0 | OCTd |
| | $3.55 \times 10^{-6}$ | Class 0 | OCTe |
| | $1.89 \times 10^{-6}$ | Class 0 | OCTf |
| | $2.20 \times 10^{-6}$ | Class 0 | OCTg |
| KmP1 | $7.2 \times 10^{-5}$ | Class 2 | |
| KmP2 | $8.7 \times 10^{-5}$ | Class 2 | |
| KiS1 | $1.1 \times 10^{-5}$ | Class 2 | |
| KiP2 | $8.7 \times 10^{-5}$ | Class 2 | |
| Keq | 160.98 | Class 3 | |
| KcF | 137.86 | Class 0 | Vma x 178000 Da |
| | 137.86 | Class 0 | OCTb, value for 16Oxoacyl-CoA |
| | 253.52 | Class 0 | OCTc |
| | 272.94 | Class 0 | OCTd |
| | 277.38 | Class 0 | OCTe |
| | 264.07 | Class 0 | OCTf |
| | 80.244 | Class 0 | OCTg |
| KcR | 87.253 | Class 2 | |
| | 87.253 | Class 2 | OCTb, value for 16Oxoacyl-CoA |
| | 160.46 | Class 2 | OCTc |
| | 172.75 | Class 2 | OCTd |
| | 175.56 | Class 2 | OCTe |
| | 167.13 | Class 2 | OCTf |
| | 51.615 | Class 2 | OCTg |

Source for parameter estimation: Figure 5B with 200 μM Acetyl-CoA in reference 33.

**Supporting Table 29. The kinetic properties of OGC**

| | | | |
|---|---|---|---|
| Reaction | | OG(IMS) + Mal(MAT) ⇔ OG(MAT) + Mal(IMS) | |
| Mechanism | | Rapid equilibrium random Bi Bi[23] | |
| Rate equation | | Eqn. 12 | |
| Species, organ | | Bovine heart mitochondria | |
| **Parameter** | | **Class** | **Notice** |
| KiS1 | $0.3 \times 10^{-3}$ | Class 0 | |
| KiS2 | $0.7 \times 10^{-3}$ | Class 2 | |
| KiP1 | $1.4 \times 10^{-3}$ | Class 0 | |
| KiP2 | $0.17 \times 10^{-3}$ | Class 2 | |
| KcF | 3.675 | Class 0 | |
| KcR | 4.83 | Class 0 | |
| Alpha | 1.0 | Class 0 | |
| Beta | 1.0 | Class 0 | |
| Gamma | 1.0 | Class 0 | |
| Delta | 1.0 | Class 0 | |

Source for parameter estimation: Figure 2 with 20 mM malate in reference 23.

**Supporting Table 30. The kinetic properties of OGDC**

| | | | |
|---|---|---|---|
| Reaction | | $OG + NAD^+ + CoA \rightarrow SCoA + NADH + CO_2$ | |
| Mechanism | | Multisite ping-pong[22,52] | |
| Rate equation | | Eqn. 7 | |
| Species, organ | | Pig heart mitochondria | |
| **Parameter** | | **Class** | **Notice** |
| KmA | $0.22 \times 10^{-3}$ | Class 0 | Pig heart ref. 22 |
| KmB | $0.025 \times 10^{-3}$ | Class 0 | Pig heart ref. 22 |
| KmC | $0.050 \times 10^{-3}$ | Class 0 | Pig heart ref. 22 |
| KmP | $3 \times 10^{-4}$ | Class 2 | |
| KmR | $6 \times 10^{-4}$ | Class 2 | |
| Kia | $7.2 \times 10^{-4}$ | Class 2 | $0.75 \times 10^{-3}$, Dictyostelium, |
| Kib | $7.4 \times 10^{-4}$ | Class 2 | |
| Kic | $1 \times 10^{-4}$ | Class 2 | |
| Kip | $1.1 \times 10^{-6}$ | Class 2 | |
| Kiq | $81 \times 10^{-6}$ | Class 0 | Human heart ref. 53 |
| Kir | $25 \times 10^{-6}$ | Class 0 | Human heart ref. 53 |
| KcF | 177 | Class 2 | Estimated, 270 at MW = 2700000 Da |

Source for parameter estimation: Figure 1A with 0.010 mM CoA, (B) with 0.20 mM $NAD^+$, (C) with 0.10mM oxoglutarate in reference 22.

***Supporting Table 31. The kinetic properties of PC***

| | | | |
|---|---|---|---|
| Reaction | | Pyr + ATP + $CO_2$ ⇔ OXA + ADP + Pi | |
| Mechanism | | Ref. 13 | |
| Rate equation | | Eqn. 10 | |
| Species, organ | | Chicken liver | |
| **Parameter** | | **Class** | **Notice** |
| KmA | $0.11 \times 10^{-3}$ | Class 0 | ATP, Table III, inhibitor = MgADP |
| KmB | $1.63 \times 10^{-3}$ | Class 0 | $HCO_3$ , Table III, inhibitor = OXA |
| KmC | $0.37 \times 10^{-3}$ | Class 0 | Pyr, Table III, inhibitor = OXA |
| KmP | $16 \times 10^{-3}$ | Class 0 | Pi, Table III, inhibitor = MgATP |
| KmQ | $0.24 \times 10^{-3}$ | Class 0 | ADP, Table III, inhibitor = MgATP |
| KmR | $0.051 \times 10^{-3}$ | Class 0 | OXA, Table III, inhibitor = Pyr |
| Keq | 9.0 | Class 0 | |
| Kia | $0.15 \times 10^{-3}$ | Class 0 | ATP, Table I |
| Kib | $1.6 \times 10^{-3}$ | Class 0 | HCO3 , Table I |
| Kic | $0.13 \times 10^{-3}$ | Class 0 | Pyr, Table III, vs OXA |
| Kip | $7.9 \times 10^{-3}$ | Class 0 | Pi, Table I |
| Kiq | $0.19 \times 10^{-3}$ | Class 0 | ADP, Table I |
| Kir | $0.24 \times 10^{-3}$ | Class 0 | OXA, Table III, vs Pyr |
| KcF | 200 | Class 0 | Specific activity = 20, MW = 600000 |
| KcR | 20 | Class 0 | V1/V2 = 10 |

***Supporting Table 32. The kinetic properties of PDC***

| | | | |
|---|---|---|---|
| Reaction | | Pyr + $NAD^+$ + CoA ⇔ Acetyl-CoA + NADH + $CO_2$ | |
| Mechanism | | Multisite ping-pong[22,52] | |
| Rate equation | | Eqn. 7 | |
| Species, organ | | Pig heart mitochondria | |
| **Parameter** | | **Class** | **Notice** |
| KmA | $25 \times 10^{-6}$ | Class 0 | Ref. 53 |
| KmB | $13 \times 10^{-6}$ | Class 0 | Ref. 53 |
| KmC | $50 \times 10^{-6}$ | Class 0 | Ref. 53 |
| KmP | $5.9 \times 10^{-7}$ | Class 2 | |
| KmR | $6.9 \times 10^{-7}$ | Class 2 | |
| Kia | $5.5 \times 10^{-4}$ | Class 2 | Dictyostelium, ref. 54 |
| Kib | $3.0 \times 10^{-4}$ | Class 2 | |
| Kic | $1.8 \times 10^{-4}$ | Class 2 | |
| Kip | $6.0 \times 10^{-5}$ | Class 2 | |
| Kiq | $35 \times 10^{-6}$ | Class 0 | Human heart, ref. 53 |
| Kir | $36 \times 10^{-6}$ | Class 0 | Human heart, ref. 53 |
| KcF | 856 | Class 1 | Specific activity = 4.8 U/mg protein ref. 53 |

Source for parameter estimation: Figure 2A with 0.015 mM CoA, (B) with 0.050 mM $NAD^+$, (C) with 0.050 mM pyruvate in reference 22.

***Supporting Table 33. The kinetic properties of PIC***

| | | | |
|---|---|---|---|
| Reaction | | $Pi(IMS) + H^+(IMS) \Leftrightarrow Pi(MAT) + H^+(MAT)$ | |
| Mechanism | | Rapid equilibrium random Bi Bi[38] | |
| Rate equation | | Eqn. 12 | |
| Species | | Rat heart mitochondria | |
| **Parameter** | | **Class** | **Notice** |
| KiS1 | 0.87 | Class 2 | |
| KiS2 | $1.86 \times 10^{-8}$ | Class 2 | |
| KiP1 | $32.84 \times 10^{-9}$ | Class 0 | Fig. 4, ref. 38 |
| KiP2 | $11.12 \times 10^{-3}$ | Class 0 | Fig. 4, ref. 38 |
| KcF | 37.9 | Class 0 | Fig. 4, ref. 38 |
| KcR | 37.0 | Class 0 | Fig. 4, ref. 38 |
| Alpha | 1.0 | Class 0 | |
| Beta | 1.0 | Class 0 | |
| Gamma | 1.0 | Class 0 | |
| Delta | 1.0 | Class 0 | |

Source for parameter estimation: Figure 4A with pH5.85, (B) with 4 mM phosphate in reference 38.

***Supporting Table 34. The kinetic properties of PYC***

| | | | |
|---|---|---|---|
| Reaction | | $Pyr(IMS) + H^+(MAT) \Leftrightarrow Pyr(MAT) + H^+(IMS)$ | |
| Mechanism | | Rapid equilibrium random Bi Bi ("Sequential Mechanism" in ref. 55) | |
| Rate equation | | Eqn. 12 | |
| Species, organ | | Rat liver mitochondria | |
| **Parameter** | | **Class** | **Notice** |
| KiS1 | $6.1 \times 10^{-4}$ | Class 2 | |
| KiS2 | $5.9 \times 10^{-4}$ | Class 2 | |
| Kip1 | $2.6 \times 10^{-4}$ | Class 2 | |
| Kip2 | $4.1 \times 10^{-4}$ | Class 2 | |
| KcF | 0.84 | Class 1 | 0.67 ref. 56 |
| KcR | 0.78 | Class 0 | 0.61 ref. 56 |
| Alpha | 1.0 | Class 0 | |
| Beta | 1.0 | Class 0 | |
| Gamma | 1.0 | Class 0 | |
| Delta | 1.0 | Class 0 | |

Source for parameter estimation: Figure 3 in reference 56.

***Supporting Table 35. The kinetic properties of SCS***

| | | | |
|---|---|---|---|
| Reaction | | SCoA + GDP + Pi ⇔ Suc + CoA + GTP | |
| Mechanism | | See ref. 57 | |
| Rate equation | | Eqn. 13 | |
| Species, organ | | Pig heart | |
| **Parameter** | | **Class** | **Notice** |
| KmA | $5 \times 10^{-6}$ | Class 0 | GDP ($2–8 \times 10^{-6}$) |
| KmB | $3.5 \times 10^{-5}$ | Class 0 | Succinyl-CoA ($1–6 \times 10^{-5}$) |
| KmC | $4.5 \times 10^{-4}$ | Class 0 | Pi ($2–7 \times 10–4$) |
| KmP | $6 \times 10^{-4}$ | Class 0 | Succinate ($4–8 \times 10^{-4}$) |
| KmQ | $7.5 \times 10^{-6}$ | Class 0 | GTP ($5–10 \times 10^{-6}$) |
| KmC2 | $4.5 \times 10^{-4}$ | Class 0 | Pi ($2–7 \times 10^{-4}$) |
| KmP | $2\ 6 \times 10^{-4}$ | Class 0 | Succinate ($4–8 \times 10^{-4}$) |
| Keq | 8.375 | Class 0 | From haldane relationships |
| Kia | $4 \times 10^{-4}$ | Class 0 | GDP (Table II) |
| Kib | $2 \times 10^{-5}$ | Class 0 | Succinyl-CoA, (vs CoA, Fig. 7) |
| Kic | $3 \times 10^{-5}$ | Class 0 | Pi (Table II) |
| Kip | $7 \times 10^{-2}$ | Class 0 | Succinate (Table II) |
| Kiq | $5 \times 10^{-6}$ | Class 0 | GTP (Table II) |
| Kir | $6.7 \times 10^{-6}$ | Class 0 | CoA, from a haldane relationship, Kq × Kir = Kiq × Kr |
| Kc1 | 100 | | Where Kr (CoA) = $10 \times 10^{-6}$ M |
| Kc2 | 100 | Class 0 | Kcat = Kc2 = 25 to 287.5 (20 to 230 U/mg × 75000 dalton) |
| Kia | $4 \times 10^{-4}$ | Class 3 | Guess, V1/V2 = 0.20, V2'/V1' = 30 |

***Supporting Table 36. The kinetic properties of SDH***

| | | | |
|---|---|---|---|
| Reaction | | Suc + Q ⇔ Fum + $QH_2$ | |
| Mechanism | | Ping-pong Bi Bi[20] | |
| Rate equation | | Eqn. 11 | |
| Species, organ | | Bovine heart mitochondria | |
| **Paramenter** | | **Class** | **Notice** |
| KmS1 | $30 \times 10^{-6}$ | Class 0 | |
| KmS2 | $69 \times 10^{-6}$ | Class 0 | $30–130 \times 10^{-6}$ |
| KmP1 | $0.3 \times 10^{-6}$ | Class 0 | |
| KmP2 | $1.5 \times 10^{-6}$ | Class 0 | |
| KiS1 | $4.1 \times 10^{-6}$ | Class 2 | Ki for carbo x in = $3.0 \times 10^{-6}$ M |
| KiP2 | $5.6 \times 10^{-6}$ | Class 2 | Ki for carbo x in = $3.0 \times 10^{-6}$ M |
| Keq | 0.037 | Class 0 | From Haldane relationship |
| KcF | 69.3 | Class 0 | MW = 104000 Da |
| KcR | 1.73 | Class 0 | MW = 104000 Da |

Source for parameter estimation: Figure 2B in reference 20.

## Rate Equations

### *AAC*

$$v = \frac{\dfrac{k^D_{\rightarrow}(\Delta\psi)[E_{total}][ADP_{out}]}{1+\dfrac{k^D_{\rightarrow}(\Delta\psi)}{k^D_{\leftarrow}(\Delta\psi)}\left(1+\dfrac{K^{D'}}{[ADP_{in}]}\right)}}{\dfrac{K^{D'}}{1+\dfrac{k^D_{\rightarrow}(\Delta\psi)}{k^D_{\leftarrow}(\Delta\psi)}\left(1+\dfrac{K^{D'}}{[ADP_{in}]}\right)}+[ADP_{out}]} \quad (1)$$

where $k^D_{\rightarrow}(\Delta\psi) = k^D_{0\rightarrow}e^{\phi \cdot C_f} \cdot normalize$

$k^D_{\leftarrow}(\Delta\psi) = k^D_{0\leftarrow}e^{\phi \cdot C_r} \cdot normalize$

$\phi = \dfrac{RT}{F}\ln\dfrac{[H_{IMS}]}{[H_{MAT}]}$

### *Complex III*

$$v = \frac{K_{cF}[Et][A][B]}{Denom} \quad (2)$$

$$\begin{aligned} Denom &= (K_{mA}K_{q2}K_{b2} + K_{mA}K_{q2} + \frac{K_{cF}}{k_8}K_{q1}[A]K_{b1} + \frac{K_{cF}}{k_8}K_{q1}[A][B])[Q] \\ &+ K_{mA}[B] + K_{mB}[A] + [A][B] \end{aligned}$$

### *Complex V*

$$v = \frac{K_{cF}[E]\left\{\dfrac{[ADP][Pi]}{K_dK_p}klt_f \cdot e^{-3(\beta-\alpha_x)\phi}\left(\dfrac{[H^+_{IMS}]}{Khx \cdot e^{ax\phi}}\right)^3 - \dfrac{[ATP]}{K_t}K_{eq}\cdot klt_r \cdot e^{3(1-\beta-\alpha_y)\phi}\left(\dfrac{[H^+_{MAT}]}{Khy \cdot e^{-ay\phi}}\right)^3\right\}}{\left(1+\dfrac{[H^+_{IMS}]}{Khx \cdot e^{ax\phi}}+\dfrac{[H^+_{MAT}]}{Khy \cdot e^{-ay\phi}}\right)^3\left(3+\dfrac{[ADP][Pi]}{K_dK_p}+\dfrac{[ATP]}{K_t}\right)} \quad (3)$$

where $\phi = \ln\dfrac{[H_{IMS}]}{[H_{MAT}]}$

### *IDHa*

$$v = \frac{k_{cat}[E]\left([IsoCit]^2 + b[ADP][IsoCit]\right)}{[IsoCit]^2 + c[IsoCit] + d[ADP] + e[ADP][IsoCit] + f} \quad (4)$$

### *IDHb*

$$v = \frac{[E][NADP][IsoCit]}{Denom1} - \frac{[E][NADPH][OG][CO_2]}{Denom2} \quad (5)$$

$$\begin{aligned} Denom1 &= \phi_0[NADP][IsoCit] + \phi_1[IsoCit] + \phi_2[NADP] + \phi_{12} \\ Denom2 &= \phi_0'[NADPH][OG][CO_2] + \phi_1'[OG][CO_2] + \phi_2'[NADPH][CO_2] \\ &+ \phi_3'[NADPH][OG] + \phi_{12}'[CO_2] + \phi_{13}'[OG] + \phi_{23}'[NADPH] + \phi_{123}' \end{aligned}$$

### Michaelis-Menten

$$v = \frac{K_{cF}[E][S]}{K_s + [S]} \tag{6}$$

### Multisite Ping-Pong

$$v = \frac{k_{cat}[E_{total}][A][B][C]}{Denom} \tag{7}$$

$$\begin{aligned} Denom = {} & K_{mC}[A][B] + K_{mB}[A][C] + K_{mA}[B][C] + [A][B][C] + \frac{K_{mA}K_{mP}K_{ib}K_{ic}[Q][R]}{K_{mR}K_{ip}K_{iq}} \\ & \frac{K_{mC}[A][B][R]}{K_{ir}} + \frac{K_{mB}[A][C][Q]}{K_{iq}} + \frac{K_{mA}K_{mP}K_{ib}K_{ic}[A][Q][R]}{K_{mR}K_{ip}K_{ia}K_{iq}} \end{aligned}$$

### Ordered Bi Bi (1)

$$v = \frac{K_{cF}K_{cR}[E]\left([S1][S2] - \frac{[P1][P2]}{K_{eq}}\right)}{Denom} \tag{8}$$

$$\begin{aligned} Denom = {} & K_{cR}K_{iS1}K_{mS2} + K_{cR}K_{mS2}[S1] + K_{cR}K_{mS1}[S2] + \frac{K_{cF}K_{mP2}[P1]}{K_{eq}} + \frac{K_{cF}K_{mP1}[P2]}{K_{eq}} \\ & + K_{cR}[S1][S2] + \frac{K_{cF}K_{mP2}[S1][P1]}{K_{eq}K_{iS1}} + \frac{K_{cF}[P1][P2]}{K_{eq}} + \frac{K_{cR}K_{mS1}[S2][P2]}{K_{iq}} + \frac{K_{cR}[S1][S2][P1]}{K_{iP1}} \\ & + \frac{K_{cF}[S2][P1][P2]}{K_{iS2}K_{eq}} \end{aligned}$$

### Ordered Bi Bi (2)

$$v = \frac{\left(\frac{KcF[S1][S2]}{K_{iS1}K_{mS2}} - \frac{KcR[P1][P2]}{K_{mP1}K_{iP2}}\right)\cdot[E]}{Denom} \tag{9}$$

$$\begin{aligned} Denom = {} & 1 + \frac{[S1]}{K_{iS1}} + \frac{K_{mS1}[S2]}{K_{iS1}K_{mS2}} + \frac{K_{mP2}[P1]}{K_{mP1}K_{iP2}} + \frac{[P2]}{K_{iP2}} + \frac{[S1][S2]}{K_{iS1}K_{mS2}} + \frac{K_{mP2}[S1][P1]}{K_{iS1}K_{mP1}K_{iP2}} \\ & + \frac{K_{mS1}[S2][P2]}{K_{iS1}K_{mS2}K_{iP2}} + \frac{[P1][P2]}{K_{mP1}K_{iP2}} + \frac{[S1][S2][P1]}{K_{iS1}K_{mS2}K_{iP1}} + \frac{[S2][P1][P2]}{K_{iS2}K_{mP1}K_{iP2}} \end{aligned}$$

***PC***

$$v = \frac{V_1V_2[A][B][C] - \dfrac{V_1V_2[P][Q][R]}{K_{eq}}}{Denom} \tag{10}$$

$$\begin{aligned} Denom = {} & K_{ia}K_{mB}V_2[C] + K_{mC}V_2[A][B] + K_{mA}V_2[B][C] + K_{mB}V_2[B][C] + K_{mB}V_2[A][C] + V_2[A][B][C] \\ & + \frac{K_{ip}K_{mQ}V_1[R]}{K_{eq}} + \frac{K_{mQ}V_1[P][R]}{K_{eq}} + \frac{K_{mP}V_1[Q][R]}{K_{eq}} + \frac{K_{mR}V_1[P][Q]}{K_{eq}} + \frac{V_1[P][Q][R]}{K_{eq}} \\ & + \frac{K_{ia}K_{mB}V_2[C][P]}{K_{ip}} + \frac{K_{ia}K_{mB}V_2[C][Q]}{K_{ip}} + \frac{K_{iq}K_{mP}V_1[B][R]}{K_{ib}K_{eq}} + \frac{K_{iq}K_{mP}V_1[A][R]}{K_{ia}K_{eq}} \\ & + \frac{K_{ia}V_2[A][B][R]}{K_{ir}} + \frac{K_{mR}V_1[C][P][Q]}{K_{ic}K_{eq}} + \frac{K_{mA}V_2[B][C][Q]}{K_{iq}} + \frac{K_{mA}V_2[B][C][P]}{K_{ip}} \\ & + \frac{K_{mP}V_1[B][Q][R]}{K_{ib}K_{eq}} + \frac{K_{mQ}V_1[B][P][R]}{K_{ib}K_{eq}} \end{aligned}$$

***Ping-Pong Bi Bi***

$$v = \frac{K_{cF}K_{cR}[E]\left([S1][S2] - \dfrac{[P1][P2]}{K_{eq}}\right)}{Denom} \tag{11}$$

$$\begin{aligned} Denom = {} & K_{cR}K_{mS2}[S1] + K_{cR}K_{mS1}[S2] + \frac{K_{cF}K_{mP2}[P1]}{K_{eq}} + \frac{K_{cF}K_{mP1}[P2]}{K_{eq}} + K_{cR}[S1][S2] \\ & + \frac{K_{cF}K_{mP2}[S1][P1]}{K_{eq}K_{iS1}} + \frac{K_{cF}[P1][P2]}{K_{eq}} + \frac{K_{cR}K_{mS1}[S2][P2]}{K_{iq}} \end{aligned}$$

***Rapid Equilibrium Random Bi Bi***

$$v = \frac{\dfrac{[A][B]}{\alpha K_{iA}K_{iB}} k_{cat}^{f}[E]_{total} - \dfrac{[P][Q]}{\beta K_{iP}K_{iQ}} k_{cat}^{r}[E]_{total}}{1 + \dfrac{[A]}{K_{iA}} + \dfrac{[B]}{K_{iB}} + \dfrac{[P]}{K_{iP}} + \dfrac{[Q]}{K_{iQ}} + \dfrac{[A][B]}{\alpha K_{iA}K_{iB}} + \dfrac{[P][Q]}{\beta K_{iP}K_{iQ}} + \dfrac{[B][Q]}{\gamma K_{iB}K_{iQ}} + \dfrac{[A][P]}{\delta K_{iA}K_{iP}}} \tag{12}$$

***SCS***

$$v = \frac{\left([A][B][C] - \frac{[P][Q][R]}{K_{eq}}\right)\left\{V_1 + V_2\left(\frac{K_{mC}[P]}{K_{mC2}K_{ip}} + \frac{[C]}{K_{mC2}}\right)\right\}}{Denom} \tag{13}$$

$$\begin{aligned} Denom = \; & K_{ia}K_{mB}[C] + K_{mB}[A][C] + K_{mA}[B][C] + K_{mC}[A][B] + [A][B][C] \\ & + \frac{[A][B][C]^2}{K_{mC2}} + \frac{K_{ia}K_{mB}K_{mC}[P]}{K_{ip}} + \frac{K_{ia}K_{mB}K_{mC}[P][Q]}{K_{ip}K_{iq}} + \frac{K_{ia}K_{mB}K_{mC}[P][R]}{K_{ip}K_{ir}} \\ & + \frac{K_{ia}K_{mB}K_{ic}[Q][R]}{K_{mQ}K_{ir}} + \frac{K_{ia}K_{mB}K_{mC}[P][Q][R]}{K_{ip}K_{mQ}K_{ir}} + \frac{K_{ia}K_{mB}K_{mC}[P]^2[Q][R]}{K_{ip}K_{mP2}K_{mQ}K_{ir}} \\ & + \frac{K_{ia}K_{mB}[C][Q]}{K_{iq}} + \frac{K_{ia}K_{mB}[C][R]}{K_{ir}} + \frac{K_{ia}K_{mB}[C][Q][R]}{K_{mQ}K_{ir}} + \frac{K_{ia}K_{mB}[C][P][Q][R]}{K_{mP2}K_{mQ}K_{ir}} \\ & + \frac{K_{mB}K_{mC}[A][P]}{K_{ip}} + \frac{K_{mA}K_{mC}[B][P]}{K_{ip}} + \frac{K_{mC}[A][B][P]}{K_{ip}} + \frac{K_{mC}[A][B][C][P]}{K_{mC2}K_{ip}} \\ & + \frac{K_{mA}[B][C][Q]}{K_{iq}} + \frac{K_{mB}[A][C][R]}{K_{ir}} + \frac{K_{mA}K_{mC}[B][P][Q]}{K_{ip}K_{iq}} + \frac{K_{mB}K_{mC}[A][P][R]}{K_{ip}K_{ir}} \end{aligned}$$

***Uni Uni Reversible***

$$v = \frac{\left(K_{cF}K_p[S] - K_{cR}K_s[P]\right)[E]}{K_s[P] + K_p[S] + K_sK_p} \tag{14}$$

# Chapter 9

# A Computational Model of the Hepatic Lobule

**Yasuhiro Naito***

## Abstract

While many inter-organ and intra-organ gene regulations have been found recently, *raison d'être* of such regulations are hardly explicated. We aimed liver ammonia detoxification as a prospective target because of its simple histological structure and adopted systems biology approach to elucidate the question. In the mammalian liver, many metabolic systems including ammonia metabolism are heterogeneously processed among hepatocyte position in the lobule.[1-5] Three enzymes that are incorporated in ammonia metabolism are expressed gradually between the periportal zone (influx side) and the pericentral zone (efflux side) in the lobule.[6,7] To investigate the cause of the heterogeneous gene expression, a simple eight-compartments model, in which each compartment represented hepatocellular ammonia metabolism by largely enzyme kinetics equations, was developed as a lobule model.[8] In silico simulation indicated that regulated enzyme gradient reduced ATP requirement for ammonia detoxification, suggesting that these enzyme gradients by gene regulations improve the fitness of organism by saving energy (ATP consumption).

## Introduction

Gene regulation seems to be an important device for functional specialization among cells, tissues and organs. Detection of numerous inter/intra-organ differential gene regulations (e.g., the expression rate and the alternative splicing, etc.) support this argument. Many technological innovations (e.g., genome sequencing, microarray, full-length cDNA library, histochemistry, etc.) accelerate the accumulation of these discoveries, but the raison d'être of such regulations remains almost unclear. Regulation of gene expression is a highly energy consuming process because many macromolecules are involved. Therefore, it is thought that the gene regulation improves the fitness of the host individual as a payment of the energy cost. Various explanations for each regulation are proposed, but most of them are no better than the thought experiments despite the fact that many data that back up the explanations are quite solid and accurately quantitative.

At present, the greater part of the biological data and information is limited to the molecular and cellular (microscopic) level. While the explosive development of molecular and cellular biology has yielded both copious and precise information at the subcellular level, biology for higher-level (mesoscopic or macroscopic) structures has lagged far behind. Anatomy and histology illustrate a multicellular individual in a hierarchical classification scheme, namely of, tissues, organs and individual, going from the microscopic to macroscopic. The store of knowledge built up at each level of the hierarchy is at present excessively disproportionate. The knowledge accumulated in the

*Yasuhiro Naito—Institute for Advanced Biosciences, Keio University, Tsuruoka, Japan and Bioinformatics Program, Graduate School of Media and Governance and Department of Environment and Information Studies, Keio University, Fujisawa, Japan.
Email: ynaito@sfc.keio.ac.jp

*E-Cell System: Basic Concepts and Applications*, edited by Satya Nanda Vel Arjunan, Pawan K. Dhar and Masaru Tomita. 

last decade at higher-levels than the cell is undoubtedly less than that at the cellular and subcellular levels. A major constraint is the currently limited technology, which for the tissue or organ level presents greater difficulties in all aspects of sample preparation, cultivation and measurement than required for the single-cell level.

To overcome this situation, we adopted systems biology approach and focused on the ammonia detoxification in the liver as a competent model. In the mammalian hepatic lobule, many metabolic systems including ammonia metabolism are processed heterogeneously. This zonation of function seems to depend on the gradual existences of metabolic substrates, oxygen and hormones and the structural factors such as nerves, biomatrix and receptors. Some enzymes are not distributed uniformly in the lobule. Among ammonia metabolism relating enzymes, carbamoylphosphate synthetase (CPS), glutamine synthetase (GS) and ornithine aminotransferase (OAT) have steep gradual expression in the lobule. Its significance is unclear now.

It is assumed that gradual gene expressions of the three enzymes in the lobule affect the efficiency of ammonia metabolism in the liver. To elucidate the significance of gradual gene expressions in the lobule, it should be evaluated that how strong the differential expressions of enzymes affect the metabolic dynamics in each hepatocyte and what the total effects of heterogeneous hepatocytes on the liver is. Both of the amount of ATP required and the velocity for ammonia detoxification are useful as indices to evaluate the metabolic efficiency.

The liver has relatively simple histological structure among mammalian organs. However, it is still a complex system, since hepatocytes queue along the sinusoidal capillary in the lobule then metabolic change in sinusoidal upstream perturbs downstream hepatocytes. In vivo and in vitro investigations have hardly techniques to measure the fraction of ATP consumed for ammonia detoxification exactly among whole ATP consumption. Moreover, it is almost impossible to grasp the metabolic states of both of the whole liver and each hepatocyte in it. Meanwhile, approximately 15% of ATP is consumed by urea cycle in rat hepatocyte,[9] indicating that a stir in urea cycle can enormously affect the energetics not merely of hepatocyte but also of the liver and the individual. In silico study using mathematical models suggested that gradual gene regulations of ammonia metabolism relating enzymes save the energy required for the metabolism.

## The Single Hepatocyte Model

We started by construction of a model for ammonia detoxification in single hepatocyte and asking how well the mathematical model simulates the actual hepatocyte. We then assemble multiple cell models to a sinusoid model, which is used to address the advantage of the gene regulations in hepatic ammonia metabolism.

The single hepatocyte model included 67 substances and 29 reactions (Fig. 1A, see Appendix for details), most reactions are related with urea cycle and largely reproduced the metabolic states described in previous reports for mammalian hepatocyte. The liver is a giant bunch of the lobules and the lobule is a cluster of the sinusoids, which connect in parallel each other. Thus, we assumed that an appropriate model for sinusoidal metabolism linearly approximates the liver metabolism.

## The Sinusoid Model

To construct the sinusoidal metabolism model, no difference among hepatocytes along sinusoid without the gradual gene expressions of CPSI, GS and OAT was assumed and single hepatocyte models were joined up in series along a model of sinusoidal material flow (Fig. 1B). A simple model that consists of eight hepatocellular compartments roughly reproduced the metabolic zonation of ammonia detoxification in the lobule.[8]

The active pathways were quite different between the periportal and the pericentral zones in the model (Fig. 2). Urea production, urea exportation and creatine generation were pronouncedly predominant in the periportal zone (light gray/red arrows in Fig. 2), while glutamine formation and exportation were predominantly seen in the pericentral zone (dark gray/blue arrows in Fig. 2). Because mitochondrial ornithine aminotransferase is mainly expressed in the pericentral zone, the concentration of glutamate, which is a reaction product of ornithine aminotransferase, was

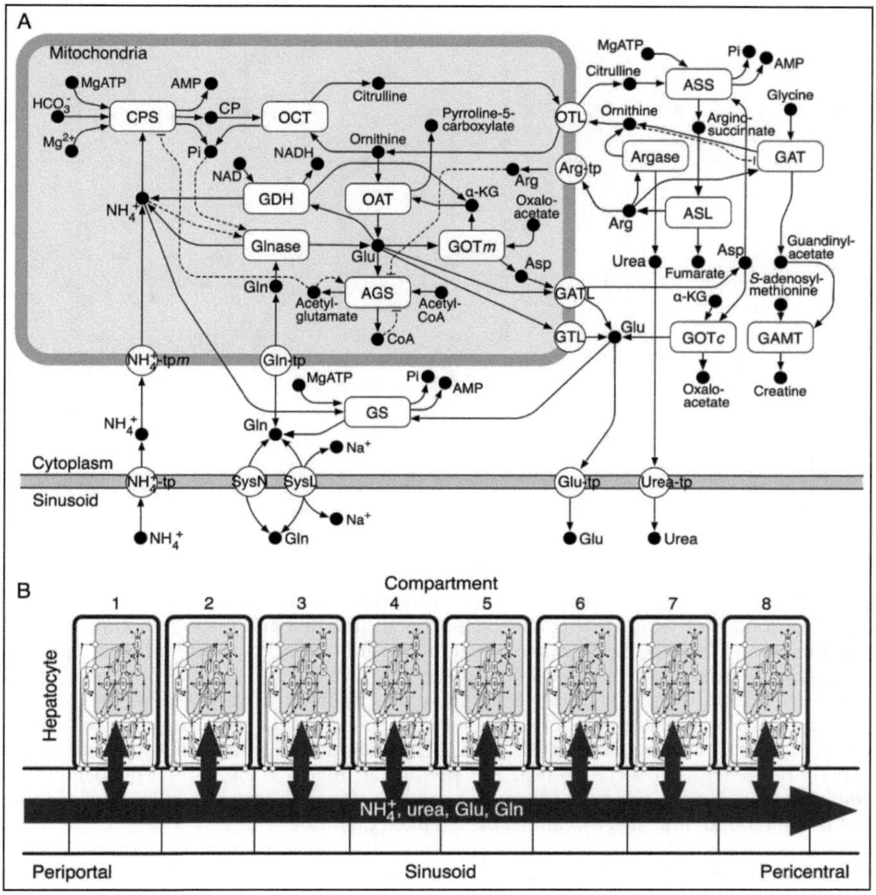


Figure 1. Schematic representation of the model. A) The model describing ammonia metabolism in single zone model. Filled circles, open round rectangles and open circles represent substances, enzymes and transporter, respectively. Solid line arrows represent reactions and transportations. Broken line with a triangular arrowhead and a bar at the end represent positive and negative feedback, respectively. AGS, *N*-acetylglutamate synthetase; Argase, arginase; ASL, argininosuccinate lyase; ASS, argininosuccinate synthetase; CPS, carbamoylphosphate synthetase; GAMT, guanidinoacetate methyltransferase; GAT, arginine:glycine amidinotransferase; GDH, glutamate dehydrogenase; Glnase, phosphate-dependent glutaminase; GOT*c*, glutamate:oxaloacetate transaminase in the cytoplasm; $GOT_m$, glutamate:oxaloacetate transaminase in the mitochondria; GS, glutamine synthetase; OAT, ornithine aminotransferase, OCT, ornithine carbamoyltransferase; Arg-tp, arginine transporter; GATL, glutamate-aspartate translocase; Gln-tp, glutamine transporter in mitochondrial membrane; Glu-tp, glutamate transporter; GTL, glutamate translocase; $NH_4^+$-tp, ammonia transporter in the cell membrane; $NH_4^+$-$tp_m$, ammonia transporter in the mitochondrial membrane; OTL, ornithine-citrulline translocase; SysL, system L; SysN, system N; Urea-tp, urea transporter; Arg, arginine; Asp, aspartate; CP, carbamoylphosphate; Gln, glutamine; Glu, glutamate; α-KG, α-ketoglutarate. The entity abbreviation may be used with an index variable which represents the location of the entity. The indices *c*, *m* and *s* indicate the cytoplasm, mitochondria and sinusoid, respectively. B) Schematic of eight cellular compartments model with sinusoidal compartments. PP and PC represent the periportal end and the pericentral end, respectively. Ammonia ($NH_4^+$), urea, glutamate (Glu) and glutamine (Gln) flow from the periportal inflow compartment to the pericentral outflow compartment interacting with cellular compartments.

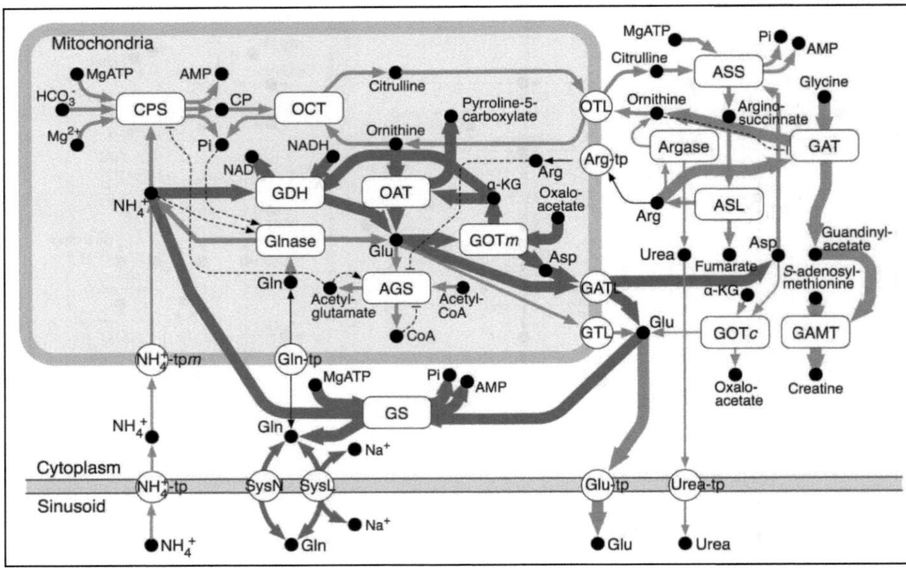


Figure 2. Flux disparities between both ends of the porto-central axis. The width of each arrow proportionally reflects the flux ratio at both ends (the first and the eighth compartment). The thickest line indicates the flux disparity to be ten-fold or more. Light (red) and dark (blue) arrows indicate fluxes predominant in the periportal and the pericentral zone, respectively. Fluxes with a disparity of less than 1.5 are indicated by the black arrow. The size of the arrows is proportional to the level of fluxes except for extremely high level fluxes: ornithine aminotransferase, Mitochondrial GOT and GATL. Pronounced urea production, urea export and creatine generation were seen in the periportal region while pronounced glutamine formation and reactions which mediate glutamate in the pericentral. A color version of this figure is available online at www.landesbioscience.com/curie.

higher in the pericentral than the periportal zone. The glutamate concentration in mitochondria was increased from 6.97E-3 M to 8.70E-2 M along the porto-central axis. Consequently, the velocity of glutamate dehydrogenase, which catalyzes glutamate, was larger in the pericentral than the periportal zone. Glutamate-aspartate translocase and mitochondrial GOT also exhibited higher activities in the pericentral zone, while cytoplasmic GOT showed an opposite trend of flux between the periportal and the pericentral zone (Fig. 2).

To address the functional meaning of the gradual gene expressions, we developed a model without the enzyme gradients. In the no-gradient model, the lobule consumed more ATP to detoxify ammonia than the original model with gradual expressions. Most of the chemical reactions and transportation exhibited larger fluxes in the periportal zone than the pericentral zone. Due to the high affinity for ammonia of glutamine synthetase, i.e., 1/10 of *Km* of carbamoylphosphate synthetase, ammonia predominantly converted to glutamine in the periportal zone. The fluxes gently changed from the periportal to the pericentral zone while dramatic alterations were seen in the sixth or seventh compartment in the model with the gradual gene expressions, revealing that the pericentral hepatocytes played a lesser role in metabolism in the no-gradient model.

GS and OAT are co-expressed in hepatocyte and no co-expression of these genes is seen in other tissues. This raises a hypothesis that the co-expression of GS and OAT benefits the liver metabolism. Activities of both enzymes, which are parallel to gene expressions, were variously perturbed in the mathematical model to enquire whether the co-expression advantages ammonia detoxification in the lobule. Consequently, cooperative gradient of GS and OAT was suggested to improve the energy efficiency of ammonia detoxification.

Four intermediate models were constructed. The first intermediate model included only GS gradient, the second one included GS and CPS gradients, the third one included only OAT gradient and the last one included GS and OAT gradients. Our study using mathematical models suggested that the gene regulation in hepatic ammonia metabolism contributed for energy conservation. Although regulation of gene expression itself should spend much energy, the returning energy save is conceivable to overcome the break-even point. Co-expression of GS and OAT was also suggested to improve the energy efficiency of ammonia metabolism. These support the aspect that intra-tissue gradual gene expression has evolved in a direction to upgrade metabolic efficiency. To compare the metabolic aspects in the periportal zone and that in the pericentral zone, the flux distributions were examined. To evaluate the effects of the enzyme slope along the lobule metabolic state, the following rates were calculated and used as the indexes.

$$\text{Rate of ammonia degradation: } J_{\mathrm{NH_4^+},deg} = v_{\mathrm{CPS}} + v_{\mathrm{GS}} \tag{1}$$

$$\text{Rate of ammonia generation: } J_{\mathrm{NH_4^+},gen} = v_{\mathrm{Glnase}} + v_{\mathrm{GDH}} \tag{2}$$

$$\text{Rate of ammonia detoxification: } J_{\mathrm{NH_4^+},detox} = J_{\mathrm{NH_4^+},deg} - J_{\mathrm{NH_4^+},gen} \tag{3}$$

$$\text{Rate of ATP consumption: } J_{\mathrm{ATP},consum} = 2v_{\mathrm{CPS}} + v_{\mathrm{ASS}} \tag{4}$$

$$\text{Energy efficiency } \eta := \frac{J_{\mathrm{NH_4^+},detox}}{J_{\mathrm{ATP},consum}} \tag{5}$$

$$\text{Rate of bicarbonate consumption: } J_{\mathrm{HCO_3^-},consum} = v_{\mathrm{CPS}} \tag{6}$$

$R_{\mathrm{NH_4^+},detox}$ and $v_{\mathrm{NH_4^+}\text{-tp}}$ are nearly equal under the assumption of steady-state. The model with all of gene expression gradients ranks higher among six models in the rate and energy efficiency of ammonia detoxification. The mean rate of elimination of ammonia from the sinusoid was 11.8% faster in the model with full-gradients than the no-gradient model. Although the rate of degradation of ammonia in all eight compartments was 20.0% slower in the with full-gradients model than the no-gradient model, the rate of ammonia generation was also 53.8% slower than the control model, showing that the full-gradients model was able to remove ammonia more efficiently than the control. The mean rate of ATP consumption in the full-gradients model was 9.5% less than the no-gradient model. Energy efficiency $\eta$, which means the number of consumed ATP molecules required for the elimination of one ammonia molecule, was smaller in the full-gradients model than the no-gradient model ($3.59 \pm 0.22$ vs $4.47 \pm 0.49$). Two intermediate models also demonstrated smaller $\eta$ while the other intermediate models demonstrated greater $\eta$ than the control.

On the other hand, the urea cycle in the liver also strongly contribute to maintain acid-base balance, but our model did not considered it this time. Since available quantitative data on acid-base balance was fewer and less precise than that on ammonia detoxification, we judged that a model of just ammonia metabolism could be more effective than that including both of ammonia metabolism and acid-base balance. For further discussion about the raison d'être of gene regulations, the mechanism of acid-base balance should be implemented to the model.

## Conclusion

We evaluated that how strong the totality of heterogeneous metabolic changes in each cell influence the fitness of tissue and organ through systems biology techniques. Such approach can link molecular processes at subcellular level and macroscopic functions at tissue, organ, or individual level together, not by statistical correlation but by concrete causal relationship. Coming biosciences should piece together the huge data (e.g., genome sequence, expression profile, protein structure, etc.,) to gain integrated comprehension of life. Generally, in vivo and in vitro approaches do not have integrability but precision and in silico approach has vice versa, thus they surely function complementally and accelerate the progress of biological sciences.

# Appendix: Details of the Mathematical Model

## *1. Carbamoylphosphate Synthetase (EC. 6.3.4.16)*

The enzyme catalyzes

$$2ATP + NH_4^+ + HCO_3^- \rightarrow 2AMP + 2Pi + CP$$

in mitochondria. The kinetic model was obtained from previous literature.[10,11]

$$v_{CPS} = \frac{k_{cat,CPS}[CPS]}{\text{denominator}_{CPS}}$$

where

$$\begin{aligned}
\text{denominator}_{CPS} = {} & 1 + \frac{K_{mATP_1,CPS} + K_{mATP_2,CPS}}{[ATP]} + \frac{K_{mHCO_3^-,CPS}}{[HCO_3^-]} + \frac{K_{mNAG,CPS}}{[NAG]} + \frac{K_{mNH_4^+,CPS}}{[NH_4^+]} \\
& + \frac{K_{sATP_1,CPS}K_{m'HCO_3^-,CPS} + K_{sHCO_3^-,CPS}\left(K_{mATP_2,CPS} + K_{m'ATP_2,CPS}\right)}{[ATP]} + \frac{K_{sNAG,CPS}K_{mATP_1,CPS}}{[ATP][NAG]} \\
& + \frac{K_{sMg^{2+},CPS}K_{mATP_1,CPS}}{[ATP][Mg^{2+}]} + \frac{K_{sATP_2,CPS}K_{mNH_4^+,CPS}}{[ATP][NH_4^+]} + \frac{K_{sNAG,CPS}K_{m'HCO_3^-,CPS}}{[NAG][HCO_3^-]} \\
& + \frac{K_{sNAG,CPS}K_{sMg^{2+},CPS}K_{mATP_1,CPS}}{[ATP][Mg^{2+}][NAG]} \\
& + \frac{K_{sATP_1,CPS}K_{sNAG,CPS}K_{m'HCO_3^-,CPS} + K_{sNAG,CPS}K_{sHCO_3^-,CPS}K_{m'ATP_2,CPS}}{[ATP][NAG][HCO_3^-]} \\
& + \frac{K_{sATP_1,CPS}K_{sMg^{2+},CPS}K_{m'HCO_3^-,CPS}}{[ATP][Mg^{2+}][HCO_3^-]} + \frac{K_{sATP_2,CPS}K_{sHCO_3^-,CPS}K_{m'HCO_3^-,CPS}\left(K_{mNH_4^+,CPS} + K_{m'NH_4^+,CPS}\right)}{[ATP][HCO_3^-][NH_4^+]} \\
& + \frac{K_{sATP_1,CPS}K_{sMg^{2+},CPS}K_{sNAG,CPS}K_{m'HCO_3^-,CPS}}{[ATP][Mg^{2+}][NAG][HCO_3^-]} + \frac{K_{sATP_2,CPS}K_{sNAG,CPS}K_{sHCO_3^-,CPS}K_{m'NH_4^+,CPS}}{[ATP][NAG][HCO_3^-][NH_4^+]} \\
& + \frac{K_{sATP_1,CPS}K_{sHCO_3^-,CPS}K_{m'ATP_2,CPS}}{[ATP]^2[HCO_3^-]} + \frac{K_{sATP_1,CPS}K_{sNAG,CPS}K_{sHCO_3^-,CPS}K_{m'ATP_2,CPS}}{[ATP]^2[NAG][HCO_3^-]} \\
& + \frac{K_{sATP_1,CPS}K_{sMg^{2+},CPS}K_{sHCO_3^-,CPS}K_{m'ATP_2,CPS}}{[ATP]^2[Mg^{2+}][HCO_3^-]} + \frac{K_{sATP_1,CPS}K_{sATP_2,CPS}K_{sHCO_3^-,CPS}K_{m'NH_4^+,CPS}}{[ATP]^2[HCO_3^-][NH_4^+]} \\
& + \frac{K_{sATP_1,CPS}K_{sMg^{2+},CPS}K_{sNAG,CPS}K_{sHCO_3^-,CPS}K_{m'ATP_2,CPS}}{[ATP]^2[Mg^{2+}][NAG][HCO_3^-]} \\
& + \frac{K_{sATP_1,CPS}K_{sATP_2,CPS}K_{sMg^{2+},CPS}K_{sHCO_3^-,CPS}K_{m'NH_4^+,CPS}}{[ATP]^2[Mg^{2+}][HCO_3^-][NH_4^+]} \\
& + \frac{K_{sATP_1,CPS}K_{sATP_2,CPS}K_{sNAG,CPS}K_{sHCO_3^-,CPS}K_{m'NH_4^+,CPS}}{[ATP]^2[NAG][HCO_3^-][NH_4^+]} \\
& + \frac{K_{sATP_1,CPS}K_{sATP_2,CPS}K_{sMg^{2+},CPS}K_{sNAG,CPS}K_{sHCO_3^-,CPS}K_{m'NH_4^+,CPS}}{[ATP]^2[Mg^{2+}][NAG][HCO_3^-][NH_4^+]}
\end{aligned}$$

## 2. *N-Acetylglutamate Synthetase (EC. 2.3.1.1)*

The enzymes catalyze AcCoA + Glu → CoA + NAG.

The reaction mechanism is a nonreversible rapid equilibrium random bi-bi mechanism.[12]

$$v_{\mathrm{AGS}} = \frac{\dfrac{k_{\mathrm{cat,AGS}}[\mathrm{AGS}][\mathrm{AcCoA}][\mathrm{Glu}]}{\left(1+\dfrac{K_{\mathrm{aArg,AGS}}}{[\mathrm{Arg}]}\right)}}{\mathrm{denominator}_{\mathrm{AGS}}}$$

where

$$\begin{aligned}{}_{\mathrm{AGS}} = {} & K_{\mathrm{iAcCoA,AGS}} K_{\mathrm{mGlu,AGS}} \left(1+\frac{[\mathrm{CoA}]}{K_{\mathrm{iCoA,AGS}}}\right)\left(1+\frac{[\mathrm{NAG}]}{K_{\mathrm{iNAG,AGS}}}\right) \\ & + K_{\mathrm{mGlu,AGS}}\left(1+\frac{[\mathrm{NAG}]}{K_{\mathrm{iNAG,AGS}}}\right)[\mathrm{AcCoA}] \\ & + K_{\mathrm{mAcCoA,AGS}}\left(1+\frac{[\mathrm{CoA}]}{K_{\mathrm{iCoA,AGS}}}\right)[\mathrm{Glu}] + [\mathrm{AcCoA}][\mathrm{Glu}]\end{aligned}$$

## 3. *Glutamine Synthetase (EC. 6.3.1.2)*

The enzyme catalyzes ATP + Glu + $NH_4^+$ → AMP + Pi + Gln.

$$v_{\mathrm{GS}} = \frac{k_{\mathrm{cat,GS}}[\mathrm{GS}][\mathrm{Glu}][\mathrm{ATP}][\mathrm{NH_4^+}]}{(K_{\mathrm{mGlu,GS}}+[\mathrm{Glu}])(K_{\mathrm{mATP,GS}}+[\mathrm{ATP}])(K_{\mathrm{mNH_4^+,GS}}+[\mathrm{NH_4^+}])}$$

## 4. *Phosphate-Dependent Glutaminase (EC. 3.5.1.2)*

The enzyme catalyzes Gln + Pi → Glu + $NH_4^+$. It is activated by the product: ammonia.[13] Cooperativity of glutamine and Pi, which is an essential activator for phosphate-dependent glutaminase, were modeled by the Hill equation.[14]

$$v_{\mathrm{Glnase}} = \frac{\dfrac{k_{\mathrm{cat,Glnase}}[\mathrm{Glnase}]}{1+\dfrac{K_{\mathrm{a,Glnase}}}{[\mathrm{NH_4^+}]}}[\mathrm{Gln}]^{n_{\mathrm{Gln,Glnase}}}}{[\mathrm{Gln}]_{0.5}^{n_{\mathrm{Gln,Glnase}}}\left(1+\dfrac{[\mathrm{Pi}]_{0.5}^{n_{\mathrm{Pi,Glnase}}}}{[\mathrm{Pi}]^{n_{\mathrm{Pi,Glnase}}}}\right)+[\mathrm{Gln}]^{n_{\mathrm{Gln,Glnase}}}\left(1+\dfrac{[\mathrm{Pi}]_{0.5}^{n_{\mathrm{Pi,Glnase}}}}{[\mathrm{Pi}]^{n_{\mathrm{Pi,Glnase}}}}\right)}$$

### 5. *Ornithine Carbamoyltransferase (EC. 2.1.3.3)*

The enzyme catalyzes CP + Orn ↔ Pi + Cit. The reaction mechanism is an ordered bi-bi sequential mechanism.[15]

$$v_{\mathrm{OCT}} = \frac{\left(k_{1,\mathrm{OCT}}k_{3,\mathrm{OCT}}k_{5,\mathrm{OCT}}k_{7,\mathrm{OCT}}[\mathrm{CP}][\mathrm{Orn}] - k_{2,\mathrm{OCT}}k_{4,\mathrm{OCT}}k_{6,\mathrm{OCT}}k_{8,\mathrm{OCT}}[\mathrm{Cit}][\mathrm{Pi}]\right)[\mathrm{OCT}]}{\mathrm{denominator}_{\mathrm{OCT}}}$$

where

$$\begin{aligned}\mathrm{denominator}_{\mathrm{OCT}} = {} & k_{2,\mathrm{OCT}}k_{7,\mathrm{OCT}}\left(k_{4,\mathrm{OCT}} + k_{5,\mathrm{OCT}}\right) + k_{1,\mathrm{OCT}}k_{7,\mathrm{OCT}}\left(k_{4,\mathrm{OCT}} + k_{5,\mathrm{OCT}}\right)[\mathrm{CP}] \\ & + k_{2,\mathrm{OCT}}k_{8,\mathrm{OCT}}\left(k_{4,\mathrm{OCT}} + k_{5,\mathrm{OCT}}\right)[\mathrm{Pi}] + k_{3,\mathrm{OCT}}k_{5,\mathrm{OCT}}k_{7,\mathrm{OCT}}[\mathrm{Orn}] \\ & + k_{2,\mathrm{OCT}}k_{4,\mathrm{OCT}}k_{6,\mathrm{OCT}}[\mathrm{Cit}] + k_{1,\mathrm{OCT}}k_{3,\mathrm{OCT}}\left(k_{5,\mathrm{OCT}} + k_{7,\mathrm{OCT}}\right)[\mathrm{CP}][\mathrm{Orn}] \\ & + k_{6,\mathrm{OCT}}k_{8,\mathrm{OCT}}\left(k_{2,\mathrm{OCT}} + k_{4,\mathrm{OCT}}\right)[\mathrm{Pi}][\mathrm{Cit}] + k_{1,\mathrm{OCT}}k_{4,\mathrm{OCT}}k_{6,\mathrm{OCT}}[\mathrm{CP}][\mathrm{Cit}] \\ & + k_{1,\mathrm{OCT}}k_{3,\mathrm{OCT}}k_{6,\mathrm{OCT}}[\mathrm{CP}][\mathrm{Orn}][\mathrm{Cit}] + k_{3,\mathrm{OCT}}k_{5,\mathrm{OCT}}k_{8,\mathrm{OCT}}[\mathrm{Orn}][\mathrm{Pi}] \\ & + k_{3,\mathrm{OCT}}k_{6,\mathrm{OCT}}k_{8,\mathrm{OCT}}[\mathrm{Orn}][\mathrm{Pi}][\mathrm{Cit}]\end{aligned}$$

### *6. Argininosuccinate Synthetase (EC. 6.3.4.5)*

The enzyme catalyzes ATP + Cit + Asp ↔ AMP + Pi + ASA. The reaction mechanism is an ordered ter-ter mechanism.[15]

$$v_{\mathrm{ASS}} = \frac{\begin{pmatrix} k_{1,\mathrm{ASS}}k_{3,\mathrm{ASS}}k_{5,\mathrm{ASS}}k_{7,\mathrm{ASS}}k_{9,\mathrm{ASS}}k_{11,\mathrm{ASS}}[\mathrm{Cit}][\mathrm{Asp}][\mathrm{ATP}] \\ -k_{2,\mathrm{ASS}}k_{4,\mathrm{ASS}}k_{6,\mathrm{ASS}}k_{8,\mathrm{ASS}}k_{10,\mathrm{ASS}}k_{12,\mathrm{ASS}}[\mathrm{ASA}][\mathrm{AMP}][\mathrm{Pi}] \end{pmatrix}[\mathrm{ASS}]}{\mathrm{denominator}_{\mathrm{ASS}}}$$

where

$$\begin{aligned}
\mathrm{denominator}_{\mathrm{ASS}} = {} & k_{2,\mathrm{ASS}}k_{4,\mathrm{ASS}}k_{9,\mathrm{ASS}}k_{11,\mathrm{ASS}}\left(k_{6,\mathrm{ASS}}+k_{7,\mathrm{ASS}}\right) \\
& +k_{1,\mathrm{ASS}}k_{4,\mathrm{ASS}}k_{6,\mathrm{ASS}}k_{8,\mathrm{ASS}}k_{11,\mathrm{ASS}}[\mathrm{Cit}][\mathrm{Pi}] \\
& +k_{1,\mathrm{ASS}}k_{4,\mathrm{ASS}}k_{9,\mathrm{ASS}}k_{11,\mathrm{ASS}}\left(k_{6,\mathrm{ASS}}+k_{7,\mathrm{ASS}}\right)[\mathrm{Cit}] \\
& +k_{2,\mathrm{ASS}}k_{5,\mathrm{ASS}}k_{7,\mathrm{ASS}}k_{9,\mathrm{ASS}}k_{12,\mathrm{ASS}}[\mathrm{Asp}][\mathrm{ASA}] \\
& +k_{2,\mathrm{ASS}}k_{5,\mathrm{ASS}}k_{7,\mathrm{ASS}}k_{9,\mathrm{ASS}}k_{11,\mathrm{ASS}}[\mathrm{Asp}] \\
& +k_{1,\mathrm{ASS}}k_{3,\mathrm{ASS}}k_{6,\mathrm{ASS}}k_{8,\mathrm{ASS}}k_{11,\mathrm{ASS}}[\mathrm{Cit}][\mathrm{ATP}][\mathrm{Pi}] \\
& +k_{1,\mathrm{ASS}}k_{3,\mathrm{ASS}}k_{9,\mathrm{ASS}}k_{11,\mathrm{ASS}}\left(k_{6,\mathrm{ASS}}+k_{7,\mathrm{ASS}}\right)[\mathrm{Cit}][\mathrm{ATP}] \\
& +k_{1,\mathrm{ASS}}k_{4,\mathrm{ASS}}k_{6,\mathrm{ASS}}k_{8,\mathrm{ASS}}k_{10,\mathrm{ASS}}[\mathrm{Cit}][\mathrm{AMP}][\mathrm{Pi}] \\
& +k_{1,\mathrm{ASS}}k_{5,\mathrm{ASS}}k_{7,\mathrm{ASS}}k_{9,\mathrm{ASS}}k_{11,\mathrm{ASS}}[\mathrm{Cit}][\mathrm{Asp}] \\
& +k_{3,\mathrm{ASS}}k_{5,\mathrm{ASS}}k_{7,\mathrm{ASS}}k_{9,\mathrm{ASS}}k_{12,\mathrm{ASS}}[\mathrm{ATP}][\mathrm{Asp}][\mathrm{ASA}] \\
& +k_{3,\mathrm{ASS}}k_{5,\mathrm{ASS}}k_{7,\mathrm{ASS}}k_{9,\mathrm{ASS}}k_{11,\mathrm{ASS}}[\mathrm{ATP}][\mathrm{Asp}] \\
& +k_{2,\mathrm{ASS}}k_{5,\mathrm{ASS}}k_{7,\mathrm{ASS}}k_{9,\mathrm{ASS}}k_{12,\mathrm{ASS}}[\mathrm{AMP}][\mathrm{Asp}][\mathrm{ASA}] \\
& +k_{2,\mathrm{ASS}}k_{4,\mathrm{ASS}}k_{9,\mathrm{ASS}}k_{12,\mathrm{ASS}}\left(k_{6,\mathrm{ASS}}+k_{7,\mathrm{ASS}}\right)[\mathrm{ASA}] \\
& +k_{1,\mathrm{ASS}}k_{3,\mathrm{ASS}}k_{6,\mathrm{ASS}}k_{8,\mathrm{ASS}}k_{10,\mathrm{ASS}}[\mathrm{Cit}][\mathrm{ATP}][\mathrm{AMP}][\mathrm{Pi}] \\
& +k_{1,\mathrm{ASS}}k_{3,\mathrm{ASS}}k_{5,\mathrm{ASS}}\left(k_{7,\mathrm{ASS}}k_{9,\mathrm{ASS}}+k_{7,\mathrm{ASS}}k_{11,\mathrm{ASS}}+k_{9,\mathrm{ASS}}k_{11,\mathrm{ASS}}\right)[\mathrm{Cit}][\mathrm{ATP}][\mathrm{Asp}] \\
& +k_{1,\mathrm{ASS}}k_{3,\mathrm{ASS}}k_{5,\mathrm{ASS}}k_{8,\mathrm{ASS}}k_{11,\mathrm{ASS}}[\mathrm{Cit}][\mathrm{Asp}][\mathrm{ATP}][\mathrm{Pi}] \\
& +k_{2,\mathrm{ASS}}k_{4,\mathrm{ASS}}k_{6,\mathrm{ASS}}k_{8,\mathrm{ASS}}k_{11,\mathrm{ASS}}[\mathrm{Pi}] \\
& +k_{1,\mathrm{ASS}}k_{3,\mathrm{ASS}}k_{5,\mathrm{ASS}}k_{7,\mathrm{ASS}}k_{10,\mathrm{ASS}}[\mathrm{Cit}][\mathrm{Asp}][\mathrm{ATP}][\mathrm{AMP}] \\
& +k_{2,\mathrm{ASS}}k_{4,\mathrm{ASS}}k_{6,\mathrm{ASS}}k_{8,\mathrm{ASS}}k_{10,\mathrm{ASS}}[\mathrm{AMP}][\mathrm{Pi}] \\
& +k_{3,\mathrm{ASS}}k_{5,\mathrm{ASS}}k_{7,\mathrm{ASS}}k_{10,\mathrm{ASS}}k_{12,\mathrm{ASS}}[\mathrm{Asp}][\mathrm{ATP}][\mathrm{ASA}][\mathrm{AMP}] \\
& +k_{2,\mathrm{ASS}}k_{4,\mathrm{ASS}}k_{6,\mathrm{ASS}}k_{8,\mathrm{ASS}}k_{12,\mathrm{ASS}}[\mathrm{ASA}][\mathrm{Pi}]
\end{aligned}$$

### *7. Argininosuccinate Lyase (EC. 4.3.2.1)*

The enzyme catalyzes ASA ↔ Fum + Arg. The reaction mechanism is an ordered uni-bi mechanism.

$$v_{\mathrm{ASL}} = \frac{\left(k_{1,\mathrm{ASL}}k_{3,\mathrm{ASL}}k_{5,\mathrm{ASL}}[\mathrm{ASA}] - k_{2,\mathrm{ASL}}k_{4,\mathrm{ASL}}k_{6,\mathrm{ASL}}[\mathrm{Fum}][\mathrm{Arg}]\right)[\mathrm{ASL}]}{\begin{array}{l} k_{5,\mathrm{ASL}}\left(k_{2,\mathrm{ASL}} + k_{3,\mathrm{ASL}}\right) + k_{1,\mathrm{ASL}}\left(k_{3,\mathrm{ASL}} + k_{5,\mathrm{ASL}}\right)[\mathrm{ASA}] + k_{2,\mathrm{ASL}}k_{4,\mathrm{ASL}}[\mathrm{Fum}] \\ + k_{6,\mathrm{ASL}}\left(k_{2,\mathrm{ASL}} + k_{3,\mathrm{ASL}}\right) + k_{4,\mathrm{ASL}}k_{6,\mathrm{ASL}}[\mathrm{Fum}][\mathrm{Arg}] + k_{1,\mathrm{ASL}}k_{4,\mathrm{ASL}}[\mathrm{ASA}][\mathrm{Fum}] \end{array}}$$

### *8. Arginase (EC. 3.5.3.1)*

The enzyme catalyzes Arg → urea + Orn. The reaction is an irreversible process and inhibited by ornithine.

$$v_{\mathrm{Argase}} = \frac{k_{1,\mathrm{Argase}}k_{3,\mathrm{Argase}}k_{4,\mathrm{Argase}}[\mathrm{Arn}][\mathrm{Argase}]}{k_{4,\mathrm{Argase}}\left(k_{2,\mathrm{Argase}} + k_{3,\mathrm{Argase}}\right) + k_{5,\mathrm{Argase}}\left(k_{2,\mathrm{Argase}} + k_{3,\mathrm{Argase}}\right)[\mathrm{Orn}] + k_{1,\mathrm{Argase}}\left(k_{3,\mathrm{Argase}} + k_{4,\mathrm{Argase}}\right)[\mathrm{Arn}]}$$

### *9. MetaNet Model*

OTL, GTL, GATL, OAT, $\mathrm{GOT_m}$, $\mathrm{GOT_c}$, GDH, GAT and GAMT were modeled using MetaNet.[16] Reaction stoichiometries were defined as follows:

| | |
|---|---|
| OTL: | $\mathrm{Cit}_m + \mathrm{Orn}_c \leftrightarrow \mathrm{Cit}_c + \mathrm{Orn}_m$ |
| GTL: | $\mathrm{Glu}_c \leftrightarrow \mathrm{Glu}_m$ |
| GATL: | $\mathrm{Glu}_c + \mathrm{Asp}_m \leftrightarrow \mathrm{Glu}_m + \mathrm{Asp}_c$ |
| OAT: | Orn+AKG ↔ Pyrroline-5-carboxylate + Glu |
| $\mathrm{GOT}_m$: | Glu + OAA ↔ Asp + AKG |
| $\mathrm{GOT}_c$: | Asp + AKG ↔ Glu + OAA |
| GDH: | $\mathrm{Glu} + \mathrm{NAD^+} \leftrightarrow \mathrm{AKG} + \mathrm{NH_4^+} + \mathrm{NADH}$ |
| GAT: | Gly + Arg ↔ Orn + GAA |
| GAMT: | SAM + GAA → Cre |

Although MetaNet is not guaranteed to accurately reproduce enzyme kinetics, it was used in our model with the expectation it would roughly estimated the rates of reactions. Velocities of reactions were calculated as follows:

$$v_x = \frac{V_{\max,x}\left(1 - \dfrac{V_{r,x}}{V_{f,x}}\dfrac{\prod_{j_x}\left(\dfrac{c_{j_x}}{K'_{j_x,x}}\right)}{\prod_{i_x}\left(\dfrac{c_{i_x}}{K'_{i_x,x}}\right)}\right)}{1+\sum_{i_x}\left(\dfrac{c_{i_x}}{K'_{i_x,x}}\right)^{n_{i_x,x}}\left(1+\sum_{j_x}\left(\dfrac{c_{j_x}}{K'_{j_x,x}}\right)^{n_{j_x,x}}\right)\left(1+\sum_{k'_x}\left(\dfrac{K_{k'_x,x}}{c_{k'_x}}\right)^{n_{k'_x,x}}+\sum_{h'_x}\left(\dfrac{c_{h'_x}}{K_{h'_x,x}}\right)^{n_{h'_x,x}}\right)}$$

where

$$K'_{s,x} = K_{s,x}\left(1+\sum_{k_x}\left(\frac{K_{k_x,x}}{c_{k_x}}\right)^{n_{k_x,x}}+\sum_{h}\left(\frac{c_{h_x}}{K_{h_x,x}}\right)^{n_{h_x,x}}\right)$$

$K_{s,x}$ and $n_{s,x}$ is the binding constant and the "cooperativity index" (essentially a Hill exponent) of substance (or effecter) *s* of enzyme *x* (equilibrium constant for dissociation of the enzyme-ligand complex), respectively and $K'_{s,x}$ is the former's effective binding constant, which reflects the activities of the competitive activators $k_x$ and the competitive inhibitors $h_x$. $c_s$ is the concentration of substance $s$. $k'_x$ and $h'_x$ are noncompetitive activators and noncompetitive inhibitors of the reaction catalyzed by enzyme $x$, respectively.[13]

### 10. System N

Glutamine is transported into the cytoplasm by a sodium-dependent transport mechanism. This process is inhibited by histidine.[17]

$$v_{\mathrm{SysN}} = V_{\mathrm{max,SysN}} \left( \left( \frac{[\mathrm{Na}^+]_e}{[\mathrm{Na}^+]_e + K_{\mathrm{mNa,SysN}}} \right) \left( \frac{[\mathrm{Glu}]_e}{[\mathrm{Glu}]_e + K_{\mathrm{mGlu,SysN}} \left( 1 + \frac{[\mathrm{His}]_e}{K_{\mathrm{iHis,SysN}}} \right)} \right) - \left( \frac{[\mathrm{Na}^+]_c}{[\mathrm{Na}^+]_c + K_{\mathrm{mNa,SysN}}} \right) \left( \frac{[\mathrm{Glu}]_c}{[\mathrm{Glu}]_c + K_{\mathrm{mGlu,SysN}} \left( 1 + \frac{[\mathrm{His}]_c}{K_{\mathrm{iHis,SysN}}} \right)} \right) \right)$$

### 11. System L

Glutamine is transported into the cytoplasm by a sodium-independent transport mechanism. This process is inhibited by tryptophan.[17]

$$v_{\mathrm{SysL}} = V_{\mathrm{max,SysL}} \left( \frac{[\mathrm{Glu}]_e}{[\mathrm{Glu}]_e + K_{\mathrm{mGlu,SysL}} \left( 1 + \frac{[\mathrm{Trp}]_e}{K_{\mathrm{iTrp,SysL}}} \right)} - \frac{[\mathrm{Glu}]_c}{[\mathrm{Glu}]_c + K_{\mathrm{mGlu,SysL}} \left( 1 + \frac{[\mathrm{Trp}]_c}{K_{\mathrm{iTrp,SysL}}} \right)} \right)$$

### 12. Ammonia Transport between Sinusoid and Cytoplasm

Ammonia transport between the sinusoid and cytoplasm was modeled based on the general mass action law.

$$v_{\mathrm{NH_4^+\,4\text{-}tp}} = k_{\mathrm{NH_4^+\,4\text{-}tp}} \left( [\mathrm{NH_4^+}]_c - [\mathrm{NH_4^+}]_e \right)$$

### 13. Transportation of Glutamine, Arginine and Ammonia between Cytoplasm and Mitochondria

Transports of glutamine, arginine and ammonia across the mitochondrial membrane were presumed to rapidly attain equilibrium.

$$K_{\mathrm{eq},x} \left( [\mathrm{S}]_c - v_x \right) = ([\mathrm{S}]_m + v_x)$$

### 14. Urea Transport to Sinusoid

Excretion of urea in the sinusoidal space was modeled based on the general mass action law.

$$v_{\mathrm{Urea\text{-}tp}} = k_{\mathrm{Urea\text{-}tp}} \left( [\mathrm{urea}]_c - [\mathrm{urea}]_e \right)$$

### 15. Glutamate Transport between Sinusoid and Cytoplasm

Glutamate transport between the sinusoid and cytoplasm was modeled as Michaelis-Menten reversible kinetics.

$$v_{\mathrm{Glu\text{-}tp}} = V_{mF,\mathrm{Glu\text{-}tp}} \left( \frac{[\mathrm{Glu}]_e}{[\mathrm{Glu}]_e + K_{m\mathrm{Glu,Glu\text{-}tp}}} \right) - V_{mR,\mathrm{Glu\text{-}tp}} \left( \frac{[\mathrm{Glu}]_c}{[\mathrm{Glu}]_c + K_{m\mathrm{Glu,Glu\text{-}tp}}} \right)$$

### 16. Glutamate Flux from the Outside Pathways

Glutamate flux from the outside pathways of the model was represented by the difference between zero-order influx and efflux based on the general mass action law.

$$v_{\text{Glu-spp}} = J_{\text{Glu-spp}} - k_{\text{Glu-spp}}[\text{Glu}]_c$$

### 17. Degradation of Metabolites

Degradation of $N$-acetylglutamate, Pi and CoA were modeled based on the general mass action law under the assumption of steady-state.

$$v_{deg,s} = k_{deg,s}[s]$$

where $s$ is a substance.

### 18. Ornithine Inflow from Other Reactions

To hold the steady-state, ornithine inflow from other reactions was presumed to be equal to the flux of ornithine aminotransferase, $v_{\text{OAT}}$.

### 19. Metabolites Flows in Sinusoid

Flows of ammonia, glutamine, glutamate and urea from $n$th sinusoidal compartment to $n$ + 1th compartment, $v_{e,s_n}$, were modeled based on the general mass action law.

$$J_{e,s_n} = k_e[s_n]_e$$

where $s_n$ represents a substance in the $n$th compartment of the sinusoid.

### 20. Heterogeneous Gene Expression in Hepatic Lobule

To describe the regulated gene expression of three enzymes, carbamoylphosphate synthetase, glutamine synthetase and ornithine aminotransferase along the porto-central axis, we adopted the mechanistic model proposed by Christoffel et al.[18] The model is based on simple receptor-ligand kinetics and the parameters are fitted by experimental values. $[F_x^*]$ is the concentration of the active transcription factor $F$ of enzyme $x$ and assumed as follows[18]:

Carbamoylphosphate synthetase: $[F_{CPS}^*]$ 0.2 – 0.01$X$

Glutamine synthetase and ornithine aminotransferase: $[F_{GS}^*] = [F_{OAT}^*]$ 0.1$X$

$X$ is the radius of the hepatic lobule: $X = 0$ corresponds to the portal tracts and $X = 10$ corresponds to the central vein. Thus, $X$ was defined as follows in our model:

$$X = 10 \times \frac{n}{\text{the total of sinusoidal compartments}}$$

$n$ is the number of compartment out of eight compartments: $n = 1$ corresponds to the compartment adjacent to the portal tracts and $n = 8$ corresponds to the compartment adjacent the central vein. The total of sinusoidal compartments is eight in our model. $R_{\text{GX},x}$ is the relative rate of transcription, assumed to correspond to the transcription rate in our model. $R_{\text{GX},x}$ is calculated using the fractional saturation $Y_{\text{GX},x}$, the discussion constant $K_{\text{GX},x}$ and the Hill coefficient $n_{\text{GX},x}$ as follows:[18]

$$Y_{\text{GX},x} = \frac{[F_x^*]^{n_{\text{GX},x}}}{[F_x^*]^{n_{\text{GX},x}} + K_{\text{GX},x}{}^{n_{\text{GX},x}}}$$

$$R_{\text{GX},x} = R_{\max,\text{GX},x} Y_{\text{GX},x}$$

Carbamoylphosphate synthetase was fitted with high-affinity ($Y_{GX,CPS,h}$) and low-affinity ($Y_{GX,CPS,l}$) units as follow:[18].

$$R_{\text{GX,CPS}} = R_{\max,\text{GX,CPS}}\left(Y_{\text{GX,CPS},h} + Y_{\text{GX,CPS},l}\right)$$

## References


1. Jungermann K, Katz N. Functional specialization of different hepatocyte populations. Physiol Rev 1989; 69(3):708-764.
2. Gebhardt R. Metabolic zonation of the liver: regulation and implications for liver function. Pharmacol Ther 1992; 53(3):275-354.
3. Jungermann K, Kietzmann T. Zonation of parenchymal and nonparenchymal metabolism in liver. Annu Rev Nutr 1996; 16179-203.
4. Haussinger D. Liver and systemic pH-regulation. Z Gastroenterol 1992; 30(2):147-150.
5. Meijer AJ, Lamers WH, Chamuleau RA. Nitrogen metabolism and ornithine cycle function. Physiol Rev 1990; 70(3):701-748.
6. Kuo FC, Darnell JE Jr. Evidence that interaction of hepatocytes with the collecting (hepatic) veins triggers position-specific transcription of the glutamine synthetase and ornithine aminotransferase genes in the mouse liver. Mol Cell Biol 1991; 11(12):6050-6058.
7. Kuo FC, Hwu WL, Valle D et al. Colocalization in pericentral hepatocytes in adult mice and similarity in developmental expression pattern of ornithine aminotransferase and glutamine synthetase mRNA. Proc Natl Acad Sci USA 1991; 88(21):9468-9472.
8. Ohno H, Naito Y, Nakajima H et al. Construction of biological tissue model based on single-cell model: A computer simulation of metabolic heterogeneity in the liver lobule. Artif Life 2008; 14(1):3-28.
9. Schneider W, Siems W, Grune T. Balancing of energy-consuming processes of rat hepatocytes. Cell Biochem Funct 1990; 8(4):227-232.
10. Elliott KR, Tipton KF. Product inhibition studies on bovine liver carbamoyl phosphate synthetase. Biochem J 1974; 141(3):817-824.
11. Elliott KR, Tipton KF. Kinetic studies of bovine liver carbamoyl phosphate synthetase. Biochem J 1974; 141(3):807-816.
12. Bachmann C, Krahenbuhl S, Colombo JP. Purification and properties of acetyl-CoA:L-glutamate N-acetyltransferase from human liver. Biochem J 1982; 205(1):123-127.
13. Kohn MC. Propagation of information in MetaNet graph models. J Theor Biol 1992; 154(4):505-517.
14. Segel IH. Enzyme Kinetics: Behavior and Analysis of Rapid Equilibrium and Steady State Enzyme Systems. New York: John Wiley and Sons, 1993.
15. Kuchel PW, Roberts DV, Nichol LW. The simulation of the urea cycle: correlation of effects due to inborn errors in the catalytic properties of the enzymes with clinical-biochemical observations. Aust J Exp Biol Med Sci 1977; 55(3):309-326.
16. Kohn MC, Tohmaz AS, Giroux KJ et al. Robustness of MetaNet graph models: predicting control of urea production in humans. Biosystems 2002; 65(1):61-78.
17. Low SY, Salter M, Knowles RG et al. A quantitative analysis of the control of glutamine catabolism in rat liver cells. Use of selective inhibitors. Biochem J 1993; 295(Pt2)617-624.
18. Christoffels VM, Sassi H, Ruijter JM et al. A mechanistic model for the development and maintenance of portocentral gradients in gene expression in the liver. Hepatology 1999; 29(4):1180-1192.

## Chapter 10

# Decoding the Signaling Mechanism of Toll-Like Receptor 4 Pathways in Wild Type and Knockouts

**Kumar Selvarajoo***

**Guest Editor: Sankar Ghosh**

## Abstract

The Myeloid Differentiation Primary-Response Protein 88 (MyD88)-dependent and—independent pathways induce proinflammatory cytokines when toll-like receptor 4 (TLR4) is activated through lipopolysaccharide (LPS) stimulus. Recent studies have implicated a crosstalk mechanism between the two pathways. However, the exact location and nature of this interaction is poorly understood. Using my previous ordinary differential equations-based computational model of the TLR4 pathway, I investigated the roles played by the various proposed crosstalk mechanisms by comparing in silico nuclear factor κB (NF-κB) and Mitogen-Activated Protein (MAP) kinases dynamic activity profiles with experimental results under various conditions in macrophages to LPS stimulus (MyD88 deficient, TRAF-6 deficient etc.). The model that best represents the experimental findings suggests that the pathways interact at more than one location: (i) TRIF to TRAF-6, (ii) TRIF-RIP1-IKK complex and (iii) TRIF to cRel via TBK1.

## Introduction

The Toll-like receptors (TLRs) are key elements of the innate immune system. These receptors recognize conserved pathogen-associated molecular patterns related to micro-organisms, such as lipopolysaccharide (LPS) and double-stranded RNA and trigger both microbial clearance and the induction of immunoregulatory chemokines and cytokines. There are a total of 13 known TLRs to date, of which TLR4 has received particular attention.[1,2] Upon LPS ligation, TLR4 activates the MyD88-dependent and MyD88-independent pathways. The MyD88-dependent pathway, which is common to all TLRs except TLR3, activates NF-κB and activator protein-1 (AP-1) resulting in the induction of proinflammatory chemokines and cytokines such as Tumour-Necrosis-Factor α (TNF-α) and interleukin-1β (IL-1β). The MyD88-independent pathway, on the other hand, activates Interferon (IFN) Regulatory Factor 3 (IRF-3) and induces IFN-β and other chemokines like CCL5 and CXCL10.[1,2]

*Kumar Selvarajoo—Bioinformatics Institute, A*STAR, Biopolis, Singapore 138-671; Institute for Advanced Biosciences, Keio University, Tsuruoka, 997-0035, Japan. Email: kumar@ttck.keio.ac.jp

*E-Cell System: Basic Concepts and Applications*, edited by Satya Nanda Vel Arjunan, Pawan K. Dhar and Masaru Tomita. 

Studies of signaling cascades mediated through the MyD88-dependent and -independent pathways have so far been predominantly performed in a nonconstitutive manner. That is, the two pathways have been studied independently of each other. More recently there have been implications that the components of the two pathways may indeed interact downstream of TRIF and, therefore, may be dependent on each other in the activation of transcription factor NF-κB. For example, the interaction of TRIF with TNF-Receptor-Associated Factor 6 (TRAF6) has been suggested by Sato et al (2003).[3] This leads to the question whether TRAF6 binding to TRIF could lead to the activation of NF-κB in a MyD88-independent manner. However, other studies involving the LPS-induced activation of TLR4 in TRAF-6 deficient mice have also shown the induction of NF-κB.[4,5] Collectively, these studies indicate a possible link between the MyD88-dependent and -independent pathways in the activation of NF-κB in both MyD88 and TRAF-6 deficient mice. However, the suggestion of signaling crosstalk occurring by the binding of TRAF-6 to TRIF seems controversial.[3,5]

I approached this issue in a systemic manner. Previously, I developed a computational model of the MyD88-dependent and -independent pathways.[6] The model showed the possible signaling mechanism for the delayed NF-κB kinetics observed in MyD88-deficient mice. Using this model with careful modifications, I investigated several in silico crosstalk mechanisms between the MyD88-dependent and -independent pathways and compared the model simulations with experimental findings for NF-κB and MAP kinases activity in wild type and various knock-out conditions.

## Materials and Methods

The details of the modeling strategy and the original computational model (reference model) have been previously published.[6] In short, the development of our model includes selecting appropriate signaling reaction networks and determining associated kinetic parameters. As the TLR field is relatively new, we do not know the kinetic details of each signaling process. In addition,

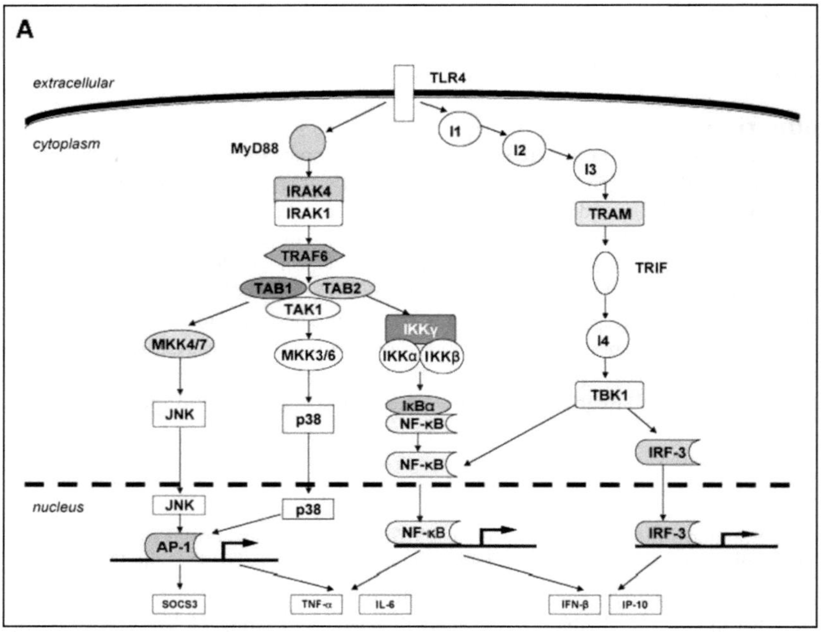


Figure 1. Figure and legend continued on following page.

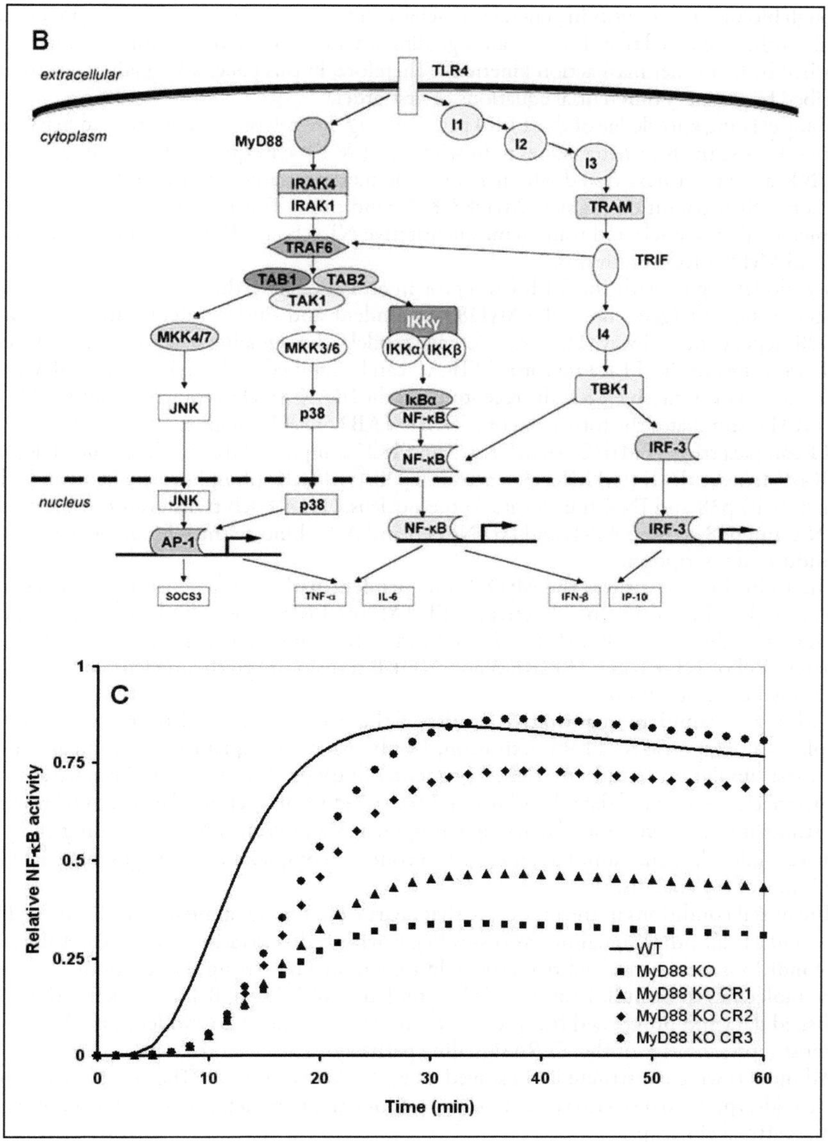


Figure 1. A, viewed on previous page) Reference TLR4 model. The MyD88-dependent and MyD88-independent signaling pathways with hypothetical intermediates, adapted from Selvarajoo, 2006. B) The addition of a crosstalk mechanism between TRIF and TRAF6 molecules (Model A); see Appendix A for details. C) The simulated time course of the relative activity of NF-κB for various reactions rates of TRIF to TRAF6 crosstalk in MyD88 KO conditions using Model A. The x-axis represents the time in minutes and the y-axis represents the relative activity of NF-κB. WT (line) and MyD88 KO (squares) profiles were generated using Model A. MyD88 KO- CR1 to CR3 refers to simulation with TRIF/TRAF6 rate constant at 0.1/min (triangles), 0.5/min (diamonds), and 1.0/min (circles), respectively. Note: For all figures, the relative activities have been normalized to a maximum unit value.

although biological networks in general can behave in nonlinear fashion, in my original model I and also others, showed that downstream signaling reaction events to receptor activation can be described by first order mass action kinetics.[7,8] Therefore, in this paper all signaling reactions are described by ordinary differential equations of first order.

Using existing knowledge of the TLR4 pathway (Fig. 1A, reference pathway) and mass-action kinetics, I chose the parameter values to fit wild-type (WT) semi-quantitative profiles of NF-κB and JNK activity.[9] I next tested whether the same model parameters also performed well in a knockout (KO) condition, namely MyD88 KO condition.[9] This is an iterative process where parameter values are selected using semi-quantitative NF-κB and JNK activity profiles in both WT and MyD88 KO conditions.[6]

My model begins with the TLR4 receptor in an active state through the binding of LPS. The active signal triggers both the MyD88-dependent and -independent pathways. For the MyD88-dependent pathway (Fig. 1A, reference model), the signaling reactions are (i) MyD88/MAL associates to the TLR4 receptor (TIRAP can be lumped with MyD88), (ii) IRAK1 and IRAK4 associate with MyD88 at the receptor, (iii) the IRAK-MyD88 complex activates TRAF6, (iv) TRAF6 stimulates the formation of a TAB1/TAB2/TAK1 complex, (v) the TAB1/TAB2/TAK1 complex triggers MKK3/6, MKK4/7 and IKK complexes (IKKα, IKKβ and IKKγ), (vi) MKK4/7 activates JNK (vii) MKK3/6 activates p38, (vii) IKKs phosphorylate IκBα and release NF-κB, (viii) p38 and JNK translocate to the nucleus, (ix) NF-κB translocates to the nucleus, (x) JNK and p38 activate AP-1, and (xi) NF-κB and AP-1 bind to the relevant gene promoters and induces transcription.

The following constitutes the MyD88-independent pathway: (a) TLR4 stimulates intermediate 1 (I1), I2 and I3, (b) I3 activates TRAM, (c) TRIF is recruited to the TIR domain of TLR4 together with TRAM, (d) TRIF binds TBK1 and activates IRF-3, (e) TBK1 also activates cRel of NF-κB and (f) IRF-3 and NF-κB translocate to the nucleus and induce the relevant gene transcription.

Although I simulate quantitative results of the various activated proteins and protein complexes in response to TLR4 activation, I only make semi-quantitative comparisons between the simulation results and the experimental findings. This is due to the general lack of quantitative experimental data. In addition, I restricted my model simulations to 60 min after LPS stimulation, to ignore secondary signaling such as autocrine TNF-α signaling and IκBα negative feedback regulation. I assume such secondary complexities are negligible within the time frame of my analysis.[5,10]

The initial conditions in the model are that apart from the signaling step TLR4 to MyD88/MAL and I1, all other signaling processes begin with null activation (at $t = 0$). The various KO conditions were generated from the wild-type model by setting the reaction(s) upstream of the molecules to be null. I compared the simulation of JNK, p38 and NF-κB activity with published data and progressed from reference model to Model A to Model B, the latter being the most representative of the TLR4 signaling pathway.

All models were constructed and solved using E-Cell version 3.[11] The complete computational wild-type Model B with the kinetic expressions and parameters is available upon request (kumar@ttck.keio.ac.jp).

## Results

### *TRAF-6 Independent NF-κB Activation in MyD88 KO Is Possible*

To test the proposed mechanism of crosstalk between TRAF-6 and TRIF that leads to the NF-κB activation in the MyD88-independent manner,[3] I inserted, in silico, a signaling reaction between TRIF and TRAF-6 in the original reference model and labeled the updated model as Model A (Fig. 1B and Appendix A). Using this model, I simulated the NF-κB activity profile for WT and MyD88 KO conditions, initially setting the TRIF to TRAF-6 reaction null, and checked whether the model simulation mimics the experimental observation of Kawai et al, 1999 (Fig. 1C, WT & MyD88 KO).

It is well known that for wild type macrophages the MyD88-dependent pathway is the key pathway for early phase NF-κB activation. Therefore, to investigate the importance of TRIF and TRAF-6 crosstalk, I performed the NF-κB simulation at various rates of reaction between TRIF and TRAF-6 in MyD88 KO conditions (Fig. 1C, MyD88 KO- CR1 etc.). Interestingly, we observed that as the rate constant between TRIF-TRAF-6 is increased, the peak levels of NF-κB activity approaches the WT profile, even in MyD88 KO conditions, although with a time-delay response. This implies that TRIF to TRAF-6 crosstalk can result in MyD88-independent activation of NF-κB; however, it may not be dominant.

### *MyD88-Independent Pathway also Interacts Downstream of TRAF-6 but Upstream of TBK1*

In TRAF6-deficient mice, delayed activation of MAP kinases has been reported.[5] This observation indicates that in addition to TRIF to TRAF-6 and TRIF to cRel via TBK1 (Fig. 1B) there exists other crosstalk mechanisms, intuitively, upstream of MAP kinases and downstream of TRAF-6. I next tested my model in silico by making interactions between TRIF and signaling molecules/complexes downstream of TRAF-6 but upstream of JNK. This reduced the possibility of crosstalk of TRIF with either the TAK/TAB complex or MKK3/6 and MKK4/7 (Fig. 1B).

Recently, Transforming-Growth-Factor-β-Activated Kinase (TAK1) has been shown to play a vital role in multiple signaling pathways.[12] TAK1 KO studies revealed that TAK1 is essential for the TLR-induced JNK activity[12] and the activation of MAP kinases in response to IL-1β.[13] To test whether TRIF and the TAK/TAB complex interact, I once again included the relevant in silico interaction in Model A and performed WT and MyD88 KO simulations to LPS stimulus. In order to generate the delayed activation of MAP kinases observed in MyD88 KO conditions, I added at least two hypothetical intermediates between TRIF and the TAK/TAB complex (Fig. 2A, Model B, Appendix A) in the same manner I performed earlier.[6] Using the modified model I simulated in silico TAK1 KO for JNK activation in TLR4 activation. The model simulation showed complete abolition of JNK activation (Fig. 2B). Similar result for TAK1 KO cells was reported by Shim et al, 2005. Next, I performed in silico TRAF-6 KO simulations and reproduced p38 and NF-κB activity profile in accordance with Gohda et al, 2004 (Fig. 2C,D).

A computational model is acceptable only if it is able to predict multiple perturbation studies. The updated Model B is also able to predict the NF-κB activation for various types of available KO studies (MyD88 KO, TRAF-6-KO and TRIF KO) in macrophages (Fig. 2D).[5,9,14] In all conditions and also for JNK and p38 relative activity, I observed the simulation profiles yield consistent result with experimental observations (Fig. 2B-D).

## Discussion

Recent studies have shown that the MyD88-dependent and -independent signaling cascades may interact and thereby possibly coregulate NF-κB and MAP kinases. For instance, blocking the MyD88 pathway through MyD88 KO in TLR4 stimulus also leads to JNK and NF-κB activation, albeit with delayed kinetics.[4,9] There have been other reports that TRAF-6 binds to TRIF and may thus activate NF-κB in a MyD88-independent manner.[3] However, cells deficient of TRAF-6 still showed JNK and NF-κB activation.[4,5]

Previously I reported a computational model (MyD88-dependent and -independent pathways) that demonstrated the probable reasons for the delayed NF-κB activation observed in MyD88-deficient mice.[6] I used this model, with appropriate modifications, to first test the idea whether TRAF-6 binding to TRIF activates NF-κB (Model A, Fig. 1B). By performing in silico simulations and comparing the results with reported experimental findings, I showed that this mechanism is possible. However it may not be sufficient to concur that this is the only other MyD88-independent activator of NF-κB on top of TRIF to cRel via TBK1 mentioned in my previous model (Fig. 1A).

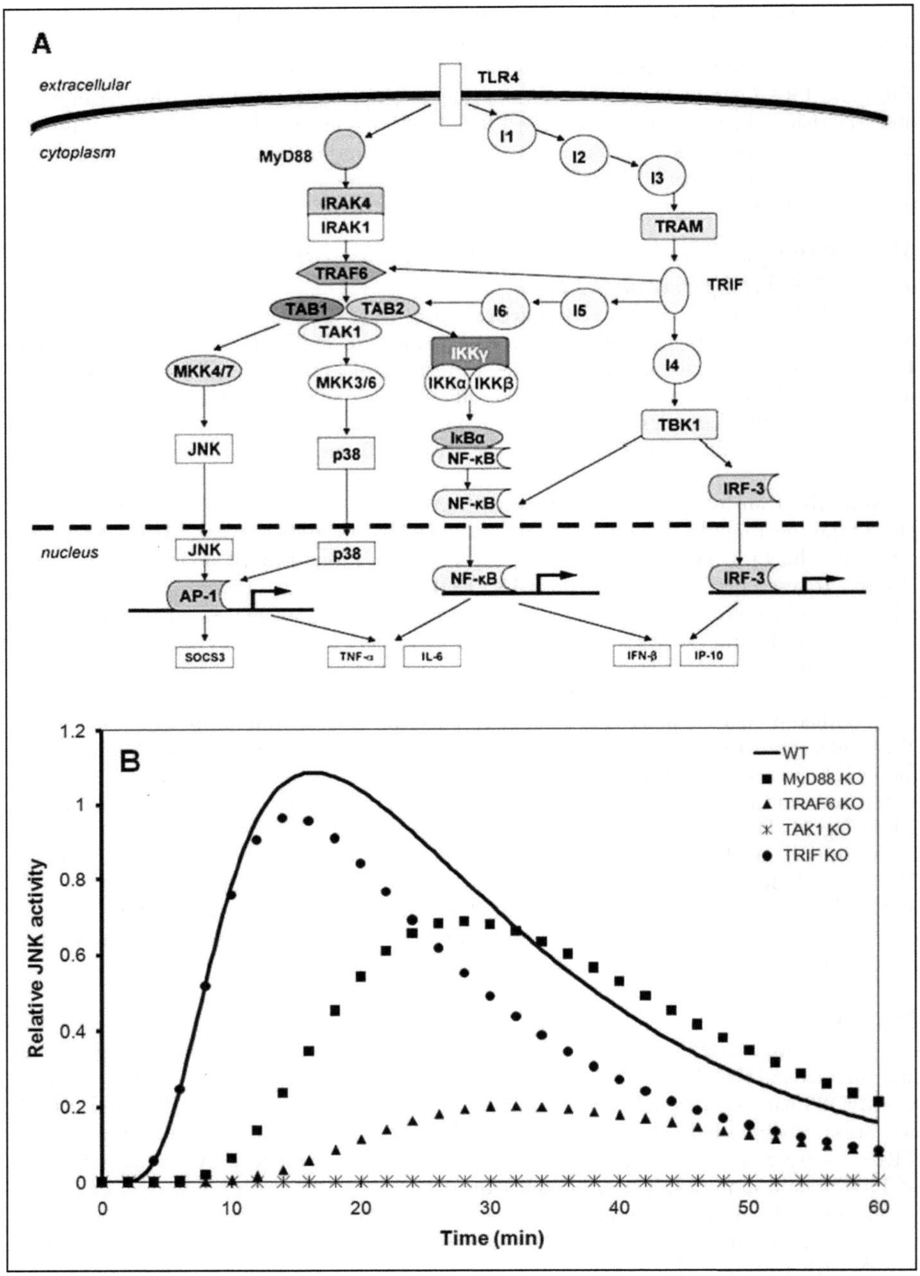


Figure 2. Figure and legend continued on following page.

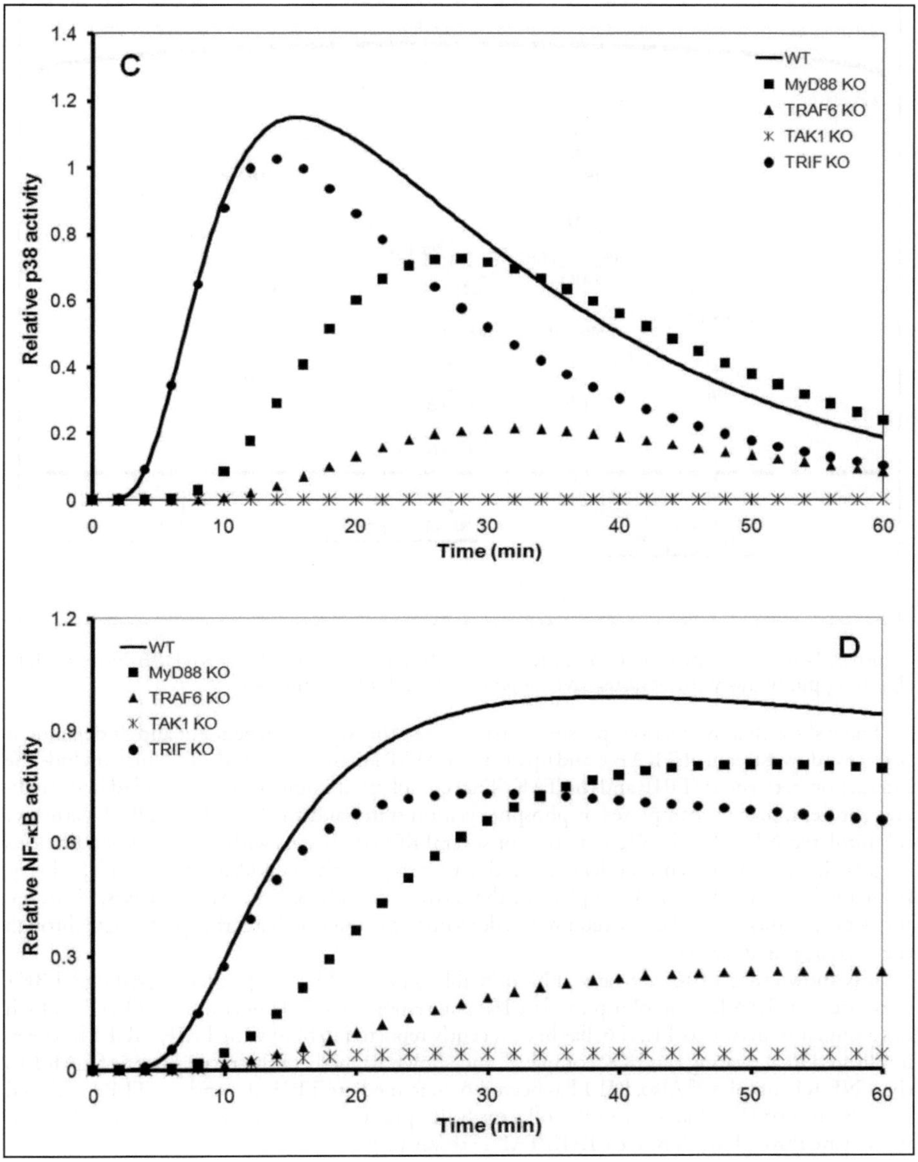


Figure 2. A) Model B. The MyD88-dependent and MyD88-independent signaling pathways with the crosstalk mechanism between TRIF and TAK/TAB complex via a few hypothetical intermediates (protein, protein complexes or phosphorylation step). See Appendix A for details. The simulated time course of the relative activity of (B) JNK, (C) p38 and (D) NF-κB for the WT (line), MyD88 KO (squares), TRAF-6 KO (triangles), TAK1 KO (crosses) and TRIF KO (circles) in Model B. The x-axis represents the time in minutes and the y-axis represents the relative activity of JNK (B), p38 (C) and NF-κB (D).

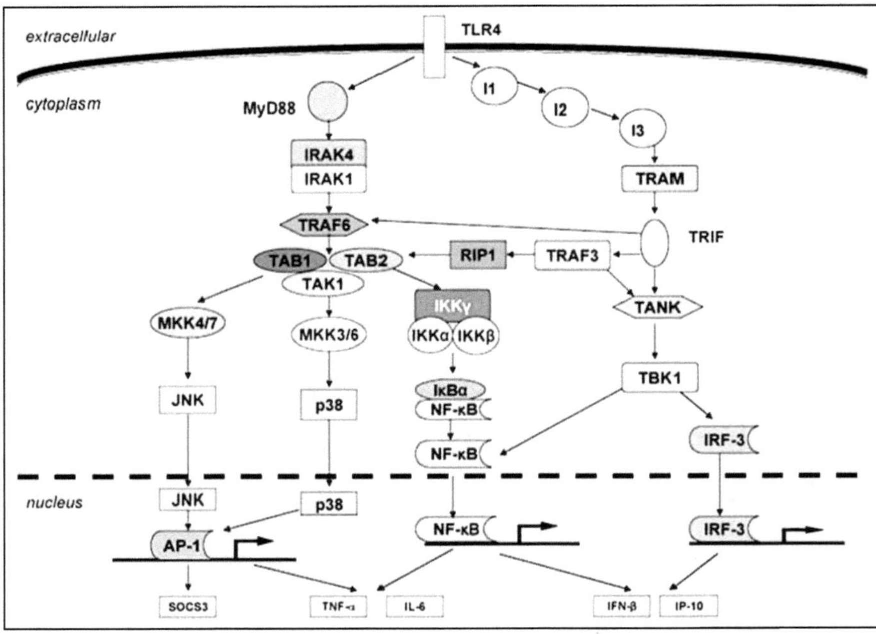


Figure 3. The new proposed TLR4 pathway. The MyD88-dependent and MyD88-independent signaling pathways with various investigated crosstalk mechanisms.

I next show that interactions possibly exist between the MyD88-dependent and -independent pathways downstream of TRAF-6 and upstream of MAP kinases. The Model B (which include the interaction between (i)TRIF and the TAK/TAB complex with numerous unclassified intermediates (protein, protein complexes or phosphorylation state) and the (ii)TRIF/ TBK1 pathway) recapitulated NF-κB and JNK activities for several KO conditions with reasonable simulations (Fig. 2B-D). In summary, my model suggests that there is possibly one additional crosstalk pathway, from TRIF to the TAK/TAB complex, for the activation of NF-κB and MAP kinases. However, further experimental studies are required to determine the intermediates that participate through the two suggested pathways.

It is known that TBK1 activates IFN-inducible genes via TRIF-dependent signaling.[3] TBK1 associate with TANK[15] and phosphorylate IRF3 in response to viral infection.[16,17] TRAF3, which has a similar structure to TRAF6, has been recently reported to bind with TRIF.[18] RIP1 has been implicated in activating the IKK complex[19] and shown to mediate the recruitment of TAK1 to the TNF-R1 complex.[20] Also, RIP1 has been shown to mediate TRIF-dependent, TLR4-induced NF-κB but not IRF-3 activation.[21] Collectively, it appears that both TRAF3 and RIP1 might participate through the TRIF to TAK/TAB pathway (Fig. 3).

## Conclusion

The TLR field is rapidly evolving and many time-course experiments are being performed to understand the regulatory roles of various signaling adaptors and molecules. Without the use of appropriate analytical tools, like the computational TLR4 pathway models, it is a daunting challenge for biologists to analyse and interpret the complex information generated by the various experiments. In this paper, I have shown the utility of in silico models to put together and test various hypotheses regarding the TLR signaling mechanism. I investigated, through various simulations, the crosstalk mechanisms between the MyD88-dependent and -independent pathways at early time signaling to LPS stimulus, without assuming too many details of the TLR4 signaling pathways from literature. The final Model B is consistent across several literature observations, showing how computer models can help us understand the mechanistic process behind the complex signaling dynamics. Such result from systemic work will surely provide hints to the wet-bench experimentalist to perform more targeted research that will eventually, but at an increasing pace, lead to the discovery of novel intracellular targets, say, for the TLR signaling in disease conditions.

## *Acknowledgments*

Koichi Matsuo, Masa Tsuchiya (Keio University) and Shizuo Akira (Osaka University) are thanked for their critical reading of the manuscript. I would also like to thank my funding agency, Biomedical Research Council of Singapore.

## References

1. O'Neill LA. TLRs: Professor Mechnikov, sit on your hat. Trends Immunol 2004; 25:687-693.
2. Akira S, Takeda K. Toll-like receptor signalling. Nat Rev Immunol 4(7), 499-511.
3. Sato S, Sugiyama M, Yamamoto M et al. Toll/IL-1 receptor domain-containing adaptor inducing IFN-beta (TRIF) associates with TNF receptor-associated factor 6 and TANK-binding kinase 1 and activates two distinct transcription factors, NF-kappa B and IFN-regulatory factor-3, in the Toll-like receptor signaling. J Immunol 2003; 171(8):4304-4310.
4. Kawai T, Takeuchi O, Fujita T et al. Lipopolysaccharide Stimulates the MyD88-Independent Pathway and Results in Activation of IFN-Regulatory Factor 3 and the Expression of a Subset of Lipopolysaccharide-Inducible Genes. J Immunol 2001; 167(10):5887-5894.
5. Gohda J, Matsumura T, Inoue J. Cutting edge: TNFR-associated factor (TRAF) 6 is essential for MyD88-dependent pathway but not toll/IL-1 receptor domain-containing adaptor-inducing IFN-beta (TRIF)-dependent pathway in TLR signaling. J Immunol 2004; 73(5):2913-2917.
6. Selvarajoo K. Discovering differential activation machinery of the Toll-like receptor 4 signaling pathways in MyD88 knockouts. FEBS Lett 2006; 580(5):1457-1464.
7. Covert MW, Leung TH, Gaston JE et al. Achieving stability of lipopolysaccharide-induced NF-kappaB activation. Science 2005; 309(5742):1854-1857.
8. Yamada S, Shiono S, Joo A et al. Control mechanism of JAK/STAT signal transduction pathway. FEBS Lett 2003; 534(1-3);190-196.
9. Kawai T, Adachi O, Ogawa T et al. Unresponsiveness of MyD88-deficient mice to endotoxin. Immunity 1999; 11(1):115-122.
10. Hoffmann A, Levchenko A, Scott ML et al. The IκB-NF-κB Signaling Module: Temporal Control and Selective Gene Activation. Science 2002; 298(5596):1241-1245.
11. Takahashi K, Ishikawa N, Sadamoto Y et al. E-Cell 2: multi-platform E-Cell simulation system. Bioinformatics 2003; 19:1727-1729.
12. Shim JH, Xiao C, Paschal AE et al. TAK1, but not TAB1 or TAB2, plays an essential role in multiple signaling pathways in vivo. Genes Dev 2005; 19(22):2668-2681.
13. Sato S, Sanjo H, Takeda K et al. Essential function for the kinase TAK1 in innate and adaptive immune responses. Nat Immunol 2005; 6(11):1087-1095.
14. Hoebe K, Du X, Georgel P et al. Identification of Lps2 as a key transducer of MyD88-independent TIR signalling. Nature 2003; 424(6950):743-748.
15. McWhirter SM, Fitzgerald KA, Rosains J et al. IFN-regulatory factor 3-dependent gene expression is defective in Tbk1-deficient mouse embryonic fibroblasts. Proc Natl Acad Sci USA 2004; 101(1):233-238.
16. Fitzgerald KA, McWhirter SM, Faia KL et al. IKKepsilon and TBK1 are essential components of the IRF3 signaling pathway. Nat Immunol 2003; 4(5):491-496.
17. Sharma S, tenOever BR, Grandvaux N et al. Triggering the interferon antiviral response through an IKK-related pathway. Science 2003, 300(5622):1148-1151.
18. Hacker H, Redecke V, Blagoev B et al. Specificity in Toll-like receptor signalling through distinct effector functions of TRAF3 and TRAF6. Nature 2005; 439(7073):204-207.
19. Poyet JL, Srinivasula SM, Lin JH et al. Activation of the Ikappa B kinases by RIP via IKKgamma / NEMO-mediated oligomerization. J Biol Chem 2000; 275(48):37966-37977.
20. Blonska M, Shambharkar PB, Kobayashi M et al. TAK1 is recruited to the tumor necrosis factor-alpha (TNF-alpha) receptor 1 complex in a receptor-interacting protein (RIP)-dependent manner and cooperates with MEKK3 leading to NF-kappaB activation. J Biol Chem 2005; 280(52):43056-43063.
21. Cusson-Hermance N, Khurana S, Lee TH et al. Rip1 mediates the Trif-dependent toll-like receptor 3- and 4-induced NF-{kappa}B activation but does not contribute to interferon regulatory factor 3 activation. J Biol Chem 2005; 280(44):36560-36566.

# Appendix A

## *Model A*

| No. | Reaction | Kinetic Formula | Parameter Values (1/min) |
|---|---|---|---|
| | *MyD88-dependent pathway* | | |
| 1 | TLR4 ↔ MyD88 | $k_{f1}$*TLR4—$k_{b1}$*MyD88 | $k_{f1} = 1.0$, $k_{b1} = 0.0001$ |
| | | | $k_{f1} = 0$, $k_{b1} = 0$ (MyD88 KO) |
| 2 | MyD88 ↔ IRAK4/1 | $k_{f2}$* MyD88—$k_{b2}$* IRAK4/1 | $k_{f2} = 1.0$, $k_{b2} = 0.0001$ |
| 3 | IRAK4/1 ↔ TRAF6 | $k_{f3}$* IRAK4/1—$k_{b3}$* TRAF6 | $k_{f3} = 1.0$, $k_{b3} = 0.0001$ |
| | | | $k_{f3} = 0$, $k_{b3} = 0$ (TRAF-6 KO) |
| 4 | TRAF6 ↔ TABTAK | $k_{f4}$* TRAF6—$k_{b4}$* TABTAK | $k_{f4} = 1.0$, $k_{b4} = 0.0001$ |
| 5 | TABTAK ↔ MKK4 | $k_{f5}$ * TABTAK—$k_{b5}$* MKK4 | $k_{f5} = 0.1$, $k_{b5} = 0.0001$ |
| 6 | TABTAK ↔ MKK3/6 | $k_{f6}$ * TABTAK—$k_{b6}$* MKK3/6 | $k_{f6} = 0.1$, $k_{b6} = 0.0001$ |
| 7 | TABTAK ↔ IKKαβγ | $k_{f7}$ * TABTAK—$k_{b7}$* IKKαβγ | $k_{f7} = 0.21$, $k_{b7} = 0.0001$ |
| 8 | MKK4 ↔ JNK | $k_{f8}$ * MKK4—$k_{b8}$* JNK | $k_{f8} = 0.34$, $k_{b8} = 0.0001$ |
| 9 | JNK ↔ JNK_n | $k_{f9}$ * JNK—$k_{b9}$* JNK _n | $k_{f9} = 1.0$, $k_{b9} = 0.0001$ |
| 10 | MKK3/6 ↔ p38 | $k_{f10}$ * MKK3/6—$k_{b10}$* p38 | $k_{f10} = 0.4$, $k_{b10} = 0.0001$ |
| 11 | p38 ↔ p38_n | $k_{f11}$ * p38—$k_{b11}$* p38_n | $k_{f11} = 1.0$, $k_{b11} = 0.0001$ |
| 12 | p38_n AP-1_n | $k_{f12}$* AP-1_n | $k_{f12} = 0.054$ |
| 13 | IKKαβγ ↔ IkBα/NF-κB | $k_{f13}$ * IKKαβγ—$k_{b12}$* IkBα/NF-κB | $k_{f13} = 1.0$, $k_{b12} = 0.0001$ |
| 14 | IkBα/NF-κB ↔ NF-κB_c | $k_{f14}$ * IkBα/NF-κB—$k_{b13}$* NF-κB_c | $k_{f14} = 0.2$, $k_{b13} = 0.0001$ |
| 15 | NF-κB_c NF-κB_n | $k_{f15}$* NF-κB_c | $k_{f15} = 1.0$ |
| | *MyD88-independent pathway* | | |
| 16 | TLR4 ↔ IND1 | $k_{f16}$*TLR4—$k_{b14}$* IND1 | $k_{f16} = 0.57$, $k_{b14} = 0.0001$ |
| 17 | IND1 ↔ IND2 | $k_{f17}$* IND1—$k_{b15}$* IND2 | $k_{f17} = 0.6$, $k_{b15} = 0.0001$ |
| 18 | IND2 ↔ IND3 | $k_{f18}$* IND2—$k_{b16}$* IND3 | $k_{f18} = 0.6$, $k_{b16} = 0.0001$ |
| 19 | IND3 ↔ TRAM | $k_{f19}$* IND3—$k_{b17}$* TRAM | $k_{f19} = 0.6$, $k_{b17} = 0.0001$ |
| 20 | TRAM ↔ TRIF | $k_{f20}$* TRAM—$k_{b18}$* TRIF | $k_{f20} = 0.6$, $k_{b18} = 0.0001$ |

*continued on next page*

***Model A. Continued***

| No. | Reaction | Kinetic formula | Parameter values (1/min) |
|---|---|---|---|
| 21 | TRIF ↔ TRAF6 | $k_{f21}$* TRIF—$k_{b19}$* TRAF6 | $k_{f21} = 0.32$, $k_{b19} = 0.0001$<br>$k_{f21} = 0$, $k_{b19} = 0$ (TRAF-6 KO) |
| 22 | TRIF ↔ IND4 | $k_{f22}$* TRIF—$k_{b20}$* IND4 | $k_{f22} = 1.0$, $k_{b20} = 0.0001$ |
| 23 | IND4 ↔ TBK1 | $k_{f23}$* IND4—$k_{b21}$* TBK1 | $k_{f23} = 0.5$, $k_{b21} = 0.0001$ |
| 24 | TBK1 ↔ NF-κB_c | $k_{f24}$* TBK1—$k_{b22}$* NF-κB_c | $k_{f24} = 0.036$, $k_{b22} = 0.0001$ |
| 25 | TBK1 ↔ IRF3_c | $k_{f25}$* TBK1—$k_{b23}$* IRF3_c | $k_{f25} = 0.2$, $k_{b23} = 0.0001$ |
| 26 | IRF-3_c → IRF-3_n | $k_{f26}$* IRF-3_c—$k_{b24}$* IRF-3_n | $k_{f26} = 0.01$, $k_{b24} = 0.0001$ |

***Model B (The modifications/additions made for Model A)***

| No. | Reaction | Kinetic formula | Parameter values (1/min) |
|---|---|---|---|
| 27 | TRIF ↔ IND5 | $k_{f27}$* TRIF—$k_{b24}$* IND5 | $k_{f27} = 0.6$, $k_{b24} = 0.0001$ |
| 28 | IND5 ↔ RIP1 | $k_{f28}$* IND5—$k_{b25}$* RIP1 | $k_{f28} = 0.1$, $k_{b25} = 0.0001$ |
| 29 | RIP1 ↔ TABTAK | $k_{f29}$* RIP1—$k_{b26}$* TABTAK | $k_{f29} = 0.6$, $k_{b26} = 0.0001$ |

I have assumed, throughout the paper, that the translocation of NF-κB and AP-1 into the nucleus will increase the binding activity of NF-κB and JNK onto the DNA respectively. Hence, the activity of NF-κB is proportionate to the NF-κB expression and the activity of JNK is proportionate to the AP-1 expression in the nucleus. JNK_n means concentration of activated JNK in the nucleus etc.

# Chapter 11

# Modeling of Hsp70-Mediated Protein Refolding

**Bin Hu,* Matthias P. Mayer and Masaru Tomita**

## Abstract

In this work, we used E-Cell, a software package aiming at large-scale modeling with full object-oriented modeling support, to analyze the 70kDa heat shock protein (Hsp70) chaperone mediated protein folding. We analyzed the kinetic characteristics of this chaperone system during folding of an unfolded protein using computer simulations. Our simulation results are consistent with reported laboratory experiments and support the kinetic partitioning hypothesis. Our model suggests that although the DnaK chaperone system is robust in assisting protein folding, this robustness is limited by the availability of ATP. Based on this model, we also discuss why object-oriented modeling is needed to reduce the complexity of large-scale biochemical models.

## Introduction

Although the entire information for the precise three-dimensional structure of a protein is encoded in its amino acid sequence, in vivo many proteins depend on the assistance of molecular chaperones such as Hsp70 (DnaK) and Hsp60 (GroEL) heat shock proteins for folding from a nascent or denatured state into their correct structure.[1,2] It is known that in *Escherichia coli* the DnaK, DnaJ and GrpE chaperone machinery can efficiently repair misfolded *Photinus pyralis* luciferase both in vivo and in vitro but cannot protect it from heat induced unfolding.[3] Experimental findings suggest that this refolding process is achieved through ATP-dependent interaction between the DnaK chaperone and the substrate protein or peptides.[4] DnaJ and GrpE function as regulators in this system by stimulating DnaK's ATP hydrolysis activity and subsequent nucleotide exchange.[5-8]

The kinetics of the DnaK chaperone system has been studied extensively.[9,10] Different mechanisms have been suggested to explain the steps in chaperone action. The mechanism suggested by Schröder et al[3] has been widely accepted. In this proposed mechanism, an unfolded protein substrate (e.g., *Photinus pyralis* luciferase) first associates with DnaJ, which will present it to DnaK.ATP and induce the formation of a trimeric DnaK.ATP.DnaJ.substrate complex. DnaJ and substrate synergistically stimulate ATP hydrolysis by DnaK and thereby trigger the transition of DnaK from the ATP state with low affinities for substrates to the high-affinity ADP state. GrpE will bind to the latter complex and catalyze the release of ADP. Subsequent ATP binding induces conformational changes in the ATPase domain and substrate binding domain leading to a rapid dissociation of GrpE and substrate from the complex. These steps form a cycle of the DnaK-assisted folding. With enough ATP and all the chaperone molecules, after many cycles, the substrate can be refolded back to its active state (Fig. 1, see also ref. 3). Here we describe a kinetic model for DnaK chaperone action in protein refolding based on Figure 1. The rate constants were derived from literature or completed by our experiments. Our model is shown to simulate correctly the

*Corresponding Author: Bin Hu—Institute for Advanced Biosciences, Keio University. Tsuruoka, 997-035, Japan. Current address: Genome Sciences Group (B-6), Bioscience Division, Los Alamos National Laboratory, M888, Los Alamos, NM 87544. Email: binhu@lanl.gov

*E-Cell System: Basic Concepts and Applications*, edited by Satya Nanda Vel Arjunan, Pawan K. Dhar and Masaru Tomita. 

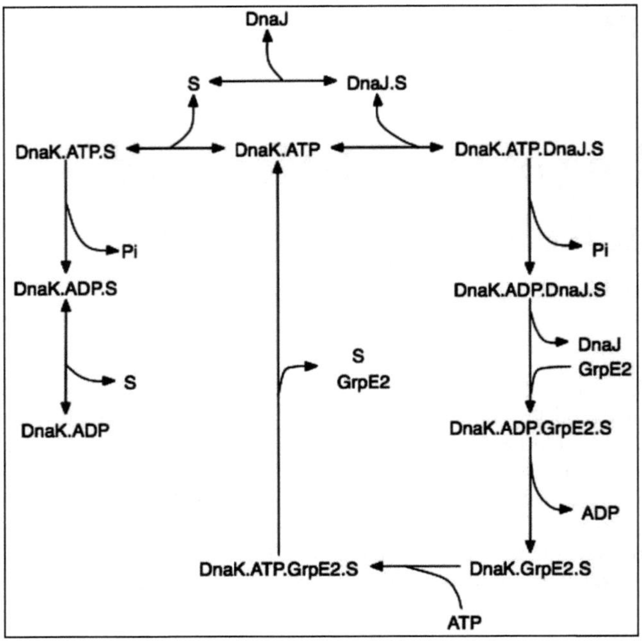


Figure 1. Kinetic model of the DnaK chaperone system in protein refolding. Arrows indicate the reaction direction. S is an abbreviation for substrate. GrpE2 stands for dimer.[25] Pi stands for inorganic phosphate. Dot (.) in between molecules indicates a molecule complex. The substrate first interacts with DnaJ. The DnaJ-substrate complex binds to DnaK.ATP and substrate and DnaJ stimulate the ATP hydrolysis by DnaK, leading to a stable DnaK.ADP.substrate.DnaJ complex. DnaJ may leave and the GrpE dimer enters the complex, catalyzing ADP dissociation. ATP binding to the nucleotide-free DnaK triggers dissociation of substrate and GrpE2, thereby completing the chaperone cycle.

behavior of *E. coli* DnaK chaperone action. The kinetic partition hypothesis proposed for protein refolding, the sensitivity of refolding productivity to alterations in activity and concentration of the chaperones and ATP consumption are discussed.

## Materials and Methods

### *Reaction and Parameters*

The model is based on the rate equations derived from the kinetic model in Figure 1. All the reactions and parameters used in this computer model were either based on published literatures or measured in the M.P.M. lab. For each substrate protein passing through a cycle of refolding process, a probability is assigned for it to be fully refolded. Protein aggregation is not included in our model. This is because of: (1) Lack of quantified data on aggregation; (2) The model is developed to test the property of the DnaK chaperone system at physiologically optimal growing temperatures, where the probability of protein aggregation is small. Please refer to Table1 for a reaction list for DnaK chaperone kinetic model.

### *Simulation and Plotting*

The simulation was based on an improved version of Gillespie's exact stochastic simulation algorithm[21] by Gibson and Bruck,[22] as implemented in E-Cell v3, an open source computer software package for large scale cellular events simulation,[22,24] developed at Keio University (www.e-cell.

***Table 1. Reaction list for DnaK chaperone kinetic model***

| Reaction | Parameter | References |
|---|---|---|
| S + DnaJ -> DnaJ.S | $3.3 \cdot 10^5\ M^{-1}s^{-1}$ | [1] |
| DnaJ.S -> S + DnaJ | $6.2 \cdot 10^{-3}\ s^{-1}$ | [1] |
| DnaJ.S + DnaK.ATP -> DnaK.ATP.DnaJ.S | $1.0 \cdot 10^6\ M^{-1}s^{-1}$ | * |
| DnaK.ATP.DnaJ.S -> DnaK.ATP + DnaJ.S | $2\ s^{-1}$ | ** |
| DnaK.ATP.DnaJ.S -> DnaK.ADP.DnaJ.S + Pi | ca. $1.8\ s^{-1}$ | [2] |
| DnaK.ADP.DnaJ.S + GrpE2 -> DnaK.ADP.GrpE2.S | $3.0 \cdot 10^4\ M^{-1}s^{-1}$ | [3] |
| DnaK.ADP.GrpE2.S -> DnaK.GrpE2.s + ADP | $127\ s^{-1}$ | [4] |
| DnaK.GrpE2.S + ATP -> DnaK.ATP.GrpE2.S | $1.3 \cdot 10^5\ M^{-1}s^{-1}$ | [5] |
| DnaK.ATP.GrpE2.S -> S+ DnaK.ATP + GrpE2 | $0.0001\text{-}7.9\ s^{-1}$ | [6] |
| S + DnaK.ATP -> DnaK.ATP.S | $4.5 \cdot 10^5\ M^{-1}s^{-1}$ | [7] |
| DnaK.ATP.S -> DnaK.ATP + S | $0.0004\text{-}7.2\ s^{-1}$ | [6] |
| DnaK.ATP.S -> DnaK.ADP.S + Pi | $1\text{-}6 \cdot 10^{-3}\ s^{-1}$ | [8, 9] |
| DnaK.ADP.S -> DnaK.ADP + S | $4.7 \cdot 10^{-4}$ | [10] |

*The rate constant was estimated to be similar as the reaction:
S + DnaK.ATP -> DnaK.ATP.S.
**This rate constant was estimated to be similar as the reaction:
DnaK.ATP.S -> DnaK.ATP + S.
Abbreviations used here are the same those used in Figure 1. For reaction: DnaK.ATP.GrpE2.S -> S + DnaK.ATP + GrpE2 a probability is given for S to be fully refolded.

org). The simulation results were plotted by using GnuPlot (www.gnuplot.info). The power fitting in Figure 5 was done with the Microsoft Excel program.

### *Model Validation*

To validate our model, we compared our model results with those published in.[3] As shown in Figure 2, with a refolding probability of 1.16% in a single cycle, results from our model are consistent with laboratory results. A probability value of 1.96% could bring a result with similar dynamics with faster refolding rate.

## Results

### *Partition of the Substrate Binding*

Based on in vitro experiments, it has been proposed that the substrate binding to chaperone follows a kinetic partitioning.[9] In the fast phase, which may take seconds to minutes, more than half of the substrates are bound by chaperones. Later, in the slow phase, the rest, about 50% of the substrates, slowly associate with the chaperones. Our model accurately reproduced this phenomenon when we introduced 1000 molecules of unfolded substrates into the system and simulated the generation of refolded substrates. After about 30 minutes, more than 99% of the substrates were fully refolded (Fig. 3). This result shows the kinetic partitioning is an inherent property of this network with the parameter set we used. It also indicates that the function of DnaK.ATP being able to combine with substrate directly may provide a buffer of the subsequent refolding reactions.

### *Robustness Analysis*

Robustness can be defined as the insensitivity to changes in variables. Here we tested the robustness of the DnaK chaperone system by reducing the initial values for the numbers of DnaK, DnaJ and GrpE molecules by half. Figure 4 shows that after a 50% reduction of the amounts of these chaperone molecules, the system is still able to maintain its behavior for refolding the substrate,

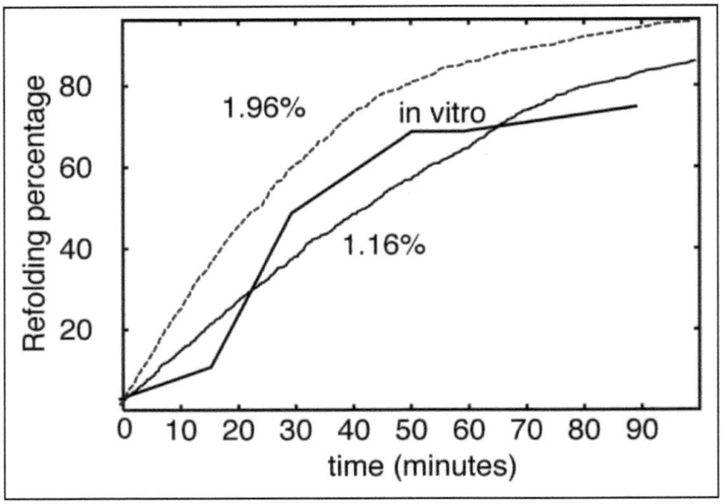


Figure 2. Model validation. In vitro experiment result as published in reference 3. With a refolding probability of 1.16%, our result fits well with their report. Different probability values can result in different refolding speed, although other parameters are the same.

which indicates that the chaperone system is robustly designed. Among the three chaperone molecules tested, a 50% reduction of DnaJ and GrpE had the strongest impact on the refolding process and no significant differences could be found in the results when DnaK and ATP was varied. This is surprising and contrasts in vitro observations. We will discuss this matter below.

### *ATP Consumption*

The function of the DnaK chaperone system depends on the hydrolysis of ATP.[12] In each cycle of the DnaK chaperone action, one molecule of ATP is hydrolyzed to drive the cycle and/or to provide the energy for the refolding process (Fig. 1). During the heat shock response, many cellular proteins will become unfolded and proteins belonging to different functional and structural groups will be affected. It is very likely that these proteins, when exposed to the DnaK machinery, require various chaperone cycles until they reach their native state. To survive heat shock, bacteria must refold as many proteins to their physiological state and as fast as possible. It is known that to achieve this, bacteria will accelerate the heat shock gene expression.[13] The increasing repair activity concomitantly increases the ATP consumption. However, some of the heat-inactivated proteins may be components of the energy generating systems. Thus it is an important question whether the ATP levels are sufficiently high to sustain the repair function. We addressed this question by using four different refolding probabilities and comparing the ATP consumption. As summarized in Figure 5, the relationship between the probabilities of refolding and ATP consumption is nonlinear. A simple power fitting results in the equation: $y = 0.9239\ x^{-1.0327}$

Therefore, the refolding of proteins with a lower refolding probability after release by DnaK consumes much more ATP than the refolding of proteins with a higher refolding probability, especially if the refolding probability is less than about 5%, which means about 20 cycles are needed on average for the unfolded protein to return to its physiological conformation. Under such conditions, cellular ATP levels may soon be exhausted and the functionality of the heat shock proteins will be limited by the quantity of ATP. ATP generation will most likely decrease with increasing temperatures above the physiologically range for which the organism adapted. At the same time, the unfolding probability for native proteins will increase and the refolding probability of proteins released after chaperoning by Hsp70 will decrease. Therefore, slowing down the ATP-consuming chaperone cycle by decreasing the activity of GrpE may be an evolutionary strategy to cope with

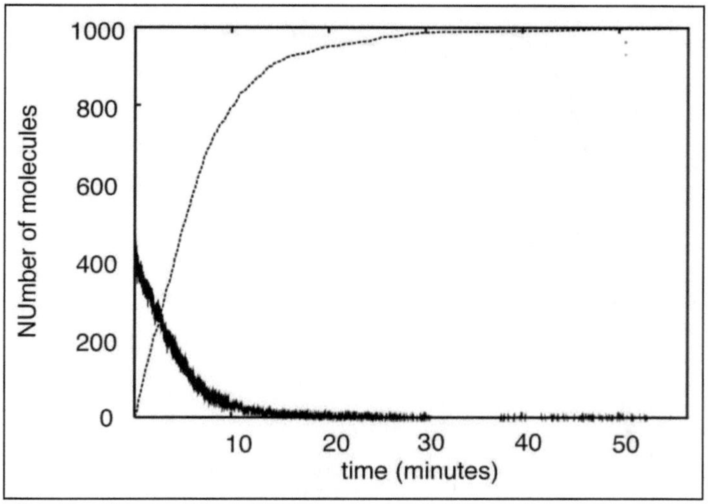


Figure 3. Partition of substrate binding. Solid curve is the number of substrate in the free unfolded state. The dashed curve is the number of refolded substrate.

such situations. Taken together we concluded that although the DnaK chaperone system is robustly designed, this robustness is limited by the cellular amount of ATP.

## Discussion and Conclusion

Based on published literature and our experimental results, we developed a kinetic model for analyzing the DnaK chaperone system in folding de novo synthesized polypeptides or refolding of unfolded proteins at ambient temperatures. Using this model, we analyzed the kinetic partitioning found in DnaK substrate binding reactions and tested the sensitivities of the system's function with respect to DnaK, DnaJ and GrpE. Our model accurately represents the laboratory findings, except the effects of decreased DnaK concentration and activity. The results of the simulations demonstrate that GrpE is the most sensitive component (data not shown) among the three chaperones, which explains the potential function of GrpE as a thermosensor.[11]

The inconsistency of the effect of DnaK concentration and activity between our model and laboratory reports in[10] can have at least two alternative explanations. (1) In our model, we have not included substrate aggregation. If luciferase aggregation is considered, the system will be much more sensitive to the DnaK concentration. This is because DnaK binding of unfolded luciferase will compete the self-aggregation of luciferase. Thus, a part of the high sensitivity of DnaK concentration found in[10] may be due to the aggregation prevention function. (2) In our model we have not considered the possibility of more than one molecule of DnaK binding simultaneously to a single substrate, since to our knowledge there is no experimental evidence published on this issue so far. However, we hypothesize that this is a possible mechanism in vivo to enhance the refolding process. Such a mechanism also would be more sensitive to a reduction of concentration and activity of DnaK. Further laboratory experiments are needed to validate this hypothesis. Protein aggregation and synergistic action of several DnaK molecules during the refolding of a single substrate shall be implemented into future versions of our model when experimental evidence will allow an estimation of the kinetic parameters involved.

One question of debate concerning the DnaK-chaperone cycle was the dissociation of DnaJ. Based on the fact that DnaJ is only 1/10th to 1/30th as abundant as DnaK in vivo[14] and can act substoichiometrically in vitro[15,8] it was assumed that DnaJ leaves the cycle just after the transfer of the substrate onto DnaK and before GrpE binds to the complex.[4] This scenario was chosen for

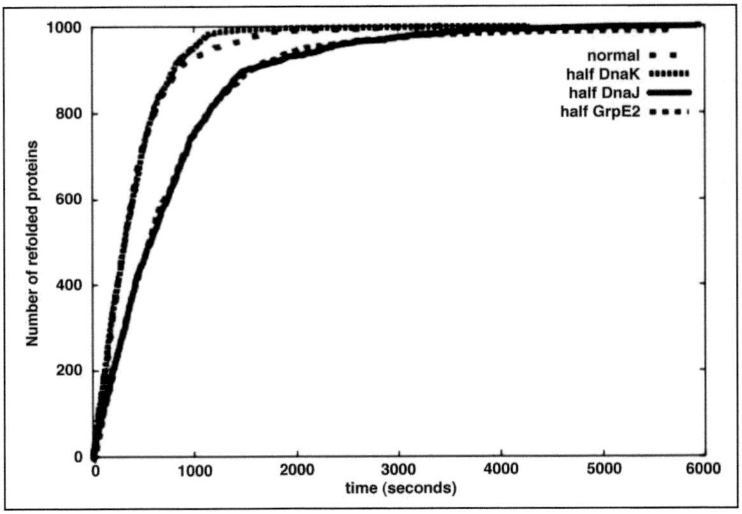


Figure 4. Robustness with respect to initial values.

our model. The elucidation of the binding sites for GrpE in the cocrystal structure with DnaK[16] and for DnaJ through genetic and biochemical analyses[17,18] indicated that both DnaJ and GrpE could eventually bind at the same time to DnaK and possibly to the DnaK-substrate complex. We therefore asked the question whether the refolding efficacy for the substrate would change when DnaJ leaves the cycle together with GrpE upon binding of ATP instead of before the binding of GrpE. However, the results did not change when only the exit point for DnaJ was varied (data not shown). Therefore, despite the substoichiometric concentration of DnaJ, the actual exit point of DnaJ is not critical for the refolding efficacy as long as a quarternary complex of DnaK with DnaJ, substrate and GrpE does not change the dissociation kinetics significantly or has any other additional effect on the refolding probability of the substrate.

Robustness, i.e., buffering relatively large alterations in system parameters, is a natural property of many biological systems and should be expected for the Hsp70 chaperone system as well. Under stress situations, the availability and activity of Hsp70 chaperones may be reduced and it is important to know how the chaperone function is affected under these conditions. Such questions are generally difficult to address experimentally (see also 14). In robustness tests of our model we found that this chaperone system is robustly built to refold proteins. A 50% reduction in the concentration (Fig. 4) did not affect the behavior of refolding dramatically. In the absence of side reactions such as aggregation, the unfolded substrates, once they enter this pathway, will complete their destiny towards refolding. Within the range tested, fluctuations in concentration or activity of the chaperones only delayed the refolding process and did not change the overall behavior. Only severe activity reductions caused significantly longer delays. Such a robust design provides the fundamentals of the heat shock response,[19] where the DnaK chaperone system assists cells to survive temperature increases by refolding heat denatured proteins. Some of this apparent robustness may be due to the exclusion of side reactions such as aggregation and will be investigated in future implementations of the model. Nevertheless, our robustness analysis emphasizes that exclusion or reversion of side reactions are major issues for the cells under stress conditions since the actual refolding reaction can cope with relatively large fluctuations in chaperone abundance and activity.

The nonlinear relationship between ATP consumption and the refolding probability (Fig. 5) is also interesting. It is known that in *ΔrpoH* mutants, which lack the heat shock transcription factor and therefore have low levels of all major cytosolic proteases and chaperones except GroEL, 5-10% and 20-30% of all total proteins aggregated at 30°C and 42°C, respectively. The aggregates contained

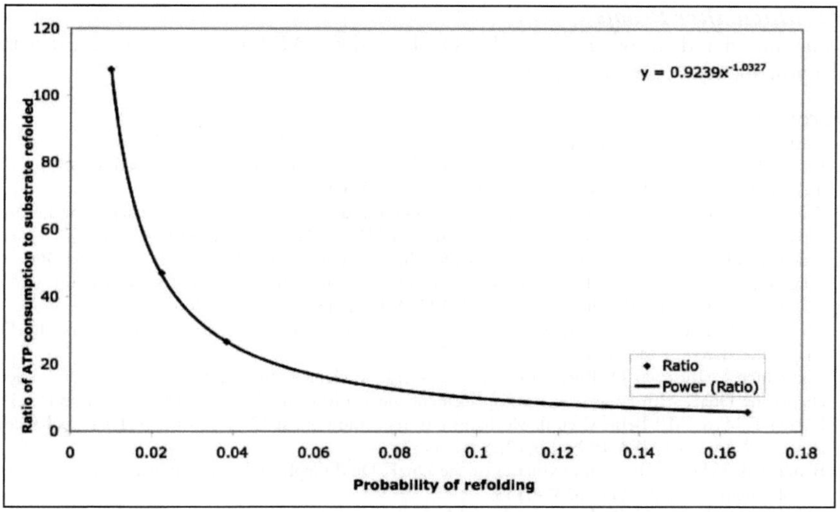


Figure 5. ATP consumption and the probability of refolding. After more than 95% of the substrate was fully refolded, ratios of ATP consumed were calculated and divided by the number of transformed substrates. Probability is the probability value of one substrate molecule after finishing exact one cycle of the chaperone system to be able to fold to natural states.

350-400 protein species.[20] Since the DnaK system is beside GroEL the only chaperone system in *E. coli* that is able to refold proteins to their native state, these protein species must be substrates for DnaK under normal conditions. These proteins may cover a wide range of probabilities of refolding, which is most likely determined by their sequence and fold. Although ATP has under optimal growth conditions a relatively high total concentration (3 mM), in stress situations the effective free concentration of ATP may nevertheless be insufficient to meet the challenge of refolding hundreds of different molecules simultaneously. Thus, we think the cellular amount of ATP may actually limit the robustness of the Hsp70 chaperone system in its protein folding function.

Currently, the complexity in the model is limited because we are focusing on the situation where only one substrate species exists. But if we are going to simulate the refolding of 100 different substrates at the same time, the complexity of model construction easily goes up and becomes hard to manage. One possible solution is to borrow the idea of object-orientation from computer science. Consider that if all the protein species have the inherent property of refolding and aggregation, etc (which is true in nature) inside the simulation software when we construct a large-scale model, we can just send the protein a message "fold" and it would find its way towards the folding process. In this way, we can replace the thousands of reactions with just 100 messages. Thus, object-oriented modeling is a prominent solution for complex biological models.

## *Acknowledgments*

The contents of this chapter were based on a previous publication by the same authors.* A more detailed model based on this work can be found in reference 26. This work is supported in part by grants from the Ministry of Education, Culture, Sports, Science and Technology of Japan(Leading Project for Biosimulation, The 21st Century COE Program and Grant-in-Aid for Scientific Research on Priority Areas) and a grant from CREST, JST. This work was also supported by the Deutsche Forschungsgemeinschaft (SFB638 to M.P.M.).

*Bin Hu, Matthias P. Mayer and Masaru Tomita (2005) HSP-mediated Prote in Refolding in the E-Cell, in The Proceedings of The 9 World Multi-Conference on Systemics, Cybernetics and Informatics VIII, Callaos N et al Ed. 377-382.

## *Note Added after Proofs*

Goloubinoff and coworkers found that DnaK used five ATPs to refold a specific denatured model protein, which does not aggregate.[27]

## References

1. Gething MJ, Sambrook J. Protein folding in the cell. Nature 1992; 355(6355):33-45.
2. Langer T, Lu C, Echols H et al. Successive action of DnaK, DnaJ and GroEL along the pathway of chaperone-mediated protein folding. Nature 1992; 356(6371):683-689.
3. Schröder H, Langer T, Hartl FU et al. DnaK, DnaJ and GrpE form a cellular chaperone machinery capable of repairing heat-induced protein damage. EMBO J 1993; 12(11):4137-4144.
4. Bukau B, Horwich AL. The Hsp70 and Hsp60 chaperone machines. Cell 1998; 92(3):351-366.
5. Liberek K, Marszalek J, Ang D et al. Escherichia coli DnaJ and GrpE heat shock proteins jointly stimulate ATPase activity of DnaK. Proc Natl Acad Sci USA 1991; (88)7:2874-2878.
6. McCarty JS, Buchberger A, Reinstein J et al. The role of ATP in the functional cycle of the DnaK chaperone system. J Mol Biol 1995; 249(1):126-137.
7. Packschies L, Theyssen H, Buchberger A et al. GrpE accelerates nucleotide exchange of the molecular chaperone DnaK with an associative displacement mechanism. Biochemistry 1997; 36(12):3417-3422.
8. Laufen T, Mayer MP, Beisel C et al. Mechanism of regulation of hsp70 chaperones by DnaJ cochaperones. Proc Natl Acad Sci USA 1999; 96(10):5452-5457.
9. Banecki B, Zylicz M. Real time kinetics of the DnaK DnaJ GrpE molecular chaperone machine action. J Biol Chem 1996; 271(11):6137-6143.
10. Mayer MP, Schroder H, Rudiger S et al. Multistep mechanism of substrate binding determines chaperone activity of Hsp70. Nat Struct Biol 2000; 7(7):586-593.
11. Grimshaw JP, Jelesarov I, Siegenthaler RK et al. Thermosensor action of GrpE. The DnaK chaperone system at heat shock temperatures. J Biol Chem 2003; 278(21):19048-19053.
12. Szabo A, Langer T, Schröder H et al. The ATP hydrolysis-dependent reaction cycle of the Escherichia coli Hsp70 system DnaK, DnaJ and GrpE. Proc Natl Acad Sci USA 1994; 91(22):10345-10349.
13. Straus DB, Walter WA, Gross CA et al. The heat shock response of E.coli is regulated by changes in the concentration of sigma 32. Nature 1987; 329(6137):348-351.
14. Tomoyasu T, Ogura T, Tatsuta T et al. Levels of DnaK and DnaJ provide tight control of heat shock gene expression and protein repair in Escherichia coli. Mol Microbiol 1998; 30(3):567-581.
15. Pierpaoli EV, Sandmeier E, Schonfeld, HJ et al. Control of the DnaK chaperone cycle by substoichiometric concentrations of the cochaperones DnaJ and GrpE. J Biol Chem 1998; 273(12):6643-6649.
16. Harrison CJ, Hayer-Hartl M, Di Liberto M et al. Crystal structure of the nucleotide exchange factor GrpE bound to the ATPase domain of the molecular chaperone DnaK. Science 1997; 276(5311):431-435.
17. Gassler CS, Buchberger A, Laufen T et al. Mutations in the DnaK chaperone affecting interaction with the DnaJ cochaperone. Proc Natl Acad Sci USA 1998; 95(26):15229-15234.
18. Suh WC, Burkholder WF, Lu CZ et al. Interaction of the Hsp70 molecular chaperone, DnaK, with its cochaperone DnaJ. Proc Natl Acad Sci USA 1998; 95(26):15223-15228.
19. Gross CA. Function and regulation of the heat shock proteins in Escherichia coli and salmonella cellular and molecular biology. Ed. N. F.C., Adobe and Mira Digital Publishing 1999.
20. Tomoyasu T, Mogk A, Langen H et al. Genetic dissection of the roles of chaperones and proteases in protein folding and degradation in the Escherichia coli cytosol. Mol Microbiol 2001; 40(2):397-413.
21. Gillespie DT. A general method for numerically simulating the stochastic time evolution of coupled chemical reactions. Journal of Computational Physics 1976; 22:403-434.
22. Gibson MA, Bruck J. Efficient exact stochastic simulation of chemical systems with many speecies and Many Channels. J Phys Chem A 2000; 104:1876-1889.
23. Tomita M, Hashimoto K, Takahashi K et al. E-CELL: software environment for whole-cell simulation. Bioinformatics 1999; 15(1):72-84.
24. Takahashi K, Kaizu K, Hu B et al. A multi-algorithm, multi-timescale method for cell simulation. Bioinformatics 2004; 20(4):538-546.
25. Schonfeld HJ, Schmidt D, Schroder H et al. The DnaK chaperone system of Escherichia coli: quaternary structures and interactions of the DnaK and GrpE components. J Biol Chem 1995; 270(5):2183-2189.
26. Hu B, Mayer MP, Tomita M. 4 Modeling hsp70-mediated protein folding. Biophys J 2006; 91(2):496-507.
27. Sharma SK, De Los Rios P, Christen P et al. The kinetic parameters and energy cost of the Hsp70 chaperone as a polypeptide unfoldase. Nat Chem Biol 2010; 6(12):914-920.

# INDEX

## H



## I



## K



## L



## M



## N



## O



## P

MIX
Papier aus verantwortungsvollen Quellen
Paper from responsible sources
FSC® C105338

If you have any concerns about our products,
you can contact us on
**ProductSafety@springernature.com**

In case Publisher is established outside the EU,
the EU authorized representative is:
**Springer Nature Customer Service Center GmbH**
**Europaplatz 3, 69115 Heidelberg, Germany**

Printed by Libri Plureos GmbH
in Hamburg, Germany